COMPLIANCE FOR CODING, BILLING & REIMBURSEMENT

A Systematic Approach to Developing a Comprehensive Program

SECOND EDITION

COMPLIANCE FOR CODING, BILLING & REIMBURSEMENT

A Systematic Approach to Developing a Comprehensive Program

SECOND EDITION

DUANE C. ABBEY

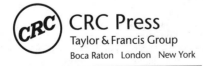

CRC Press
Taylor & Francis Group
Boca Raton London New York

CRC Press is an imprint of the
Taylor & Francis Group, an **informa** business

A PRODUCTIVITY PRESS BOOK

Productivity Press
Taylor & Francis Group
270 Madison Avenue
New York, NY 10016

Library of Congress Cataloging-in-Publication Data

Abbey, Duane C.
   Compliance for coding, billing & reimbursement : a systematic approach to developing a comprehensive program / Duane C. Abbey. -- 2nd ed.
     p. ; cm.
   Includes bibliographical references and index.
   ISBN 978-1-56327-368-1 (alk. paper)
   1. Medical fees. 2. Nosology--Code numbers. 3. Medicine--Terminology--Code numbers. 4. Health insurance claims--Code numbers. I. Title. II. Title: Compliance for coding, billing, and reimbursement.
   [DNLM: 1. Forms and Records Control--standards. 2. Classification. 3. Documentation--methods. 4. Fees and Charges. 5. Guideline Adherence. 6. Reimbursement Mechanisms. W 80 A124c 2008]
   R728.5.A25 2008
   651.5'04261--dc22

                                 2007049881

Visit the Taylor & Francis Web site at
http://www.taylorandfrancis.com

and the Productivity Press Web site at
http://www.productivitypress.com

Contents

Introduction

Overview

The past several years have seen increasing emphasis on compliance investigations of healthcare providers by federal and/or state agencies. The types and scopes of investigations vary significantly. Compliance issues arising from contractual obligations of providers and third-party payers are also escalating and triggering more reviews and audits. Little suggests a reprieve from this escalation. In fact, the numbers and types of investigations will most likely expand.

One area of great concern for healthcare providers is payment for services. The sizes of settlements have been significant enough to further fuel the fires of investigation. Thus compliance for providers is a priority. While most providers do not intend to commit fraud, file false claims, or receive overpayments, it is nearly impossible not to err because of the complexities of the delivery and payment systems, the rapid evolution of technology, and constantly changing rules and regulations. To decrease potential for fines, sanctions, and even criminal prosecutions, healthcare providers must take definitive systematic steps to address real and perceived compliance problems. This book is intended to provide a systematic approach to a major healthcare compliance area: the coding, billing, and reimbursement (CBR) process.

Three levels of CBR compliance concerns

The three levels of CBR compliance concerns addressed in this book are (1) statutorily based programs, (2) contract-based relationships, and (3) situations that do not involve formal relationships. Legislated healthcare programs represent the greatest concern because penalties often include criminal prosecution. Thus, CBR compliance personnel usually address programs such as Medicare and state Medicaid programs before considering contractual relationships. Statutorily based healthcare payment systems involve an enormous range of interlocking mechanisms. For example, Medicare follows the following information hierarchy:

- Social Security Act (SSA)
- United States Code (USC)
- *Code of Federal Regulations* (CFR)
- *Federal Register* (FR)
- *Medicare's manual system*
- *CMS transmittals and files*
- Medicare *Medlearn Matters*
- Medicare administrative contractor information

Virtually all healthcare providers have managed care contracts with third-party payers. *Managed care* can take on a variety of meanings. In theory, managed care contracts are studied, modified after negotiation, and renewed annually. In practice, however, these contracts are often signed and filed away although they impose serious obligations. CBR compliance personnel must participate in negotiation and acceptance of managed care contracts.

The third level of compliance concern relates to third-party payers with which healthcare providers have no formal relationships. If a provider must submit claims to third-party payers about which it has little information, what coding and billing requirements hold? In theory, a provider would expect full payment to be be made. However, the relationship here is between the patient and the provider. The claim is filed only as a convenience to the patient and will be paid via a default mechanism determined by the third-party payer.

The HIPAA TSC (Transaction Standard/Standard Code Sets) should ease this situation. It requires filing of standard claims in standard formats using standard code sets. In theory, a claim for a service will be consistent no matter what third-party payer is involved. To date, this is wishful thinking, as this case study illustrates.

Venipuncture Coding/Billing. Claims transaction staff at Apex Medical Center compiled a listing of the ways in which CPT Code 36415 (venipuncture for collection of specimen) is or is not to be billed. For Medicare and certain other third-party payers, the code is to be used and paid separately. Certain other third-party payers allow billing for the service but make no separate payments; payments are bundled based on a clinical laboratory fee schedule. Another third-party payer contract stipulates that the service is not to be billed; payment is treated as part of the laboratory charge. Yet another third-party payer allows a charge but the service must not appear on claim forms with CPT 36415.

This simple case illustrates the desirability of a standardized process. Perhaps the coming decades will see the achievement of the standardization goal envisaged in HIPAA TSC. Until then, CBR compliance personnel must address compliance issues at different levels of criticality, often while they attempt to cope with inconsistent external variables. They must be diligent in addressing the statutory issues because of the ever-present possibility of criminal prosecution for failure to comply.

Key learning area: Coding, billing, and reimbursement compliance activities generally address concerns at three levels: (1) statutorily established programs such as Medicare and Medicaid; (2) contractually established payment mechanisms under managed care contracts; and (3) claims filing to third-party payers with which their organizations have no formal relationship.

CBR compliance program development

Chapter 2 covers CBR compliance program development, different methods, and levels of detail based on organization size and other factors. Because CBR compliance is so specialized, a CBR program must dovetail with other compliance efforts, particularly an organization's corporate compliance program. CBR compliance issues may be integrated into a corporate plan for smaller providers. Large hospitals, multispecialty clinics, and integrated delivery systems usually require separate programs.

Systematic approach

Because CBR compliance is so broad and multifaceted, a systematic approach to identifying, analyzing, and resolving issues is paramount. Compliance personnel must approach situations systematically and act as facilitators with significant persuasive abilities to achieve full implementation of appropriate solutions. Some aspects of CBR compliance go beyond the immediate authority structure. Other personnel may have to be tactfully and logically persuaded to participate, particularly in hospitals where physicians are

independent rather than employees with line reporting relationships.

Many CBR compliance problems arise from documentation (or its lack) and medical necessity. Both issues require physicians to take or not take certain actions and fully document what was done and why. Persuading physicians, particularly those who are independent and not directly employed, to document and/or provide services in a certain way can be difficult, even for compliance purposes.

Systems theory

The *systems theory* phrase may sound academic, but it is practical for approaching and solving complex problems faced by CBR compliance personnel. This book addresses the main elements of systems theory: (1) a stepped or phased approach, (2) multiple perspectives, and (3) raised perspective. The advantage of systems theory is that it allows customization of the phases or steps depending on the context of the problem. For purposes of CBR compliance, the following steps are usual:*

- Problem/opportunity identification
- Problem/opportunity analysis
- Solution design—external
- Solution design—internal
- Solution development
- Solution implementation
- Situation monitoring and remediation

This seven-step or phased approach refines the design phase into *external* (how the solution looks) and *internal* (engineering required to achieve the solution) phases. The multiple perspective approach requires viewing a solution from different perspectives. In a hospital, different departments may view the same situation and have very different concerns. Patient accounting's perspective involves filing claims and procuring payment. Health information management is concerned with correct documentation and medical necessity. *Raised perspective* means broadening a view to make it more comprehensive. CBR compliance problems involve many layers and staff may have to raise perspectives to address all aspects of a problem. This may require a more complex investigation.

---

* This seven-step approach is an adaptation of the approach discussed in *Structured Systems Analysis and Design* by Duane C. Abbey, published by Edutronics/McGraw-Hill in 1981. See bibliography for additional books on the systems approach that can be extended to Six Sigma concepts and techniques.

> **Key learning area: The interfaces among departments and functions within a healthcare organization relative to CBR issues require careful investigation and facilitation of solutions on the part of CBR compliance personnel.**

Chunking is a powerful technique of breaking a complex situation into pieces that are reassembled after a solution is developed. Another variation on the systems approach for looking at processes and functions is the input–process–output model. Chapter 4 discusses the systems approach.

CBR policies, procedures, and infrastructure

Every healthcare compliance program should address seven key elements based on federal guidelines covered in Chapters 1 and 2. The approach of this book is to break the seven elements into: (1) policy and procedure documents and (2) program development infrastructure. Because CBR compliance may be implemented in various ways, this breakdown is logical. All compliance programs require written policies and procedures, but infrastructure development (oversight, delegation, monitoring, etc.) may differ significantly based on a provider's needs.

Preparing for external audits

Healthcare providers may decide to use external consultants and/or legal counsel when conducting audits and assessing results. Federal or state regulatory agencies may also conduct audits or order independent audits. The best preparation for audits is to charge, bill, and document correctly at all times. This is easier said than done.

The preferred approach is to conduct internal audits before formal ones are required. Even if informal audits are not conducted on statistical bases, they can identify problems before external auditors do. An even better approach is to mimic external audits by incorporating case selection that approximates or reflects statistical criteria used by outside auditors. Chapter 8 discusses auditing more fully.

Information resources

Assuming that most coding, billing, and reimbursement personnel want to produce correct claims, it is vital to deliver good information to the right people at the right time. Continuous changes in the CBR area, even for a modest sized organization, can make this almost a full-time job. CBR compliance staff should develop sources of information, network with associates, and read newsletters and the *Federal Register*. Thought should be given to monitoring and maintaining the flow of information. The Internet is one of the most valuable and immediate sources of information. CBR compliance personnel must develop an intimate knowledge of its use.

Obtaining the information is only half of the task. The remainder is ensuring the information is distributed to the right people in a timely fashion. Coding and billing personnel may review critical information, but what about service area personnel? Their priority is directed elsewhere—at providing services. Methods of keeping them informed must be tailored to their needs. The reverse is also true. Because service area people know what services are provided and the service organization, they can help coding and billing personnel do better jobs.

Hospital chargemasters serve as direct and indirect targets of compliance issues. A general rule in chargemaster development and maintenance is that "form follows function." In other words, the way the system is constructed (form) should follow from the way a service is provided (function). Service area changes such as a new service or a reorganization should be reported to the chargemaster coordinator before they are implemented. This also applies to new drugs, new procedures, and other changes. A chargemaster coordinator can be proactive and regularly visit service areas, but only service personnel know about changes in their areas.

Conducting research

CBR compliance personnel must develop knowledge bases of areas affecting their work. They may develop personal databases to reflect changes over the years. It is important for them to understand how coding and billing compliance issues have developed historically. A personal database will allow a staff member to maintain data about payment system changes, litigation and court rulings, the OIG's work plans, expansions of coding systems, and other critical changes.

CBR compliance personnel should also have access to extensive knowledge base beyond their personal databases. Specialized commercial services may provide vital information, particularly about Medicare. Healthcare attorneys may need even more extensive knowledge bases to support litigation activities. The CD-ROM accompanying this book can serve as a starting point for developing a knowledge base, but search capabilities that function across different types of documents may be essential.

The Internet offers one of the easiest ways to obtain information on healthcare coding, billing, and associated compliance issues. Search engines such as Google enable personnel to start learning which keywords generate which types of documents. The Internet contains an enormous volume of information. The maxim of not trusting anyone applies. It is wise to find three independent resources that give the same information or interpretation.

Healthcare computer billing systems

Healthcare computer billing systems serve as sources of information and analysis and, at the same time, a mechanism that can create CBR compliance problems. The ability to fully understand a computer system is essential. Most systems are capable of many functions. The way a system is set up determines how it works, how bills and claims are generated, and how it handles the range of information that must be available for report generation purposes.

It is important for CBR compliance personnel to fully understand the computer billing system, the way in which it is parameterized, the capabilities that are not used, and the general architecture. Large healthcare providers may have their own programming staffs; smaller operations may use vendors to obtain computer resources. A large entity may utilize a number of different systems to handle billing, medical records, decision support, and other functions. Such systems can require a great deal of resources to accomplish effective interfacing.

Small, integrated delivery systems may require a number of computer systems. A hospital may have one optimized for UB-04s, the clinic system may have one optimized for 1500s, home health will have its own special system, and skilled nursing may have yet another. Different systems can create real headaches, particularly because they can generate interface problems. For example, a clinic may provide a patient with laboratory and radiology services billed through a clinic system. Subsequent hospital admission may necessitate bundling of clinic services into the hospital's bill and claim. For effective operation, both systems must communicate with each other to cross-correlate the incident.*

CBR compliance officer and team development

The infrastructure development for CBR compliance may require the appointment of a CBR compliance officer and the development of a compliance team. The knowledge base and experience level for a CBR compliance officer and other compliance personnel are significant. In a small setting, CBR compliance may represent only one facet of the compliance officer's duties. The officer may work only part-time. In larger organizational settings, the compliance efforts can be differentiated to the point of having a full-time officer or small staff.

Whatever the size of the organization or compliance staff, one way to expand the knowledge load is to develop a compliance team. While compliance personnel may be expert in CBR matters, service area personnel are at the leading edge of healthcare delivery. Chapter 4 discusses team development in more detail. CBR compliance personnel should learn about effective team utilization and team dynamics. See the bibliography for additional resources.

Terminology, definitions, and acronyms

Mastering the terminology and acronyms used in the CBR is a major effort. Great care must be taken to fully understand the terminologies and definitions contained in directives and other materials about compliance. Keep in mind that day-to-day use of terminology may be less than precise. The examples below illustrate this point.

Hundreds of acronyms are used in CBR areas. For that reason, this book includes a list of them. When CMS issues an update in the *Federal Register*, a list of acronyms used in the update is included. Furthermore, a single acronym may have more than one meaning: MAC can mean *Medicare administrative contractor* or *monitored anesthesia care*. Likewise, the acronym NPP can refer to either Non-Physician Provider or Non-Physician Practitioner. Watch the context of the discussion for interpretations.

Certain terminology may be well defined only in a certain context. For example, CMS is careful to distinguish a provider from a supplier the conditions for payment cited in 42 CFR §424. A careful reading of the definitions reveals that a physician is considered a supplier and not a provider under Medicare, but healthcare providers include physicians in other contexts. Thus, it is vital to grasp precisely how and where certain terms are used. Interpretations may appear to be counterintuitive. However, personnel involved in CBR compliance should become accustomed to such inconsistencies, particularly under Medicare.

---

* See the DRG pre-admission window, also known as the 3-day or 72-hour rule.

Key learning area: A major task in the CBR compliance field is mastery of the hundreds of relevant acronyms along with terminology and definitions that may not seem logical. Because meanings can vary significantly, determine the context for terminology when reading or studying a particular area.

Author

Duane C. Abbey, Ph.D., CFP, is a management consultant and president of Abbey & Abbey, Consultants, Inc. Based in Ames, Iowa, Abbey & Abbey specializes in healthcare consulting and related areas.

Dr. Abbey, whose work in healthcare now spans more than 25 years, earned his graduate degrees at the University of Notre Dame and Iowa State University. Today, he spends about half his time developing and teaching workshops (for students who affectionately quip that the *Federal Register* is his favorite reading material) and making presentations to professional organizations. He devotes the other half to consulting work that involves performing chargemaster reviews, compliance reviews, providing litigation support, and conducting reimbursement studies.

Dr. Abbey also uses his mathematical and financial background to perform financial assessments, develop complex financial models, and conduct various types of statistical work. His studies in the field of neurolinguistic programming have enhanced his ability to provide organizational communication facilitation services for healthcare organizations. He also provides litigation support services for attorneys representing healthcare providers in legal proceedings.

Dr. Abbey can be contacted by e-mail at Duane@aaciweb.com.

Case study listing

one

Overview of healthcare compliance

Introduction

During the late 1980s the issue of healthcare compliance relative to fraud, abuse, false claims, and a host of other problems became a major concern for all healthcare providers. Since then, although concerns about all aspects of healthcare compliance gained momentum, those related to the highly technical areas involving coding, billing, reimbursement, and a multitude of payment systems increased even more dramatically. These concerns have now continued into the 21st century. This book is devoted to healthcare compliance concerns in the area of coding, billing, and reimbursement. Allied issues such as documentation, computer systems, payment systems, information resources, and the like are also considered. Among the many associated areas of concern are

- Federal tax laws
- State tax laws
- OSHA
- Employee- and employment-related issues
- Financial compliance
- Antitrust
- HIPAA privacy and security
- Americans with Disabilities Act
- Environmental Protection Act

Corporate compliance programs are designed to address all of the compliance areas for healthcare providers. The CBR (coding, billing, and reimbursement) compliance program concentrates on an area of great concern for statutory compliance (e.g., Medicare, Medicaid, and other government programs) and contractual compliance (e.g., managed care contracts).

Key learning area: While the various compliance aspects of a coding, billing, and reimbursement compliance program are the main topics of this book, there are many additional corporate compliance concerns.

Healthcare industry

The healthcare industry continues to grow at an incredible speed. The changes in medical technology, integration of delivery, diversification of payment mechanisms, aging population, quality of care concerns, and a host of other developments drive the rapid pace of change. The constant changes mean that providers of all types are hard pressed to provide proper care, file claims appropriately, remain financially viable, and stay within both statutory and contractual compliance guidelines. In many cases, the guidelines are in a continuing cycle of development as payment systems and organizational structures change.

From a compliance perspective, the pressures that are brought to bear on the coding, billing, reimbursement, and documentation process for any provider are:

1. Legal foundation: laws, rules, regulations, contracts
2. Payment systems: cost-based, prospective, capitated
3. Organizational structure: ownership, tax status, holding entities
4. Delivery systems: hospital systems, physician–hospital organizations, clinic networks

These four concerns or pressure points are illustrated in Figure 1.1. As various compliance issues related to the CBR process are discussed, these four points will come into focus.

It is important to note that because healthcare delivery, both in terms of delivery processes and advancing techniques, is changing so rapidly, payment systems, associated regulations, and contracts may sometime become unsynchronized. It is in this lack of synchronization that much of the conflict perceived in the healthcare industry comes into play. This can occur at a very detailed level or at a higher, organizational level. A simple example of this conflict at a detailed level is the hospital chargemaster coordinator who may have to decide whether a new supply item is a billable item or must be considered part of another billable item. At an organizational level, conflict can arise when two hospitals decide to merge or a hospital and a group of clinics decide to come under common ownership. In both examples, the underlying conflict is tied to compliance issues.

Compliance officers, in general, and CBR compliance personnel more specifically, must identify and follow trends in the four key areas illustrated in Figure 1.1. While current compliance issues are certainly of concern, those issues that will be critical concerns several years hence are of even greater interest. What truly

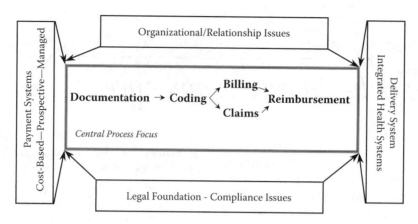

Figure 1.1   CBR compliance: Influencing factors.

matters is that changes that will meet those future compliance concerns can be effected now.

Key learning area: There are four pressures affecting CBR compliance: Legal foundation, delivery systems, organizational structuring, and payment systems.

Key learning area: While current compliance problems are of interest, it is necessary to look ahead to determine what will be a compliance concern in the future to effect changes to meet such concerns today.

Healthcare payment systems

There are many different ways for third-party payers to reimburse for services provided and items supplied. Payment systems are complex and diverse; a given type of payment system may involve significant variability, and thoroughly understanding even one of these complex payment systems is, at the very least, a formidable challenge. At the same time, it is critical for CBR compliance personnel to be intimately familiar with all payment systems used to provide reimbursement or payment to providers. This book divides the payment systems into three categories that are illustrated in Figure 1.2.

There is no unique way to categorize payment systems, and these three systems provide only a very general categorization. Occasionally, the systems overlap as in the case of a managed care company that may have a contract with a hospital to reimburse a fixed percentage of charges made. Although this is generally considered a fee-for-service payment system, it can also be categorized as a managed care payment system.

Note that the emphasis in our discussions here is with payment systems used by third-party payers and that we are interested in situations in which a claim is filed and reimbursement is based on that claim. Situations in which a provider simply charges a patient and the patient pays the bill without third party involvement seldom generate compliance concerns except in relationship to other third-party payment arrangements. For example, providing discounts to self-pay patients may generate questions about charging them less than Medicare patients are charged.

Cost-Based	⬅➡ Fee-for-Service ⬅➡	Managed Care
Cost Rules	Fee Schedules/Grouping	Contracted Amounts
Retrospective Adjustment	PPSs - DRGs, APGs, RBRVS Prospective Determination	Capitated Payments
	Coding Protocols	Care/Practice Protocols
Cost Management Interim Payments	Micro-Management Fixed Payment for Specific Services	Macro-Management Overall Payment for Global Services
Risk-Costs Over or Under Target	Risk - Market Too Few Patients	Risk-Utilization Too Many Services

Figure 1.2   Payment system development.

Cost-based systems

Cost-based systems represent one of the oldest approaches to payment for healthcare services. The healthcare industry trend is to move away from these systems, but they are still in use. Under the Medicare program, for example, Critical Access Hospitals (CAHs), Rural Health Clinics (RHCs), and Federally Qualified Health Centers (FQHCs) are all cost-based reimbursed. The basic idea is that a provider is reimbursed based upon costs incurred for the provision of services.

While the theme certainly includes many variations, a reimbursement system can be considered cost-based only if the third-party payer knows the provider's costs. For the Medicare program, this information comes in the form of a Medicare cost report. Developing cost reports is a genuine challenge: They are complex and many decisions must be made during the development process. Once completed, cost reports become sensitive elements in compliance along with associated accounting and/or work papers.

For example, proper revenue codes on the chargemaster can influence the way in which a cost report is developed. It is important that the information gathered and used to develop cost reports be well understood by the report preparers. Conversely, the personnel involved in peripheral activities that feed data to the report must be sensitive to their influence on this process.

Typically, cost-based systems begin with an interim payment arrangement, followed at a later date with a final reconciliation that takes into account costs as reported through the cost reporting process. Note also that the information provided through the cost reporting process may also be used as the basis for developing prospective payment systems (see next section). For example, with the APC (ambulatory payment classification) and DRG (diagnosis-related group) payment systems, the cost-to-charge ratios (CCRs) are used to convert charges into costs. These costs, as associated with APC or DRG categories, are then used to develop APCs and, respectively, the DRG weights.*

Note that some current fee-for-service payment systems are really one step removed from cost-based systems. For instance, hospitals typically have some third-party payer contracts that pay a percentage of charges made. Payments are generally in the 75 to 95 percent range. From the perspective of a third-party payer, the presumption is that the charges made by the hospital faithfully reflect the hospital's costs. In other words, the charges are based on a standardized

mark-up. Thus, the third-party payer is really making payment based on costs that have been uniformly converted into charges.

Key learning area: Over the past two decades there has been a significant movement away from cost-based payment systems. Critical access hospitals (CAHs) have become popular in rural areas. The cost report is critical for cost-based reimbursement. Additionally, the Medicare cost report is still important for prospective payment systems such as APCs and DRGs.

Prospective payment systems

From a compliance perspective, prospective payment systems (PPSs) are great challenges. It is not possible to discuss any one of these systems in detail because all of them are complex enough to be the subjects of separate books. Moreover, as this book is prepared for publication, most of these prospective payment systems are undergoing continuing evolution. The three PPSs briefly discussed here are

- DRGs (Hospital Inpatient Payment)
- APCs (Hospital Outpatient Payment)
- RBRVS (Physician Professional Payment)

PPSs for skilled nursing services, long-term care hospitals, home health services, and inpatient rehabilitation were all developed in a relatively short time. Although all these PPSs have common elements, complex nuances make them distinct. These nuances make them susceptible to a multitude of potential compliance issues, and CBR personnel should monitor them carefully to identify any problems.

CMS, through its Medicare program, provides the impetus for these PPSs. Other third-party payers may then follow with their own variations. With the Medicare DRG system, for example, different third-party payers in different parts of the country use the following variations:

- AP-DRGs (All Patient DRGs)
- APR-DRGs (All Patient Refined DRGs)
- SR-DRGs (Severity Refined DRGs)†
- MS-DRGs (Medicare Severity DRGs)

Note that for FY2008 CMS has implemented a three-level severity refinement to the DRG system, namely the MS-DRGs. Other third-party payers may use the old system, now referred to as CMS-DRGs, or other

---

* See the annual National Public Rulemaking process for both APCs and DRGs. Through *Federal Register* entries a proposed rule is issued, comments may be made, and then CMS issues a final rule.

---

† SR-DRGs (Severity Refined DRGs) were proposed by CMS (then HCFA) in 1994 and never implemented.

variations on DRGs. Questions surrounding DRG compliance issues will probably be more complicated with the new severity refinement.

Similarly, Medicare's APCs are derivatives of the more general APGs (Ambulatory Patient Groups) that in turn were derived from AVGs (Ambulatory Visit Groups) among other research conducted in the outpatient payment area. For hospital outpatient services and the associated coding, billing, and reimbursement, APCs have had a significant impact both on finance and compliance.

The Resource-Based Relative Value System (RBRVS) is an extended fee schedule that provides payment for Medicare services provided by physicians. RBRVS is probably the most complicated fee schedule that we have today. Among its many features is a differentiation in physician payment between "facilities" and "non-facilities" that relates back to the provider-based rule (PBR). RBRVS uses the CPT coding system as does APCs. Thus, all of the concerns about proper coding come into play on the compliance front. Additionally, RBRVS through the Medicare physician fee schedule (MPFS) also provides payment for certain non-physicians such as physical therapists and occupational therapists. A PPS that can include many fee schedules generally has the following characteristics:

1. A classification system
2. Weights or relative values based upon the classification system
3. A payment rate or conversion factor to calculate payment

PPSs are characterized by payments that are fixed in advance. Whatever payment is made is final for the given period of time. The weights and payment rates may be varied (typically on an annual basis), but for the given period of time the payment is fixed. Changes in the weights or relative values is called *recalibration*, and changes in the payment rate or conversion factor is called *rebasing*.

Beyond these basic characteristics, a given PPS may be configured in a variety of ways. The coding systems used to drive the process may also vary. For instance, with DRGs, the systems are ICD-9-CM Volume 3, procedure codes, and ICD-9-CM Volumes 1 and 2, diagnosis codes. APCs and RBRVS, use a combination of CPT and the Level II HCPCS (Healthcare Common Procedure Coding System), including various modifiers.

Note: The current ICD-9 coding system has been slated to change to ICD-10. As this book was going to press, the final date for this change was still in question and

there was even some speculation that that the United States will go directly to ICD-11.

Some of these systems allow for the coding of everything that is done with subsequent grouping of services while others have specialized coding requirements. The use or non-use of certain codes or code combinations can be quite daunting. Both CPT and CMS's HCPCS Level II (national) also have many modifiers require full understanding. CMS has developed an extensive set of edits that numbers in the range of 200,000. These edits are typically code combinations that cannot be used together unless there is some good reason to use both codes. Modifiers are needed to separate code pairs that are on the Correct Coding Initiative (CCI) list.

While the phrase *prospective payment* is used to describe this system, other arrangements such as fee schedules and discounted fee schedules may also apply.

Key learning area: CBR compliance personnel must be well versed in all the PPSs used to provide payment to a given healthcare provider. Note that these systems change constantly and thus the associated rules and regulations, both statutory and contractual, change with great frequency. Also, different third-party payers will implement a system in slightly different fashions, compounding the complexity of compliance.

PPSs are of great importance for CBR compliance activities. These systems provide a mechanism to monitor utilization and to track changes in activities. Since these systems have classifications with some sort of weights or relative values, various types of case-mix indexes can be developed and used for monitoring. Chapter 8 discusses the baseline compliance audit process that can be used over time to monitor compliance issue surrounding the use of these payment systems.

Capitated systems

While the phrase *managed care* can be interpreted in many ways, most private third-party payers use some form of a fee-for-service arrangement using cost-based, charge-based, or prospective payment systems. Capitation represents the newest of the payment systems and is a radical departure from both the cost-based systems and PPSs. The biggest difference is that the locus of risk is shifted from the third-party payer to the provider. With the cost-based, charge-based, and PPS systems the locus of risk is with the third-party payer. If there are increases in utilization, the third-party payer must bear the responsibility. Thus, third-party payers are very sensitive to proper utilization, medical necessity, and a host of other compliance concerns.

With capitated payment, the basic idea is that the provider will provide services within a fixed payment scheme, for example, a per member per month payment, for which all services (or a defined part of services) are to be provided without additional payment. While the concept is simple, the implementation of capitated payment systems can be quite complex.

Since the locus of risk is changed with capitation, compliance concerns that are normally associated with the filing of claims, development of cost reports, or documentation of medical necessity become relatively unimportant to the third-party payer. The healthcare provider has the incentive to provide the services at the lowest possible cost. Thus, the need to know costs and actuarial incidence of services for a given population become paramount. The issue with capitated programs is not compliance but the proper provision of care and satisfaction of customers, that is, the patients.

Key learning area: Payment systems are in the process of shifting from cost-based to prospective payments, which, in turn, sometimes shift to capitated arrangements. With the shift in risk from one party to another, compliance concerns change as well, depending on the payment system employed.

Healthcare delivery systems

A full discussion of healthcare delivery systems, their forms, formats, and the evolution of new models and/or relationships, are well beyond the scope of this book. It is, therefore, best to limit this discussion to the general trend in healthcare delivery systems toward integration of healthcare providers with the goal of seamless delivery or one-stop shopping. While the specifics of any particular structure of a delivery system is too much to consider, there are a number of organizational considerations that affect the CBR compliance area. Two areas that will be considered here are provider relationships and clinical, hospital, and IDS structuring.

Provider relationships address the way in which various healthcare providers relate to each other. Any number of different providers render services at, through, or in conjunction with a hospital. From a compliance perspective, the hospital's relationship with each of these providers needs to be examined and formalized in writing to ensure that both the hospital and the providers meet all compliance requirements related to coding, billing, documentation, and reimbursement.

A physician who is not an employee may periodically visit a hospital to conduct a day-long specialty clinic. The hospital may choose to charge the physician rent at fair market value (FMV) or charge a facility fee. The coding requirements for the physician are different, but also depend upon the relationship. Such a relationship should be spelled out in a written contract so that both parties know what they should do in order to meet compliance guidelines.

At the core of integrated delivery system (IDS) development are the fundamental building blocks of hospitals and clinics. The way in which the IDS structures relationships has a pronounced impact on billing and reimbursement as well as on a number of CBR compliance concerns.

A hospital may own a clinic and employ the physicians who work there.* As the owner of the clinic, and assuming that all applicable criteria are met, the hospital may decide to organize the clinic as a provider-based facility, that is, as a part of its outpatient department. In doing so the hospital can then file two claims, a 1500 for the professional component and a UB-04 for the technical, facilities component. Under certain payment systems such as Medicare's RBRVS, the physician will incur a small decrease in payment because of the "site-of-service" differential, but this loss is more than made up by the facility payment.

Note that this example involves a concern about the interface of the RBRVS payment system and APGs. The clinic may have its own laboratory or radiology services. If a patient is treated at the clinic with ancillary tests and is then admitted to the hospital, the DRG preadmission window may come into play because of the ancillary tests.† Here again, organizational structure has an impact on payment systems, resulting in CBR compliance concerns.

Note that a payment system or the interface between payment systems may drive the organization of the delivery system. If healthcare providers are organizing to optimize reimbursement, then such restructuring will certainly come under the close scrutiny of the third-party payers. This scrutiny typically results in new rules, regulations, and criteria that must be met before an organizational structure qualifies for reimbursement through a given payment system. The

---

* This is only one of many variations relative to hospital ownership of a clinic.

† This is an over-simplification. See discussion in Chapter 3.

organizational structuring, therefore, becomes a compliance issue.

Key learning area: Organizational structure for healthcare providers affects and is affected by payment systems, which, in turn, leads to significant compliance concerns.

Healthcare compliance laws, rules, and regulations

As mentioned in the chapter introduction, numerous laws, rules, and regulations apply to the coding, billing, documentation, and reimbursement areas and they change at an increasingly rapid rate. The institution of newer payment systems such as APCs ushers in a new array of claims submission requirements. HIPAA rules exert extensive impacts on virtually all aspects of coding, billing, and reimbursement. Some of the new requirements directly impact CBR processes while others are tangential but must still be considered. This book will divide the healthcare compliance laws, rules, and regulations into statutory and contractual categories.

Statutory requirements

These are the formal federal and state statutes, administrative rules, and regulations and include the Code of Federal Regulations (CFR) along with specific laws targeted at healthcare, such as EMTALA (Emergency Medical Treatment and Labor Act) or HIPAA (Health Insurance Portability and Accountability Act). These laws and subsequent administrative rules and regulations then filter down into more specialized directives from CMS, Medicaid programs, TRICARE, and the like.

The penalties of non-compliance with statutory law can be severe and range from civil monetary penalties to sanctions from specific programs to criminal prosecution. For all types of healthcare providers, this is an area of great concern; because of the complexity of the CBR systems, it is not always easy to be consistently compliant or even to know whether a provider is out of compliance.

Contractual requirements

Contractual agreements are common with private third-party payers. A contract is negotiated and signed by both payer and healthcare provider, and the provider must then meet any contractual requirements and adhere to associated rules and requirements promulgated by the third-party payer. Penalties associated with abrogation of contract requirements are generally monetary not criminal.

Key learning area: It is important for healthcare providers to review all contractual relationships carefully and ensure that all contractual obligations are met.

HIPAA 1996

The Health Insurance Portability and Accountability Act was passed by Congress in 1996 and it contains several major provisions. Of great concern to CBR compliance personnel are three initiatives:

* Fraud and Abuse Control Program (42 U.S.C. §1320a-7c)
* Medicare Integrity Program (42 U.S.C. §1395ddd), and
* Beneficiary Incentive Programs (42 U.S.C. §1395b-5)

Note that the Fraud and Abuse Control Pogram extends fraud and abuse concerns to all third-party payers.

Additionally, HIPAA provided legislation for three major healthcare rules:

* Privacy
* Security
* Transaction Standards/Standard Code Sets (TSCs)

These three rules along with the development and implementation of National Provider Identifiers (NPIs) have created major challenges for all types and levels of healthcare providers.

BBA 1997

The Balanced Budget Act of 1997 is comprehensive legislation that addressed the budget for FY1998 but, as with most budget legislation, BBA 1997 affected various federal programs. It is an enormous piece of legislation that produced significant impact on healthcares. It includes numerous provisions dealing with fraud and abuse, along with numerous changes and directives related to development and implementation of new payment systems. A study of only the healthcare-related aspects of BBA 1997 is a major project, and the impacts of BBA 1997 will be felt for many years to come.

MMA 2003

The Medicare Modernization Act of 2003 is a major, multifaceted piece of legislation. The drug benefit (Part D) is probably the most obvious provision and will be the longest remembered. However, the act contains many other provisions, some of which have direct and significant impacts on healthcare compliance concerns. Section 731, for example, addresses national coverage decisions (NCDs) and local coverage decisions (LCDs). Section 902 directs that when CMS issues a proposed rule, a three-year window during which the final rule must be published is a requirement.

DRA 2005

The Deficit Reduction Act of 2005 is a general legislative bill that also contains some healthcare provisions. This act extends to some extent the federal False Claims Act (FCA) to the state level in order to eliminate fraud and waste. Particular emphasis is placed on the Medicaid programs in various states. Also, the act addresses specific issues such as ASC (ambulatory surgery center) payments and reductions in Medicare payments for certain families of radiological services.

Key learning area: CBR compliance personnel are encouraged to study carefully newly enacted laws that affect healthcare. In recent years, major legislation has had a direct impact on healthcare compliance.

See the CD accompanying this book for additional information on federal legislation from the past 15 years.

Compliance concerns and program development

The breadth and scope of specific compliance concerns and certain situations that raise these concerns are too extensive to include in a single book, even if the discussion addressed only coding, billing, documentation, and reimbursement. A number of concerns related to these specific areas are discussed in Chapter 3. What is most important, however, is a systematic process for identifying real or potential compliance problems or opportunities as they are euphemistically called. These problems or opportunities can be identified internally or externally.

Internal identification involves reviewing claims and associated bills and documentation or by reviewing a process that contributes to the generation of claims. Claim denials and underpayments can also be indicators of problems. Specific mechanisms (e.g., the chargemaster) within the coding, billing, and reim-

bursement processes may be targets for both statutory and contractual compliance problems.

External identification involves reviewing reports of investigations and settlements, and newsletters. OIG advisory opinions along with OIG annual work plans, provide hundreds of potential areas for compliance concern, review, and investigation.* Many of these sources focus only on statutory compliance issues; similar attention in modified form should also be given to contractual compliance issues.

In the CBR area, many mistakes are simply technical errors that stem from inadequate information, misinformation, misunderstanding, or misinterpretation. A major objective of a CBR compliance program is to have (1) adequate sources of information and (2) appropriate organizational information flow.

CBR compliance personnel have a duty to *know* about compliance issues and proper billing, documentation, and claims filing rules and regulations. Thus a concerted effort must be made to ensure that adequate information is available at all levels—federal, state and local—for government or statutory programs and about contractual arrangements. Considering the vast array of private third-party payers to which hospitals, clinics, and physicians must submit claims, CBR personnel often find keeping all the coding and billing requirements in order difficult if not overwhelming.

At the national level for a program like CMS's Medicare, CBR compliance personnel must have direct connections to all CMS transmittals, Medicare manuals and updates, special memoranda, *Federal Register* and CFR updates, and similar resources. Establishing a process for obtaining and reviewing this type of information is a major project.

Take as an example Durable Medical Equipment (DME). Significant questions surround what constitutes DME and additional questions concern the proper processes of billing and filing claims for DME. The Medicare program uses regional carriers known as DMERCs (durable medical equipment regional carriers). The DMERCs have voluminous manuals that containing the rules and regulations surrounding billing the DMERC versus billing a fiscal intermediary (FI) or a carrier. If a given healthcare provider provides DME and subsequently bills and files claims under the Medicare program, then information and updates from the Medicare manual related to DME are critical.

Note: As this book is written, CMS is moving toward regional Medicare administrative contractors (MACs). While DMERCs may remain essentially the same, the FIs and carriers will most likely be combined.

---

* See the OIG website cited in the appendix to download the current and past year's work plans and additional information.

On the contractual side, the challenge sometimes involves obtaining specific guidance from a private third-party payer about special billing and claims filing requirements. CBR compliance personnel must have full access to contracts and should also be involved in the negotiation of these contracts. CBR personnel should also review any companion manuals that provide additional specific information about a given contract.

For any healthcare provider, the development of a CBR compliance program—either as a separately identifiable program or as a part of a more general corporate compliance program—is essential. The simple fact is that the CBR area of virtually every provider will be reviewed, monitored, visited, and/or audited. Even presuming that no fraud is intended and that no criminal proceedings will ensue, the monetary penalties for non-compliance can be ruinous.

Key learning area: CBR compliance personnel must have full access to the rules and regulations issued by government payers. Additionally, full knowledge of managed care contracts and all associated coding and billing directives that accompany such contracts is also essential.

Key elements for compliance programs

Seven key elements must be addressed for virtually any compliance program related to laboratory services, home health, skilled nursing, pharmacy, radiology, and corporate or CBR issues. The seven basic principles are shown in Figure 1.3 and should be evident in any compliance program. They are derived from the federal sentencing guidelines and from previous settlement agreements. They will be discussed throughout this book. We provide a brief summary below of each area as it relates to CBR compliance.

1. **Compliance standards and procedures**—Implementing written policies, procedures, and standards of conduct. For the CBR compliance program this consists of several policy and procedure

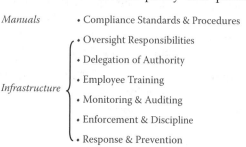

Figure 1.3   Seven key compliance principles.

manuals relative to coding, billing, and documentation. For most hospitals, two manuals are required: one covering coding policies and procedures and one covering billing policies and procedures. Medical clinics may utilize a combination of manuals that address both coding and billing. Large hospital systems and IDSs may use several different manuals from different sources that address different perspectives, for example, a utilization review policies and procedures manual or a chargemaster policies and procedures manual. The development and implementation of coding and billing policies and procedures are key to developing a CBR compliance program. After such a program is instituted, these policies and procedures must be integrated and/or interfaced into the corporate compliance program.

2. **Oversight responsibilities**—Designating a compliance officer and committee. At the corporate level, a chief compliance office and a corporate-wide compliance committee are required. At CBR compliance program level, hospitals, clinics, and IDSs can address the need for a compliance officer in a wide range of ways. For a small hospital, CBR compliance activities may simply be assigned as a part-time job. Likewise, CBR compliance activities may simply be folded into the chief compliance officer's duties. Large hospitals, clinics, and IDSs, on the other hand, may need a definitive department (e.g., Office of Billing Compliance) including a director and staff.

3. **Delegation of authority**—Staff development and preparation. As with the oversight responsibilities and depending on circumstances, it may sometimes be necessary to delegate authority. This is particularly true in a highly technical area such as coding, billing, documentation, and reimbursement. For small provider situations, such delegation of authority will be minimal. A large organization, however, may assign a specialist to each different area. At an IDS with both hospitals and clinic operations, it would be appropriate to have specialists who could address the specific billing concerns for hospital services and other specialists to do the same for clinical services.

4. **Employee training**—Developing effective lines of communication. The best written policies and procedures are of little use without mechanisms to train and communicate with employees involved in specific coding, billing, documentation, and reimbursement activities. Training programs, both at corporate compliance program level and CBR compliance program level are critical components in the implementation of compliance solutions.

5. **Monitoring and auditing**—Determining whether compliance standards are met. Monitoring the implementation of changes made to meet compliance standards and auditing for purposes of identifying potential compliance problems are critical to a CBR compliance program. The monitoring may involve various activities and targets. Computer technology and specialized programs can greatly enhance the ability to meet compliance standards and help identify potential problems. A baseline compliance audit is a tool that comes into play here. This audit is a process of "taking snapshots" of the CBR process and related areas at designated intervals over time. The snapshots are then compared to see what changes are occurring. The snapshots can also be used to identify problems or to justify changes.

6. **Enforcement and discipline**—Taking action when changes required to meet compliance standards fail to work. The greatest and most common challenge in the CBR area is not maintaining discipline. The challenge more often is the need to educate and train personnel to code, bill, and document correctly. Once this has been done, enforcement and discipline become matters of constant vigilance and taking appropriate action if and when a problem surfaces. This is particularly true in the area of documentation. Because healthcare providers are primarily interested in delivering high quality care for their patients, documentation sometimes becomes secondary. The lack of appropriate documentation can, in turn, affect the coding, billing, and reimbursement process.

7. **Response and prevention**—Taking remedial action and self-reporting. Identifying noncompliance problems with coding, billing, and reimbursement sometimes creates related or additional problems. Except for intentional fraud, most problems in this area arise from inadvertent technical mistakes or a lack of understanding. When such mistakes are identified, the first action is to correct them. This, however, does not address the possibility that the mistake has been repeated many times in the past. One common result of such mistakes is overpayment. Thus, the response now becomes two-pronged: Correcting the mistake and returning the overpayment. Both actions can be handled internally. The question then becomes whether the mistake should be reported to an external agency or authority. In other words, when is it necessary to self-report to a law enforcement agency when inadvertent mistakes have taken place? This will be discussed in Chapter 2.

Compliance program areas

As noted above, identifying compliance problems and opportunities and building the infrastructure for a CBR compliance program are critical success factors for healthcare providers. The two fundamental ways to approach this dual process are the top-down organizational approach and the bottom-up problem-driven approach. A third approach used by most healthcare providers is a combination of the top-down and bottom-up approaches and is sometimes called the "middle-in"—working from the top down and the bottom up to meet in the middle.

Chapter 9 includes a detailed discussion of the top-down and bottom-up approaches related to performing compliance baseline audits. The top-down organizational approach involves looking at the organization, its structure and the various systems and processes used for coding, billing, documentation, and reimbursement. The system has certain similarities to business process reengineering (BPR) and total quality management (TQM) also known as continuous quality improvement (CQI). Six Sigma is the latest development in the quality improvement area and incorporates certain aspects of quality improvement from the last 20 years. These disciplines along with various auditing techniques can be utilized to monitor compliance activities.

The bottom-up approach involves identifying, investigating, and resolving specific and often specialized situations. For instance, a review of physician claims may reveal that the documentation does not meet the evaluation and management (E/M) coding documentation guidelines. Remedial action may be taken, training may be provided, and a new computer-based E/M documentation system may be installed to address the specific problem. Note that the same situation may be discovered using the top-down approach through the study and review of the organization's medical records or a patient records system that includes the documentation process.

Because healthcare CBR compliance issues are so complex and diverse, it is best (and sometimes necessary) to use both approaches. Virtually every healthcare provider finds problem areas that need to be addressed, cleaned up, and monitored. At the same time, various organizational structures and systems must be reviewed for compliance purposes and to implement efficiency and/or effectiveness improvements.*

---

* The OIG recognizes that implementation of compliance programs is expensive and time consuming. Part of the justification for doing so is performance improvement.

Use of systems approach

The systems approach is a powerful tool for CBR compliance personnel. While the formal study of systems theory is mathematical (and somewhat theoretical) in nature, this tool or technique can be practically applied to address the complex and involved problems encountered with CBR compliance. This book presents the systems approach as a planned, systematic, seven-step process addressing problems (or opportunities). The seven steps used in this approach are*

1. Problem identification
2. Problem investigation
3. Problem analysis
4. External solution design
5. Internal solution design
6. Implementation
7. Monitoring and corrective action

The advantage of the systems approach is that it can be adapted to many different kinds of situations. CBR compliance personnel should feel free to modify this seven-step approach as necessary when addressing compliance situations.

Two additional features of the systems approach as used in this book are multiple and raised perspectives. The idea behind multiple perspectives is looking at a problem from different angles, from the perspectives of different departments, or from the perspectives of different people involved in a process. The idea of raising (or lowering) the perspective arises from the metaphor about looking at individual trees and missing the forest. Raising the perspective when evaluating a problem or opportunity often makes it possible to see the matter as part of a greater whole. Similarly, when tackling a problem, you may not be able to take on the whole forest and may need to lower your perspective to an individual tree or cluster.

See the foreword to this book for additional information on the systems approach. The bibliography provides a list of additional readings and references in this area. Many techniques such as root cause analysis, Six Sigma, quality function deployment, and other related methodologies can be used as adjuncts to the general systems approach.

---

* See Abbey, Duane C., *Structured Systems Approach and Design*, Edutronics/McGraw-Hill, New York, 1981.

> **Key learning area: The systems approach offers a powerful and flexible tool for addressing complex, involved CBR compliance problems and opportunities.**

Settlement agreements

The complexities of coding, billing, and reimbursement are so pervasive that many healthcare providers choose to become involved in settlement agreements with governmental programs. In some cases, this takes the form of a corporate integrity agreement (CIA). The forms and structures of individual and blanket settlement agreements should be carefully studied. Particularly in the CBR area, great care should be taken to ensure that all requirements cited in such agreements are addressed. Even if you are never involved in such agreements, you can still learn from them and follow the tenets they contain. In other words, act as if you are operating under such an agreement and pursue the activities that would normally be required under its terms. Note that some of these agreements are publicly available through the OIG website.

> **Key learning area: All types of providers can learn from the requirements contained in settlement agreements and corporate integrity agreements. Additionally, providers can use litigation concerning private third-party payer contacts as a guide to problem areas.**

Summary

Compliance is a major concern for healthcare providers. During the early years of the 21st century, the process of developing compliance programs continues to expand and grow in complexity. New payment systems, along with different types of delivery systems, continue to evolve. In the coding, billing, documentation, and reimbursement area, highly technical processes and procedures are needed to develop and maintain appropriate compliance programs. The numbers and types of compliance issues are significant, the rapid rate of change in all aspects of healthcare delivery and organization continues to increase, and new laws will increase the need for vigilance in this area.

two

Structuring CBR compliance programs

Introduction

Seven key elements must be considered with any healthcare compliance program. A CBR compliance program is specialized and must also appropriately interface with a corporate compliance program and with other specialized programs such as laboratory, pharmacy, home health, or skilled nursing. Thus, the forms and structures of a CBR compliance program and an associated written plan will vary considerably for each hospital, clinic, or integrated delivery system. For larger organizations [integrated delivery systems (IDSs) or hospital systems with multiple clinics], a CBR compliance program will most likely be relatively freestanding with all seven key elements in place. In a smaller setting, e.g., a single hospital, it is likely that a compliance program will be more closely integrated into a corporate program to the point that only certain elements are in evidence, primarily specialized policies and procedures.

Whether tightly integrated or separately organized, the elements, functions, and concerns involving coding, billing, documentation, and reimbursement issues remain essentially the same. The steps and processes are similar although the resources employed to satisfy compliance issues may vary considerably. However, because compliance is more a we-can't-afford-not-to-do-it issue than a can-we-afford-to-do-it? issue, certain basic resources and processes must always be in place.

CBR and seven key elements

The seven key elements cited in Chapter 1 are basic to a CBR compliance program. These elements represent responses to the federal sentencing guidelines. They have also been refined through litigation and various settlements and corporate integrity agreements (CIAs). While these seven elements are common to virtually all healthcare compliance plans, their application to specific areas may vary somewhat. CBR compliance concerns run a gamut of sizes and complexities from a single-physician practice all the way to a multihospital or multiclinic IDS. Interestingly, however, the compliance standards for both sized providers are the same.

Obviously, the application of these seven principles in the CBR area will vary significantly depending upon the specific issues and/or services provided. The seven areas are:

1. Compliance standards and procedures
2. Oversight responsibility
3. Delegation of authority
4. Employee training
5. Monitoring and auditing
6. Enforcement and discipline
7. Response and prevention

As shown in Figure 2.1, these elements can be broken down into two major areas: (1) manuals and written documentation including policies and procedures and (2) an infrastructure that includes personnel, processes, procedures, and various activities.

The first element is an ongoing and dynamic component of a CBR compliance program because the development and implementation of various types of procedures are critical. The remaining six elements relate to infrastructure development that must be documented and will be relatively stable. Certain elements of CBR compliance dominate but each element must be carefully considered.

Compliance standards and procedures

This first element of CBR compliance is probably the most important. *Standards and procedures* translate into *policies and procedures* in the CBR area. Key areas to consider relative to these policies and procedures are

- Coding
- Billing
- Chargemaster
- Documentation
- Utilization
- Compliance and auditing

For large organizations, these six areas may be embodied in manuals that may even be extended into specific areas, such as clinical, home health, skilled nursing, subacute care, etc. In a small or specialized setting, all these manuals may coalesce into a single volume. Note that all healthcare providers have such manuals although some may be virtual rather than absolute—that is, the policies and procedures may have developed on an ad hoc basis and are not specifically organized into a formal manual form. Moreover, distributing policies and procedures across departments and in differing

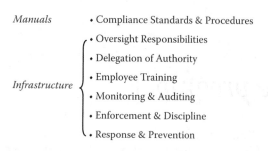

Manuals • Compliance Standards & Procedures

Infrastructure {
  • Oversight Responsibilities
  • Delegation of Authority
  • Employee Training
  • Monitoring & Auditing
  • Enforcement & Discipline
  • Response & Prevention
}

Figure 2.1 Seven key compliance principles.

formats (some paper, some electronic, some as notes, etc.) can lead to difficulties in making, changing, and maintaining consistent policies and procedures.

The simple fact is that all healthcare providers implement certain standards and procedures based upon external requirements. However, in many cases the standards, procedures, and policies may not be explicitly verbalized or organized. The compliance arena is where formalization of this process takes place. Formalization involves developing and writing policies and procedures, organizing them, disseminating them, and, finally, implementing them. After these steps are taken, monitoring can begin and thus ensure that the appropriate standards are met.

Note: Different guidelines, policies, and procedures may conflict with each other. A general example relates to the sequencing of codes. HIM coding staff may use coding guidelines that direct certain sequencing. Those filing claims for services may realize that reimbursement will be adversely affected by following the HIM sequencing of codes. Other examples of potential conflicts will be discussed in case studies throughout this book.

Key learning area: CBR compliance staff must be sensitive to conflicts that may emerge during development and application of policies and procedures.

Coding policies and procedures

Coding is a very complex process. Coding systems include CPT procedure coding and ICD-9-CM procedure and diagnosis coding. Both systems have their own guidelines along with extensive external guidelines in relation to certain payment systems and special requirements of third-party payers. Additionally, these systems are subject to constant change. For example, the present-on-admission (POA) indicator has recently been added to the hospital inpatient claims filing process as a trailing digit added to the diagnosis codes noted on UB-04 claim forms.

Although most guidelines are embedded in a given coding system or generated externally, providers have some latitude in the way these guidelines are applied. For example, for the inpatient DRG system, the principal diagnosis can become a point of contention and the contention may be magnified as additional diagnoses representing complications and/or comorbidities are added. This and similar seemingly small issues have generated compliance concerns with DRG upcoding and with the bundling of certain pre-admission outpatient services into the DRG.

Billing policies and procedures

For hospitals, the basic device for developing statements and claims forms is the chargemaster. Since different third-party payers have different requirements for billing and claims adjudication, the chargemaster and associated processes can be complex and various payment systems such as managed care and capitated contracts add to the complexity. It is little wonder that specific, written policies and procedures covering billing are necessary.

Billing personnel also become involved with coding, both directly and indirectly. For certain types of services in a hospital setting, CPT codes are developed through the chargemaster. Additionally, modifiers on outpatient technical component claims are now required. In an indirect fashion, billing personnel become involved with diagnosis coding relative to medical necessity through the adjudication process. For instance, an ER claim may be denied on the basis that the diagnosis codes did not justify emergency level services. The bill may have to be reworked as an urgent care claim within third-party payer guidelines.

Every facility or department where statements and claims are developed utilizes billing policies and procedures. However, pulling together all appropriate information and keeping it up-to-date while addressing problem areas is a challenge. For example, receipt of a cease-and-desist order from a Medicare FI or carrier certainly warrants a full investigation, changing the billing and claims filing process, and developing a written policy and procedure for area targeted.

Chargemaster policies and procedures

The chargemaster is a lynchpin in the coding, billing, and claims generation process. Many decisions must be made regarding organization and utilization of the chargemaster and several different interfaces are of significant concern. For instance, coding may be performed through charge entry. In a hospital radiology setting, the different CPT/HCPCS codes are entered (statically placed) in the chargemaster as separate line items for each radiological service. When a technician enters a charge for a service, the CPT/HCPCS code is generated through charge entry. In other cases such as general surgery, the chargemaster typically generates only a charge and no code.

The actual coding is performed dynamically outside the chargemaster. In some cases, both static and dynamic coding occur simultaneously, for example, in cardiovascular interventional radiology. Note that coding is only one interface of several that must be carefully considered, analyzed, and documented. Many of chargemaster decisions involve CBR compliance issues.

Documentation policies and procedures

The basis upon which justification for services and services actually rendered lies in documentation. The rules and regulation surrounding documentation and their effective enforcement through policies and procedures are critical. Many providers see documentation as an additional burden instead of an opportunity to excel. It is certainly true that some documentation requirements serve compliance and payment purposes rather than increasing the quality of care. However, the difference in documentation maintained by a physician prior to institution of a medical malpractice lawsuit compared with documentation maintained after suit is instituted may be dramatic.

The large number of concerns requires implementation and development of a number of policies and procedures. Questions concerning provider signatures versus initials, handwritten versus dictated and transcribed records, reviews of transcribed records, timeliness of documentation, revisions, confidentiality, and releases of records are typical, and the list goes on. The main emphasis is on the medical or patient record relative to services provided, but concerns go beyond the provision of healthcare and extend into financial areas. Claims filing, determination of primary versus secondary coverage, and collection efforts must also be documented.

From a compliance perspective, one of the more important issues is record retention. Due consideration must be given to both paper and computer-based records. Experiences with federal audits and recoupment efforts indicate that investigations may extend back as far as 10 years. The ability of a provider to retrieve and/or redevelop patient care records and associated financial records is extremely important. For this reason, careful consideration must be given to record retention polices and procedures in the CBR area. Note that the way in which financial documentation is retained may be different from retention of clinical data.

Utilization review policies and procedures

Utilization review is important for virtually all healthcare providers. In larger provider settings, the review task may be assigned to a specific person and/or department. Obviously, this is an important function because it ties into the compliance area for coding, billing, documentation, and reimbursement. In many cases, a separate set of utilization review policies is established related to certain compliance problem areas.

Consider, for example, a patient who is admitted to a hospital. Services are provided for two days and at the end of the second day, the patient is discharged. Utilization review personnel may review the case and determine that the criteria for inpatient admission were not met. The case may be reclassified to outpatient observation status, and the billing and claims may be changed using Condition Code 44. However, the documentation may not be changed. This is a case where policies and procedures should be developed to address a change process so that an auditor reviewing the case can easily see what has been done and why.

Compliance and auditing policies and procedures

A general compliance or corporate program for a healthcare provider will include a subset of CBR compliance policies and procedures. A very general categorization involves separating routine proactive activities from dynamic reactive activities. For instance, a hospital will typically have an annual inpatient and outpatient coding audit performed by an outside firm or independent review organization (IRO). A medical clinic will often have an annual E/M and procedure coding review. These are routine proactive activities to verify and ensure that compliance in ongoing problem areas is addressed.

On the other hand, certain reactive activities involve special audits and reviews. As noted, hundreds of issues may arise from a variety of sources. Special activities must be developed to resolve or accommodate these issues as compliance issues are identified internally or from external sources. The policies and procedures developed to react to different types of situations are important even if they are generalized at a basic level covering who is to do what and when. For healthcare organizations that have CIAs and settlement agreements, external requirements may be in place. These agreements generally involve reporting infractions and submitting annual reports of activities. Furthermore, these agreements, some of which may be public, can be used by other healthcare organizations to develop compliance policies and procedures.

> **Key learning area: It is critical to develop and maintain written policies and procedures in the CBR area. Significant resources and efforts are required to develop and maintain all the necessary policies and procedures.**

Oversight responsibilities

Oversight responsibilities in the CBR compliance area vary considerably, depending on the size and function of the healthcare provider. At a small hospital or medical clinic, the person designated the chief compliance officer will most likely head the CBR compliance activities as well. In larger settings, a full-time person may be designated the CBR compliance officer. Multi-facility settings may establish a separate department serving as an office of billing compliance.

Whatever the organizational approach, CBR compliance involves personnel and an organizational structure that take advantage of and integrate different disciplines. This makes a team approach logical and appropriate. The typical departments and functions involved must include at a minimum coding, billing, chargemaster, claims transactions, and information technology. Additional representation from financial, utilization review, and even corporate compliance may also be appropriate. Because compliance is considered a technical area, a small team is most effective. The individual assigned responsibility for CBR compliance oversight typically serves as coordinator of the compliance team.

The team then works with specific service areas relative to the various compliance concerns for healthcare providers. The team provides a range of expertise, a comprehensive overview of the coding, billing, documentation and reimbursement process, and synergism in general. The size and structure of a healthcare provider will dictate what personnel are used and the degree of formality accorded the organizational structure. A small hospital or a physician clinic may assign someone to CBR compliance on a part-time basis. A large hospital system or integrated delivery system will most likely have several full-time people dedicated to different aspects of compliance.

Note: The team structure represents the same system used for revenue enhancement, chargemaster reviews, and the like. The structure and the activities of the team may can be directed toward multiple objectives.

> **Key learning area: Oversight responsibilities in the CBR area generally reside with an individual who also serves as coordinator for the CBR compliance team.**

Delegation of authority

Delegation is a challenging task for CBR compliance personnel who often find themselves needing to influence or facilitate changes or implementation of policies and procedures without having line authority to do so. For the most part, personnel providing healthcare services will not be under the line authority of CBR compliance personnel. In some cases, providers (particularly physicians) may not even be employees of an organization. In the case of medical clinics, CBR personnel may be employees of the physician owners. Thus the word *authority* must be used in a slightly modified form.

The functions of a CBR compliance team outlined in the preceding section can help establish authority and credibility on a technical basis. However, with compliance issues, it is often necessary to defer to administrative authority and support in accomplishing facilitative processes. Take as an example the need for medical necessity documentation relative to observation admission. This is often a documentation issue reserved for the physician admitting the patient to observation status. CBR compliance personnel can certainly write the policies, procedures, guidelines, care paths and even provide training. However, full implementation of such policies requires the active participation of physicians. In a case of this kind, it may be more appropriate to work through upper administrative staff, the chief medical officer (CMO), and the medical staff organization (MSO) to ensure adherence to extended documentation requirements for observation services.

For another example, consider laboratory services. Many hospitals provide such services to independent physicians in the community who are not under the management control of the hospital.* When a physician orders laboratory tests, a written order must be accompanied with diagnostic information.† The whole range of medical necessity of laboratory tests and signed waivers or advance beneficiary notices (ABNs) comes into play. Even if policies and procedures relative to medical necessity are in place, it may be difficult to enforce physician compliance. Again, working through the medical staff organization, developing easy-to-use requisition forms or processes, and instituting appropriate training and education can assist in facilitating physician cooperation in meeting compliance demands in this area.

As this discussion shows, the delegation of authority in the CBR compliance area is not simply a supervisory

---

* CMS has indicated that hospitals do control physicians on their medical staffs. See *Federal Register*, April 7, 2000 (65 FR 18519) relative to using proper Place of Service (POS) on 1500 claim forms for provider-based clinics.
† This is a provision of the Balanced Budget Act (1997).

line delegation. Because many aspects involve facilitation and persuasion without line authority, alternative measures may be required.

Key learning area: Delegation of authority in the CBR compliance area requires alternative approaches involving facilitation and persuasive processes.

Employee training

The processes of coding, billing, developing documentation, and monitoring reimbursement are highly complex and constantly changing. With the exception of a small number of providers who intentionally commit fraud, most healthcare providers are simply trying to figure out how to bill correctly and be properly paid. Thus employee training and communication are prime activities for CBR compliance personnel. Training falls into several categories:

- Ongoing versus reactive
- Internal versus external
- Type and level of personnel
- Media and delivery technique

A CBR compliance training program should be carefully planned, giving due consideration to effectiveness and cost–benefit considerations. A CBR team must carefully document the various activities and, as appropriate, integrate training into the overall corporate training program, heeding continuing education unit (CEU) considerations. (Chapter 7 discusses CBR compliance training in greater detail.)

Key learning area: Training and effective communication are key elements in the development and implementation of a CBR compliance program.

Monitoring and auditing

Because of the many concerns relative to the coding, billing, documentation, claims filing and reimbursement processes, monitoring and auditing are also key elements of CBR compliance and involve computer systems, payment system interfaces, and a host of legal concerns. Both systematic processes and end products are available for review, monitoring, and auditing. Probably the biggest challenge is sheer volume. Even a modest-sized healthcare organization files tens of thousands of claims and requires methods to monitor and audit activities.

The processes of setting up systems and generating reports for review require careful analysis. The types of monitoring systems and reports generated will often emanate from problem areas; these and generalized reports can be compared to national and/or local norms. Fortunately, the various payment and associated coding systems allow us to develop and gather data. All (or nearly all) prospective payment systems involve classification systems for services provided. The DRG system that can be used for all inpatient stays classifies cases based on acuity and resource utilization, using ICD diagnosis and procedure codes. The APC system performs a similar function for outpatient services using CPT and HCPCS procedure codes.

Probably the most universal mechanism for monitoring CBR activities is reviewing payment or reimbursement. With the exception of certain contractual situations (such as capitation), most activities involving coding, billing, and reimbursement result in some form of reimbursement. Claims must be filed and adjudicated to determine payment prior to reimbursement. As third-party payers continue to refine their adjudication systems, claims rejection and/or reduced payments provide important information relative to compliance monitoring.

Another important tool for a CBR compliance team is auditing—a technique also used externally by government entities and healthcare providers. There are several levels and types of audits; on an informal level, they may be called reviews. A healthcare provider may conduct informal internal audits of 20 or 30 cases on a periodic or random basis. More comprehensive audits may be conducted internally or by outside consultants. These audits will involve samplings that are carefully chosen to be statistically valid for the audit objectives. The process of choosing an audit sample is highly dependent upon the specific service area involved.

For example, in reviewing medical charts and associated billing and claims forms for physician services relative to the proper level of E/M coding, the sampling unit will probably be based on visits. When applied to a physician, a visit is a self-contained unit that should stand on it own. However, in the area of home health, a visit becomes part of a larger process. Much of the important documentation relative to medical necessity will be at the case level of which a visit is part of a case or 60-day episode of care justified by CMS-485. In all cases, it is important to identify what objectives the audit should achieve.

Many types of errors may be uncovered in an audit. Some of the most typical are

- Incidental error affecting only reimbursement
- Incidental error resulting in non-compliance
- Systematic error affecting only reimbursement

- Systematic error resulting in non-compliance
- Other incidental and systematic errors not affecting reimbursement or compliance

One of the tools that may be developed and utilized by a CBR team to deal with such errors is a benchmark audit that can be approached from either a top-down or bottom-up perspective. Most healthcare providers use a combination of the two approaches. The basic idea is to take a snapshot of the organization (or some component of the organization) and then, at a later time, take another snapshot and compare the two to see what variations have occurred. Unusual changes or variations can then identified and analyzed. (Audits are discussed at greater length in Chapters 8 and 9.)

Key learning area: Monitoring and auditing in the CBR compliance area are critical and may be facilitated by a number of tools. The several types of audits include random, benchmarking, and organizational baseline audits.

Enforcement and discipline

As indicated, the main challenge in the CBR compliance area is to make certain everyone understands how to perform required functions correctly. Typically, enforcement and discipline are not major concerns in the CBR area. In other words, the presupposition is that personnel involved in CBR processes want to perform correctly. However, this aspect of CBR compliance cannot be omitted because employees, despite training, may not perform according to policies and procedures. Enforcement and discipline are also concerns because compliance may depend on personnel who are not employees and thus are not under the direct control of a healthcare organization in which they work.

Most of the problems in the CBR compliance area result from poor personnel performance, and disciplinary action falls within the general human resources purview. Personnel performance errors that result in non-compliance often justify disciplinary action, but it is important to remember that a lack of understanding or proper training may be the cause of a performance error.

Response and prevention

Response and prevention are ongoing processes. Response is a reactive process to a problem area. Problem areas have a number of sources including patient complaints, statistical aberrations, cease-and-desist orders, audits, reimbursement aberrations, and general situational analyses. Whatever the source of a particular

problem, it must be addressed in a systematic way to ensure that it is fully identified and resolved.

One difficult aspect of this process is the issue of self-disclosure, a significant part of corporate compliance programs. The difficulty of applying this in the CBR area is that it is not always easy to know when a situation is severe enough to warrant self-disclosure to Medicare or a law enforcement agency. A routine audit of claims, for example, may show that certain supplies have been separately charged even though they should have been bundled into the overhead cost category. The audit may also show, however, that no additional reimbursement was received. Based on these facts, does this constitute a situation requiring self-disclosure? Taking this example further, assume that the incorrect billing of supplies resulted in overpayment. Is it enough simply to refund the overpayment without self-disclosing? These and similar questions should be referred to legal counsel for guidance. Note that if a healthcare provider is under a settlement agreement or a corporate integrity agreement (CIA), the actions required may be predetermined.

Once a problem has been identified and resolved it is also necessary to take steps to prevent recurrence. One of the most important ways to prevent recurrence is to document the resolution of the problem and the ongoing steps taken.

Key learning area: CBR compliance may involve a number of different errors. The responses to and resolutions of errors that may include self-disclosure to Medicare and possibly law enforcement agencies is a sensitive area that may require advice of legal counsel.

CBR compliance officer

A CBR compliance officer (CBRCO) is a technical professional who requires a wide range of skills, capabilities, and knowledge. In some healthcare organizations, the individual assigned to this position will have a strong technical background to serve the technical needs of CBR compliance programs. In other institutions, the CBRCO may have a broad view of the compliance area and also some knowledge or training in legal and organizational matters. This person should facilitate a close working relationship between general corporate compliance level and the more detailed CBR compliance level. A job description is provided in the appendix.

Key learning area: A CBR compliance officer holds a technical position requiring extensive knowledge, experience, and skills in the

areas of coding, billing, and reimbursement. The officer may hold a part-time position in a smaller health care organization while a larger organization may require a small compliance department.

Use of investigative and review teams

The power and synergism of a team must be harnessed to achieve CBR compliance. Coding, billing, documentation, chargemaster, and reimbursement issues are complex and multidisciplinary. No one person can have full knowledge and requisite skills that can accommodate all aspects of CBR. As indicated earlier, the choice of team members is important because the team must include people with technical skills, a comprehensive perspective, and the ability to work together effectively.

A CBR compliance officer typically serves as the team coordinator or leader, depending upon the number of projects and/or teams in existence concurrently. For particularly sensitive situations, outside consultative and/or legal assistance may be required. The effective use of teams must also be coordinated at the corporate compliance level. While CBR compliance generally may be self-contained, the compliance issue may be broader in certain situations and affect the organization as well. (See the bibliography for references on team organization and effective utilization.)

Development of policies and procedures

Of the seven key elements of a compliance program, the development of policies and procedures will probably consume the most significant portion of staff time. In some cases, CBR compliance personnel will draft policies and procedures; in other cases, they will be involved only indirectly. For example, chargemaster policies and procedures will generally be developed by the chargemaster coordinator or someone with a similar title. CBR compliance personnel will review and modify such policies and procedures as appropriate in order to accommodate compliance concerns.

The application of the systems approach or other quality improvement technique relative to compliance problems (as discussed in Chapter 4) will generally result in the need to establish policies and procedures that must be carefully crafted. Multiple interlaced policies and procedures may be required. A problem may relate to the assignment of a date of service. Assume, for example, a patient arrived at 11 p.m. on a Thursday and was held as an outpatient until 1 a.m. on Friday, when he was admitted to the hospital. Health information management may want to use Thursday as the start of an episode of care. Billing personnel will want the date of service to be Friday, the second day, when the patient was given inpatient status and bundle the Thursday charges. Such differences must be discussed thoroughly appropriate policies and procedures to resolve the conflict must be put into place.

Facilitation and organizational development

Line authority for CBR compliance personnel is often not available, especially when physicians and other providers are not employees or do not serve under the direct control of the healthcare organization providing care. CBR compliance personnel must frequently be facilitators or arbitrators handling compliance issues involving different departments and/or different perspectives. Their persuasive abilities generally come from technical knowledge and a broad experience base.

Facilitation skills are also useful for CBR compliance personnel who are heavily involved in providing specialized training for a broad cross-section of personnel in a healthcare organization. The ability to train and effectively communicate with people who have highly disparate backgrounds and abilities is a highly desired skill. Training and education are keys for effectively implementing changes to meet compliance issues.

CBR and administrative decision making

While CBR compliance personnel may not have line authority in many situations, they can gain a great deal of leverage if given an administrative management mandate to develop and implement CBR compliance. In other words, CBR compliance personnel must have access to administrative management and decision-making. In fact, management support is a critical element in any CBR compliance program, and great care must be taken to integrate the infrastructure of a CBR compliance program with a corporate compliance program.

As mentioned in Chapter 1, compliance has several levels, the most important of which is statutory compliance. Many healthcare providers will focus their primary compliance efforts (including coding, billing, and reimbursement issues) on various laws, rules, regulations, directives, and interpretations that emerge from Medicare, Medicaid, and associated government programs. The next level is contractual compliance. Contractual obligations result from negotiated contract arrangements with various third-party payers, including those generically referred to as managed care contracts. It is vital for CBR compliance personnel to have full knowledge of the requirements and obligations of such contracts. Ideally, such personnel should be involved in the negotiation of these contracts.

The third level of compliance concerns relates to filing claims with third-party payers with which the organization has no contractual and/or other formal arrangements. In such situations, the coding, billing, and claims filing requirements come from state laws such as the Uniform Commercial Code or from national laws such as the HIPAA Transaction Standard/ Standard Code Set (TSR) Rule. Standard code set utilization applies, at least in theory, to all third-party payers and healthcare providers.

Compliance personnel are often viewed in a reactive mode. In actuality, however, the compliance team should be recognized as a proactive force that should have a role in the design, structuring, and organizational development of healthcare organizations. Involvement at the front end of these strategic and planning processes will enable CBR personnel to put into place the necessary arrangements and systems to prevent or inhibit potential compliance problems. It is generally easier and less expensive to design compliant service areas and associated CBR systems than to reactively fix a broken system. As noted, administrative support is critical for empowering CBR compliance teams.

Key learning area: Policies and procedures form a major element of a CBR compliance program but they are useless without a proper organizational infrastructure that facilitates their proper identification and implementation. Compliance personnel must have strong administrative support in order to identify and resolve compliance issues.

Summary and conclusion

A written CBR compliance plan will vary significantly, depending upon the size and coverage of a healthcare provider and the details of its corporate compliance plan. In all cases, however, CBR compliance planning must address the seven key elements cited above. The major areas for CBR compliance are standards and procedures, employee training, and monitoring and auditing.

A significant amount of time will be spent developing policies and procedures in the coding, billing, documentation, and utilization review areas. Coding, billing, documentation, and billing are highly complex and require significant training and education. A separate training and education plan is essential, particularly in light of the ongoing changes in payment systems and the continuing development and refinement of the supporting coding systems. Auditing in several different forms is used to assess and evaluate the overall CBR process. A particularly useful form for CBR purposes is the organizational baseline audit.

Note that CBR compliance personnel may not have line authority. Thus an administrative mandate requiring compliance is very useful to effect change.

three

Coding, billing, and reimbursement
Problem/opportunity areas

Introduction

The number, type, diversity, and complexity of CBR compliance opportunities and problems seem almost endless. The magnitude of potential compliance concerns derives directly from the complexity of coding, billing, filing claims, generating itemized statements, receiving reimbursement, and monitoring managed care activities. Moving beyond the claims filing process, the provision of healthcare in different settings has also become more complex. CMS developed the provider-based rule (PBR) in response to perceived abuses of increased payments. EMTALA was developed in response to problems encountered with providing emergency services, some of which impact coding, billing, and reimbursement. Additionally, HIPAA legislation set significant compliance requirements for privacy, the standardization of claims filing, and the use of standard code sets.

Despite the uniformity in claims filing envisaged by the HIPAA administrative simplification act, almost every third-party payer and/or payment contract is a little (sometimes a lot!) different from others. Government programs such as Medicare, Medicaid, and Tricare also have rules and regulations that must be addressed within these payment systems and in relation to interactions of these payment systems with private third-party payers. Another complicating factor is the rapid rate of change in healthcare delivery at both organizational and individual patient care levels.

This chapter reviews a number of problem/opportunity areas. The discussions are somewhat tentative because the rules and regulation and their interpretations continue to change in complex and subtle ways. Moreover, the issues involved cannot be viewed simply as hot compliance topics of today, but must be viewed in light of new topics that may arise in the coming years to become the major problems of tomorrow.

Two different mechanisms are used in this chapter. One approach is to look at a general law such as the False Claims Act or the Medicare Fraud, Abuse, and Anti-Kickback Laws, and then locate specific areas that fall under the appropriate law. The other approach is to look at specific processes and structures within the healthcare provider setting for problem/opportunity identification. The chargemaster and the documentation development process are two examples of the second approach.

Keep in mind that while the discussion in this chapter focuses primarily on statutorily related compliance issues, your healthcare organization also has many contractual obligations that must be considered. While we can all look at the relevant statutory rules and regulations, many contractual requirements are specific only to one contract and may thus differ greatly from statutory requirements.

Compliance problem and opportunity areas are addressed throughout this book. In Chapter 4 we will integrate problem identification as part of a systematic process for addressing compliance concerns. Specific compliance areas such as EMTALA, the PBR, and false claims will be discussed in more detail in later chapters.

Identifying problem/opportunity areas

As with many aspects of the coding, billing, and reimbursement process, an individual issue or problem is not the primary concern. If we know that a problem exists, we can address it. What is more important (and more challenging) is identifying unknown issues and situations. Obviously, a solution must be developed for any issue, but the first step in developing a solution is to obtain and analyze specific facts and data, about the problem at hand. This is where the question of the reliability of sources comes into play, as does the need to corroborate information and verify the interpretation of rules and regulations.*

CBR compliance personnel at any clinic, hospital, or IDS generally have little difficulty in identifying problems and/or opportunities. Often it is not even necessary to seek out areas of concern because concerns will be brought to compliance personnel in the form of questions and verification of processes. This can be viewed as a *reactive* approach because a response occurs whenever changes occur in:

- Payment systems
- Delivery systems
- Organizational structuring

---

* See discussion of the systems approach in the introduction to the book and in Chapter 4.

- Creation of new service areas
- Laws, rules, and regulations

The next step in the sequence is to carefully analyze the effects of changes on the compliance stance of the organization. A significant number of CBR compliance personnel engage in the study and analysis of such changes at both the national and local levels. It is important, especially with the rapid rate of change, that all healthcare personnel be sensitive to including compliance personnel when dealing with local changes and developments. At the national level, a careful review of payment system changes and regulatory changes is also appropriate.*

In a *proactive* approach, CBR compliance personnel seek out current compliance concerns, information about current litigation and/or OIG actions, data about impositions of sanctions, and the like. By simply referring to the OIG's Internet home page, for example, compliance personnel can download the OIG's most recent work plan showing where OIG is concentrating its efforts. These work plans generally reveal dozens of areas of concern. CBR compliance personnel can study the listing and then investigate whether the listed areas are of concern to their specific healthcare provider. The OIG categorizes areas of investigation by type of provider; however, it is wise to check for crossover areas. The topics discussed in the sections below can also serve as a general guide to potential issues of concern that should be considered.

> **Case study 3-1. Hospital to physician coding correlation.** CBR compliance personnel at the Apex Medical Center noted that the OIG listed the correlation of outpatient hospital xo physician procedure coding as an issue of concern in one of its work plans. As a simple test, Apex conducted a probe audit of 30 outpatient surgical cases. The surgeons involved were asked to share their coding so that compliance personnel could see whether a reasonable match existed between the professional and technical claims.

As might be expected, Apex found significant discrepancies between the codes in about 25 percent of the cases. Noting that CMS was in the process of developing regional Medicare administrative contractors who would easily be able to compare professional and technical claims for common services, the Apex Medical Center moved this issue up on its priority listing.

> **Key learning area: CBR personnel must often be reactive to potential and real compliance problems. The longer-term goal is to be proactive and identify and resolve situations before they become compliance problems.**

Determining real problem

In some cases, compliance problems are straightforward, for example, when an E/M code does not match the appropriate E/M coding documentation guidelines. The resolution is a matter of determining whether inappropriate levels of service were selected, either up or down, and then taking appropriate corrective action. Identification of the problem (inappropriate coding) is generally a matter of selective auditing and/or overall analysis of the frequency distribution of E/M utilization based upon specialty and/or individual physician categorization.

Other problem areas require digging deeper, asking questions, and analyzing the process or system to ensure that the real problem is identified. It does little good to resolve a problem that is only a symptom. The real solution is to resolve the underlying "real" problem or fundamental situation causing the symptom. A number of methodologies are available for this purpose. This process will be discussed more fully in Chapter 4 in connection with the systems approach.

Medical necessity

Of all the compliance issues faced by hospitals, physician, clinics, and IDSs, what constitutes medical necessity is probably the *single biggest compliance issue* (short term and long term) faced by CBR compliance personnel. Today, most payment systems are fee-for-service, that is, payments are based on the type and volume of services provided. Thus, third-party payers want to be certain that they pay only for services that are medically necessary. Their position is that they should make no payments for services that are not medically justified.

In theory, this situation should change with the development of managed care capitated contracts under which payments are fixed in advance and the risk shifts from the third-party payer to the provider of healthcare services who faces the possibility of overutilization based on prepayments. Because the provider assumes the risk, the compliance issue from the third-party payer's perspective is whether all necessary services are really provided. The basic idea behind fee-for-service arrangements is that **every claim (and associated itemized statement) filed must have medical necessity justification documented**.

---

* See Chapter 1 and the Appendix for a discussion of comprehensive informational resources in the CBR area.

While nearly everyone considers this appropriate, it is nearly impossible for any hospital, clinic, or other healthcare provider to ensure that no claim goes out the door without being medically necessary. The following two case studies show how difficult it may be to adhere to this requirement consistently and absolutely.

Case study 3-2. Post-surgery observation status. A patient presents for outpatient surgery at the Apex Medical Center. The surgery is delayed because the surgeon is running behind schedule. The patient is not taken to recovery until 3 p.m. At 4:30 p.m., the surgeon sees the patient and decides to admit her to observation status. However, the only notation placed in the record is the physician's order to admit to observation. The record contains no indication of examination, history, or medical decision making. As a result, no documentation justified provision of the service. Without such documentation, the hospital must question the appropriateness of using RC 0762 (Observation).

Case study 3-3. Emergency department: Urgent versus emergent care. An elderly patient presents to Apex Medical Center's ER at 10 p.m. His chief complaint is bowel discomfort. He is diagnosed as having a minor fecal impaction, given a laxative, and sent home with instructions. The ER claim filed is subsequently denied because no diagnosis codes indicate the situation was truly an emergency. The ensuing investigation shows that this is a typical occurrence, and that some claims are denied while others are paid. The ER coding, billing, and reimbursement system is changed, and this claim is refiled using RC 0456 (Urgent Care in the ER with Regular Office Visit or Other Outpatient Services) E/M codes. The claim is paid.

Medical necessity is more than a documentation challenge. The documentation may be appropriate, but if the diagnostic statements and subsequently developed ICD-9-CM diagnosis codes are inadequate, the claim may be denied during the adjudication process. Without appropriate diagnostic codes to justify the medical necessity of the procedures or services, requests for additional information, outright claims denial, and/or flagging for possible compliance concerns may result.

Another example related to medical necessity is tied to CMS's development of national coverage decisions (NCDs) and MACs' (Medicare administrative contractors') development of local coverage decisions (LCDs). These coverage decisions typically include extensive lists of diagnosis codes that do provide (and sometimes

do not provide) justification for medical necessity. For the Medicare program, these NCDs and LCDs lead to the further complication of issuing advance beneficiary notices (ABNs) or, for hospitals, hospital-issued notices of non-coverage (HINNs). In recent years, the numbers and types of ABNs or HINNs constitute major sources of ongoing compliance concerns.

Case study 3-4. Patient refuses to sign ABN. Apex Medical Center has been working very hard to properly use ABNs correctly in connection with laboratory services. A problem has arisen because some Medicare patients refuse to sign the ABN form even though they insist on having tests performed. Encounter personnel want to know whether they should refuse to provide the service.

ABNs have created a significant compliance issue and their proper use now involves many technical nuances. Specific modifiers* must be used on the associated claims. CBR compliance personnel must be careful to develop complete policies and procedures reflecting these nuances and must properly train service area personnel on handling sometimes delicate situations.

Key learning area: Medical necessity is the overarching compliance issue for all healthcare providers. For medical necessity, diagnosis coding is a key element from both payment system and compliance perspectives. All applicable diagnosis codes should be developed and placed on claim forms as appropriate.

False claims

False claims can be filed in many different ways, but many false claims are filed mistakenly without fraudulent intent. As in the above cases involving medical necessity, a claim can become "false" simply because the way the coding, billing, and claims filing process are set up creates problems. The following case studies further illustrate this point.

Case study 3-5. Services or supplies not rendered or used. Apex Medical Center uses charge explosion in its chargemaster for supply packs. Although all the supplies in the pack are individually billed, personnel inputting the charges need only mark off one charge code. However, on occasion some of supply items in the pack are not used and may be saved for inclusion in other packs or simply discarded. Unfortunately, the

---

* See the -GA, -G4, and -GZ modifiers.

center has no system for excluding these items from the exploded charge and is billing for supplies that are not used for the purpose intended (they are not medically necessary).

Case study 3-6. Incorrect categorization on chargemaster. The incorrect categorization of a service or supply can easily be overlooked. For instance, the ER may dispense crutches and canes, but these items are categorized as ancillary supplies (RC 0270) and not as durable medical equipment (DME), RC 0274. Similar situations occur when a chargemaster line item entry is not properly aligned, i.e., the description and/or CPT/HCPCS code and/or RC do not match.

Case study 3-7. Improper place of service or type of bill. Apex Medical Center has specialty physicians who come to the hospital on a regular basis one to four times a month. The center has no formal or written agreement with the specialty physicians although they are on the medical staff. The center makes a facility charge on a UB-04 indicating that these physicians work in provider-based clinics. The hospital is unaware that several of the physicians are filing their 1500 claim forms with incorrect place of service (i.e., office versus hospital outpatient) noted. The place of service should be hospital outpatient, but because of the Medicare site-of-service differential reduction, several of the physicians are reporting their offices as places of service.

Case study 3-8. Billing non-covered service or item as covered. This is a major problem area with self-administrable and take-home drugs and supplies. A patient may be at a hospital today for outpatient surgery and then discharged and given surgery-related drugs and/or supplies for home use. The hospital bills and files a claim as if the drugs were regular pharmacy and/or supply items instead of using RC 0253 for the drugs and RC 0623 for the take-home surgical supplies.

These four relatively simple examples illustrate how easily compliance issues can arise when incorrect or false claims are filed. Note that the discussion of these four issues is brief and shows how even simple discrepancies can create compliance issues; there is much more to consider in addressing each of these examples.

Key learning area: Numerous compliance issues can cause false claims to be unknowingly filed. Healthcare compliance personnel must be especially watchful in the coding, billing, and reimbursement area. What may appear to be appropriate may require careful investigation and analysis to make certain claims are filed in correctly.

Service area concerns

This section covers a short list of compliance concerns associated with particular departments and/or providers. This list needs to be expanded based on a specific healthcare provider's needs. See the top-down organizational approach for a baseline audit discussed in Chapter 9.

Observation status

Observation services represent a status rather than a place of service because the services can be provided anywhere in a hospital setting. How does a patient get into observation status? The following requirements should be considered:

1. A physician must order the observation status in writing.
2. The medical necessity of the patient admitted to observation status must be documented through three elements of the E/M observation codes: (a) history, (b) examination, and (c) medical decision making.

If these elements are documented, the compliance concerns surrounding admission to observation status are met and it will be easy to develop the appropriate professional E/M code for the observation services. Note that observation services represent a challenge for both hospitals and physicians relative to proper coding, billing, and payment.

This process does not mitigate the need to have care paths in place that provide guidance for the process of making a decision about admitting a patient to observation, a decision to discharge a patient from observation to acute care, home, or other service levels, and/or the decision to retain a patient in observation status. Note that observation services may be provided in a number of situations such as post-outpatient surgery, post-ER services, and direct admission from a clinic.

These themes have variations as well. Post-outpatient surgery is a distinct compliance area. Under the APC Medicare payment system, no separate payment is made because CMS believes that hospitals inappropriately use observation services. Thus, no separate payments are made for observation on a post-outpatient surgery basis. In order to have any possibility of separate payment, hospitals must be especially fastidious in documenting post-outpatient surgery services.

Observation services following ER services are relatively common. The observation services may be provided in the ER, in a dedicated observation area, or on an acute care floor. Note that distinct coding and medical staff privilege issues surround each case. For example, do the ER physicians have observation admission privileges? If they do, CPT coding guidelines do not allow an ER physician to code both an ER level of service and an observation service. However, on the hospital side, both the ER services and the observation services can be coded and billed.

It is also possible that a patient may be admitted to observation status directly from a medical clinic or physician office setting. In this case, the hospital's service may be limited to observation. This may create some coding and documentation challenges because the documentation for the admission, including the signed physician order, must be obtained directly from the physician since the main documentation may reside at the clinic.

Care should be taken to determine that true observation services are provided. It is not unusual for a pregnant woman to be observed in the context of "labor" even though she is not yet in labor. After a number of hours, she may be sent home or admitted for labor and delivery. This type of observation generally does not meet the criteria of a physician's order, history, examination, or medical decision making because a physician is not immediately involved. This type of service would probably be better described as "obstetric holding." Exceptions are observations of labor and delivery that may occur in post-accident or similar situations and thus qualify as "true observations."

Note: Although various aspects of observation services issues are discussed throughout this book, a thorough and complete discussion of the observation issue is beyond the scope of this work. A thorough discussion would require addressing a number of situations, including one-day hospitalizations, the use of Condition Code 44 on UB-04 claim forms, and documentation and medical decision making related to specific clinical pathways.

Case study 3-9. Same day inpatient admit and discharge. An elderly patient was admitted as an inpatient to Apex Medical Center in the morning. The patient exhibited an electrolyte imbalance. The patient was taking a diuretic along with supplemental potassium. However, the patient refused to take the potassium orally. In order to stabilize the electrolytic balance, potassium was given intravenously. By afternoon, the patient was ready to go home and was discharged. Unfortunately, utilization review did not get to this patient

before discharge to switch the case from inpatient to outpatient using Condition Code 44. The center is now concerned that this case cannot be billed because no medical necessity was documented.

Key learning area: Observation services continue to be major compliance problems for hospitals in many respects. The issue is exacerbated by the fact that the provision of observation services is almost totally in the hands of physicians whose primary concern is proper care for patients and not necessarily the specific documentary status relative to coding, billing, and payment.

Emergency department

The emergency room (ER) is a microcosm of hospital services, including assessments and various medical and surgical procedures. Thus, the potential for compliance problems (along with issues involving patient care) is significant. Probably the issue of greatest concern with respect to ER services is medical necessity. The simple fact is that patients present to the ER for a variety of reasons, not all of which can be classified as emergencies. Often, the precise purpose and nature of the patient visit to ER may not be known until services are provided. Even diagnostic testing, in retrospect, may have been performed unnecessarily. To accommodate these imprecise variables, a coding, billing, and documentation system that addresses various levels of care for the ER should be established. Typically, an ER provides services at three levels: (1) emergent, (2) urgent, and (3) clinic.

For CBR purposes, the three different levels of service should involve the chargemaster (both for professional and technical fee schedules), encounter and charge slips for checking off services, the documentation system, and, in some cases, the design of the delivery system. In larger hospital or IDS situations it is possible to have an ER triage process that will separate and classify patients as emergent or urgent. Distinct facilities can then be established to handle the different levels of care. In some cases, the true emergencies are addressed by physicians while the urgent cases can be addressed by mid-level or non-physician providers; clinic level cases can be referred to appropriate clinic settings.

The relationship between the hospital and ER physicians can also create concerns, although the concerns are less significant if the ER physicians are employees. If, however, the ER physicians are contracted by the hospital or, in some cases, simply cover the ER without a formal contract, certain aspects of the relationship should be reviewed. With respect to contracted

ER physicians, the primary question is how they are compensated. If any component of the compensation involves a volume incentive, contracts between the hospital and physicians must be carefully structured and reviewed. In smaller, generally rural hospitals, an ER physician may simply be an on-call community physician. How does the on-call status affect compensation? Are these physicians compensated for being on-call or do they simply handle their own billing under their own national provider identifiers?

Questions about the use of non-physician providers (NPPs) also arise. If the NPPs work under the supervision of a physician, their reimbursement comes through the technical or facilities component. If the NPPs are practitioners and have their own national provider identifiers, their services can be billed on a 1500. However, both cases involve concerns about the type and level of supervision and also about the associated documentation.

The concerns about the NPPs also extend to the ER nursing staff. In many cases, the primary services may be provided by the ER nursing staff under the direction of an ER physician. The question then becomes whether the physician can code and bill for services he or she did not personally provide. These same types of concerns can be further magnified in certain settings. For instance, for critical access hospitals (CAHs) questions about ER physicians and qualified non-physician practitioners who are on call take on added meaning due to special rules and regulations that apply to CAHs.

Coding issues abound with ER services. On the physician side, one area of concern is the global surgical package (GSP) used by Medicare and other third-party payers. ER physicians are often involved with various types of surgical services, e.g., laceration repair, fracture repair, debridement, burn care, etc. Depending on the way in which ERs are organized, post-operative care is sometimes transferred to other physicians and clinics. If ER physicians are not involved in post-operative care, it is important to make certain that the -54 (intraoperative only component) modifier is used to indicate that only the intraoperative portion of the GSP was provided. This results in lower reimbursement but keeps the physician billing within compliance guidelines and avoids false claims. Note that on the hospital side, there is no GSP, at least under APCs.

The chargemaster can also be an issue. As noted in Case study 3-6, canes and crutches are often dispensed in an ER. These are durable medical equipment (DME) items that typically must be billed differently from the way other supplies are billed. Another supply issue is whether a skin adhesive such as Dermabond is separately billable. These examples are typical and hundreds of other circumstances raise similar questions.

Documentation issues beside those related to medical necessity and legal liability also surface frequently. Typically, nursing staffs maintain records as well as dictated or handwritten notes from ER physicians. Because timing is a consideration for certain coding scenarios, the records must indicate the amount of time spent performing certain services and the documentation cannot lump certain services into a single unit. Critical care services and CPR (cardiopulmonary resuscitation) services, for example, must be separated because only critical care services are coded on a time basis.

Special laws relate to emergency services. EMTALA (Emergency Medical Treatment and Active Labor Act) guidelines specify that services must be provided in a manner that adheres to national guidelines. A number of state laws and various tax laws may also affect hospitals as not-for-profit organizations. Note that special revenue codes cover EMTALA services* and that EMTALA basically addresses refusals of service and patient transfers. For this these reasons alone, the role, function, and purpose of EMTALA should be well understood by hospitals and ER physicians.

ER physicians are in a transitional stage and are often involved in urgent care centers and clinic activities, depending upon the size of the ER and the volume of care provided. One service that ER physicians may perform is observation. As discussed above, observation is a status and can be provided virtually anywhere. Thus ER physicians, if they have admitting-to-observation privileges, can place a patient in observation and then provide ongoing observation care. This is often appropriate as a patient may need to be held for 4 to 6 hours, something that typically occurs in ER settings. Note that CPT coding guidelines do not allow ER physicians to code for both an ER visit and observation. Only one of the services will be paid. However, on the facility side, since separate resources are used for the ER and the observation, both codes should be used.†

Coding guidelines for unusual cases must also be considered. For example, an elderly patient may present to the ER late at night. The ER physician performs a medical workup and decides that the patient should be admitted as an inpatient. Since ER physicians do not normally have admitting privileges, an attending physician is called at home. The attending physician concurs and says, "Admit the patient and I'll see her in the morning." The attending physician sees the patient the next day; this may be permissible under the medical staff bylaws. However, it can lead to a compliance question: whether the attending physician can code for

---

* See RC 0451 and 0452 for further information in your state's UB-04 manual.

† Be certain to check coding guidelines for any specific requirements and/or bundling provisions.

a hospital admission since he or she did not see the patient (personally) on the date of admission.*

Other issues surround ER physicians working with consulting physicians. In some cases, both physicians are involved in care. They may both work on the same condition and at other times work on different injuries or illnesses. A consulting physician may function as a true consultant and simply advise an ER physician caring for a patient. In other cases, a consulting physician may take over the care of a patient. The complexity of such relationships and the associated coding require careful documentation as to the provider of a service and the reason for the service.

Clearly, ER services are subject to a wide range of compliance concerns. False claims, medical necessity, correct coding, use of modifiers, and organizational concerns must be carefully considered. Because the scope of the issues involved is so broad, great potential for compliance problems exists and hospitals must carefully review their policies and procedures as well as associated licensing and certification requirements.

Case study 3-10. Emergency department rib fracture coding. Emergency department (ED) coding personnel at Apex Medical Center code only the hospital technical component. Quite by accident, someone discovered that when patients present with uncomplicated rib fractures, ER physicians are coding fracture care (CPT code 21800) in addition to the E/M level. However, the hospital ED staff bundle this fracture care service into the E/M level, leading to concern that the professional and technical claims forms do not correlate. (See also Case study 3-1.)

Key learning area: The ED is a microcosm of hospital services, requiring both physician and hospital coding, billing, and reimbursement for a wide range of services. Special attention must be given to a variety of compliance concerns for the ED.

Subacute care

Subacute care covers a variety of services at different levels. Subacute care implies a level between acute and skilled nursing. In an outpatient setting, subacute care indicates a higher level of clinic care as, for example, a wound care center. In a home health setting it refers to services such as high technology infusion therapy. No matter which setting is involved, subacute care repre-sents a distinct level of care and thus deviates from the recognized standard care level that is "normal" for the given setting. Payment systems are typically geared toward well defined standard levels of care.

It is important to note that whenever healthcare providers develop additional care levels (in this case, sub-acute care) to achieve a better cost–benefit ratio, they face the risk that compliance concerns surrounding medical necessity, coding, and documentation will arise. Additionally, payment systems are slow to integrate new delivery levels into their payment algorithms.

Another problem with specialized subacute care services is that an NPP often renders the services. Some NPPs, such as PAs, NPs, CNSs, are fully recognized and can bill professionally on a 1500. Others cannot bill professionally and legitimate concerns arise about their rights to use physician-based CPT codes. Consider the example of an outpatient wound care center. The personnel providing services may be specially certified nurses (certified enterostomal nurse therapists or CENTs). As this book was going to press, this class of certified nurses had not yet been recognized as professionals for payment purposes and could not bill on 1500 forms. Similar conditions affect other personnel such as first RN surgical assistants. Payment for these specially trained staff members must come through the hospital technical component. Some non-physician provider services may have specific CPT or HCPCS codes for services and/or special modifiers that must be used.

Key learning area: Subacute care is an intermediate service level that cuts across virtually all levels of services from hospital, to outpatient, and even to home health. For this reason, subacute care presents particular compliance and reimbursement challenges.

Non-physician providers

Non-physician providers (NPPs) were mentioned in the preceding sections. As hospitals, clinics, and IDSs strive to provide correct levels of service at the lowest cost, their use of NPPs in growing. The payment system and organizational considerations for NPPs are significant, and healthcare providers must analyze the ramifications of using NPPs from management and economic perspectives and also from a compliance perspective, particularly in CBR areas. Certain NPPs can obtain their own national provider numbers and bill on 1500s. NPPs recognized for this purpose are:

- NPs (nurse practitioners)
- PAs (physician assistants)

---

* Note that the CPT code that will be used by the physician is for "initial" hospital care provided on the next date of service.

- CNSs (clinical nurse specialists)
- CRNAs (certified registered nurse anesthetists)
- Nurse midwives
- CSWs (clinical social workers)
- Psychologists

We can add registered dietitians and nutrition specialists to this list as well, although Medicare utilizes special payment processes for diabetes training and medical nutrition therapy.

Note that the scope of practice for any NPP is defined by state law that must be reviewed before any consideration of third-party payer rules and regulations. For the Medicare program, the recognition of NPPs started with the November 25, 1991 *Federal Register* and was updated via BBA 1997. Most of the major healthcare legislation since 1991 addresses NPPs to a degree. See, for example, BBRA 1999, BIPA 2002, MMA 2003, and DRA 2005.

NPPs, both those who can obtain their own national provider identifiers and those who cannot, become heavily involved in providing "incident-to" services. The idea behind incident-to services is that a physician may direct the activities of an NPP. The physician then codes and bills for the services of the NPP as if the physician actually performed the services. In order for such billing to take place, certain employment and supervision arrangements must be in place and these services must be provided in a free-standing setting as opposed to a provider-based setting. This may be referred to as incident-to billing.

In a hospital (provider-based) setting, inpatient or outpatient, incident-to services may be provided but incident-to billing is prohibited. A physician can code and bill only for personally provided services. Payment for incident-to services of NPPs in such settings occur through technical or facility payments via UB-04s. Note that this same prohibition applies to facility-based clinics and clinics organized as parts of hospital outpatient departments. Only in a free-standing clinic that is not provider-based can incident-to services be coded and billed by a supervising physician.

Of course, NPPs who qualify can obtain their own provider numbers and bill on 1500s both in hospital and free-standing clinic situations. Note that if NPPs with provider numbers are employed by a hospital and bill on 1500s, their costs should be removed from the hospital's cost report. If a healthcare provider uses NPPs of any type, careful consideration should be given to services provided, levels of supervision, billing and coding status, and licensing and/or certification.

Case study 3-11. Assistant-at-surgery conflict. A rift has developed at Apex Medical Center. It employs two FRNA (first registered nurse assis-

tants) who are specially trained as assistants-at-surgery. However, several surgeons utilize their own PAs (physician assistants) to provide this service. The PAs can bill professionally for services so that the physicians who employ them receive extra reimbursement. The FRNAs claim that the physicians are "gaming" the payment system and that this is a compliance issue.

Key learning area: The use of non-physician providers is appropriately and proportionately increasing with the growing need to provide correct levels of service with proper personnel. At the same time, coding and billing requirements continue to evolve to accommodate the changes in service personnel, giving rise to significant compliance concerns.

Medicare fraud, abuse, and anti-kickback laws

The broadly worded Medicare Fraud, Abuse, and Anti-Kickback Laws relates to giving or receiving inducements for referring or bringing patients into a service setting.* Since this legislation is so broadly worded, all healthcare providers must routinely ask themselves whether they are in a situation that might be seen as a violation of this law.

The OIG issued a number fraud alerts in this area to provide greater insight to personnel involved in situations that present potential for violations. The OIG also provides advisory opinions relative to specific sets of facts that can also be used for guidance. In addition, a number of safe harbor provisions concerning this law are available. A few examples of areas for application follow.

Case study 3-12. Free food, free training. It is not uncommon for hospitals to provide training for physicians and physician office staffs in connection with training for hospital personnel. As long as the physicians and the office staff are hospital employees, there is little problem. However, if the physicians and office staff are independent, free training and food may be construed as inducements to the physicians to refer patients to the hospital.

Case study 3-13. Specialty clinic reduced rent. Hospitals, particularly small rural hospitals, periodically have specialty physicians hold special clinics on site. One way this is approached is to

---

* See the Beneficiary Inducement Statute and the Anti-Kickback Statute reference in Chapter 1.

charge rent to the physician. The physician can then code and bill as if the specialty clinic is his or her own. The problem is in determining the amount of the rent. The calculation should include all the resources provided to the physician (nursing staff, room, equipment, supplies, transcription, etc.). The rent charged must be fair market value (FMV) and must be documented as FMV.*

Case study 3-14. Free crutches and canes. As previously noted, hospitals sometimes miscategorize certain supplies, particularly items like canes and crutches that might be listed as ancillary. When this occurs, billing and/or charging the appropriate party can become a compliance concern. One way hospitals avoid this issue, particularly with Medicare, is not to charge for such supplies, but the failure to charge may be construed as an inducement for patients to utilize the hospital. This same situation holds when hospitals do not charge Medicare patients for outpatient self-administrable drugs.

Case study 3-15. Office space for hospital-based physicians. Hospital-based physicians such as radiologists and anesthesiologists may not have offices within a hospital and may simply use hospital space available for ad hoc office needs. The hospital should charge rent for such space at FMV. Care must be taken, however, to distinguish work space from true office space. Similar considerations hold for billing staff for hospital-based physicians. It is not uncommon for a hospital to provide space for such staff and FMV rent should be charged. A reduced fee or no fee for the space could be construed as an incentive.

Case study 3-16. Incentive salary arrangements for physicians. Hospital ownership of clinics and employment of physicians or groups of physicians are growing phenomena. These arrangements may be on a W-2 or contractual basis. Incentive salary arrangements are common and may appear to meet the needs of both the hospital and the physicians. However, care must be exercised that the incentive arrangement is not based on production and particularly not based on an incentive that would induce a physician to provide unnecessary services. Such arrangements, particularly those based on a percentage

of charges or gross revenues, should be carefully reviewed. It is better to base incentive programs on net revenues.

These examples illustrate some of the more obvious and typical situations. More complex issues require more space than is available in this book. The bottom line is that all healthcare providers must be very careful to routinely ask themselves about arrangements with employees, non-employees, and patients, and about the possibility of perceived kickbacks. Both the OIG fraud alerts and advisory opinions provide additional information relative to possible problem areas.

Key learning area: The Medicare Fraud, Abuse, and Anti-Kickback Laws are among the most enduring and complex areas of compliance concerns, often because interpretation of the statutes is so broad.

Chargemaster concerns

The chargemaster† is both a direct and indirect target of various compliance concerns in the CBR area. This discussion will briefly address certain areas of concern. Note that some of these areas directly affect the chargemaster while others involve the system only peripherally.

Accurate information

The following are among the key elements for line items in the chargemaster:

- Description
- CPT/HCPCS
- Revenue center code (RCC)
- Charge

While a description may be abbreviated to fit onto a UB-04 or CMS-1450, it nonetheless must be meaningful and accurate. If a line item is a supply, the description should represent a supply and not a service or drug. A line item may or may not require a CPT and/or HCPCS code. If such a code is required, care must be taken to ensure that the code is current and accurate. Any modifier listed with a CPT or HCPCS code on the chargemaster should also be correct and accurate. For instance, the -25 modifier (significant, separately identifiable E/M service in addition to a procedure) should not be used with a surgical code.

---

* What constitutes fair market value (FMV) is a common healthcare compliance concern.

† The chargemaster term is used in a generic fashion. Service master, charge description master, and other terms may apply for a hospital accounts receivable computer system.

The revenue coding system is relatively imprecise and poorly designed and documented. The choice of revenue codes is often tied to getting a claim to go through a third-party payer's adjudication system, whether or not the codes used are consistent. For example, RCC 0360 is for an operating room and its use certainly implies that the given line item service was performed in the operating room. However, if you carefully examine a chargemaster, you may find that RCC 0360 or another code from the same series (generally referred to as 036X) was used for surgery-related services not provided in an operating room. Note that the use or misuse of revenue codes can affect the development of a Medicare cost report—a direct target of compliance audits. Such audits constitute a good reason to require use of accurate revenue codes.

Developing charges for the chargemaster is often an exercise in frustration. The basic idea is that charges should be based upon costs. However, many hospitals simply do not know their costs in various areas and must develop charges on some other basis. Often, charges are developed via educated guesses. Other charges may increase on an annual basis, an approach that can further skew charge data. Care should be taken to ensure a reasonably consistent charge structure tied to real costs and not merely a product of guesswork.

Note that charges for services as submitted on UB-04 claims are used to develop information databases that are then used to develop weights or relative values for payment systems such as DRGs and APCs. The charges may be converted to costs using cost-to-charge ratios (CCRs) from cost reports. If the charges and/or associated costs are inconsistent within the chargemasters for all hospitals, then the data used to develop these weights will be, at best, suspect.

Correlation of information

A significant compliance area for a chargemaster is proper correlation of the description, the CPT or HCPCS code, and the revenue code. If a description line lists a supply, a CPT or HCPCS code would be required only if the item is a take-home surgical supply or some unusual third-party payer requirement is involved. The revenue code should indicate a supply. Note that a number of special revenue codes apply to special situations and/or must be aligned with specific CPT or HCPCS codes. Also consider which codes correspond to therapeutic versus diagnostic services or to pharmaceuticals used in different settings.

Chargeable, separately chargeable, billable, and separately billable items

Over the past several years chargemaster coordinators have faced great difficulty in categorizing supply items and then determining how these items should or should not be charged, coded, and billed. Fundamentally, all services provided and items dispensed should be charged. However, the charges may be included in overhead costs used to generate a general mark-up. Another situation arises when an item is bundled into an associated service or item in the chargemaster and not separately charged. This is one way to handle "integral part" items discussed by CMS.

Many items will be separately charged and appear as separate line items in the chargemaster. If an item is not separately billable (or equivalently, separately reportable), there may be a separate charge but no associated CPT or HCPCS code for the item. The definitions and concepts in this area may become confusing, and this, in turn, makes it difficult to code and bill correctly through chargemaster in a manner that does not raise compliance concerns.

Case study 3-17. Conscious sedation billing. Sylvia, the Chargemaster Coordinator at Apex Medical Center, has been studying how the chargemaster should be organized to accommodate conscious sedation. As of 2005, CPT introduced the bull's eye or ⊙ notation to indicate that conscious sedation (CPT codes 99143 through 99145) is an inherent part of certain procedures (mainly endoscopic and catheterization procedures) and should not be reported separately. However, conscious sedation may be billed separately for procedures that do not have bull's eye notation. Sylvia has finally decided to use two line item entries in the chargemaster: One for conscious sedation with the CPT code and one without the CPT code. The charges are the same.

While this is an appropriate decision, the compliance issue then becomes the operational issue of whether or not service area personnel will be able to correctly distinguish between the two different line items.

A related issue is whether it is appropriate to bill for the use of equipment. For Medicare, DRG has a separate payment for capital items such as depreciable equipment. APC, the Medicare outpatient prospective payment system, currently makes no provision for capital costs. A chargemaster policy must explicitly state whether it is appropriate to charge separately for equipment. Over the past two decades, hospitals have typically decided not to bill separately for equipment although finding a specific federal rule or regulation in this area is difficult.

Key learning area: Determining whether an item should be billed separately or billed as part of another charge is sometimes difficult. Decisions on this issue should be made carefully.

Categorization of items

As mentioned earlier, certain supplies and items have special designations, for example, DME, prosthetics, and orthotics. The supply issue becomes even more convoluted because some supplies are considered to overhead or routine items associated with operating a hospital or clinic.* Distinguishing ancillary (chargeable) supplies from overhead supplies that should not be billed can be a challenge. Typically, a supply is considered ancillary when it is (1) specific to the procedure or service and (2) specific to the patient.

Drapes, cotton swabs, tongue depressors, exam gloves, and the like are all stock items and thus considered overhead. Special supplies such as sutures, catheters, and dressings are specific to a service and patient and are thus ancillary. To be classified as ancillary, an item must be disposable. If it is not disposable, then it is reusable and becomes equipment. While this may sound straightforward, it can cause confusion. For example, catheters used in a catheterization laboratory are typically discarded after one use although they are expensive. Would the ability to clean and/or refurbish them for use two or three times transform them into pieces of equipment?

Charge explosion

Some hospital billing systems allow the chargemaster to set up series or bundles of codes that can be invoked through a single line item charge. Areas where this can be useful include surgical supply bundles, sets of laboratory services, or bundles of codes from an area such as a catheterization laboratory. From a compliance perspective, it is important to ensure that when the single line item is expanded or exploded, all the supplies and/or services billed have indeed been used or provided. This requires an exception-based process that will allow personnel entering charges to indicate exceptions. A surgical supply package for performing

---

* Physician coding allows separate billing of limited range of supplies. Most supplies are bundled into RBRVS payments.

cataract surgery, for example, may be billed through a single line item on the chargemaster. A question arises when some part of a supply item is not used. It would be inappropriate to charge for the supply if it not used. We can then extend the question: Can a supply be charged if it has not been used but is disposed of as if it were used?

Coding interface

Some CPT and HCPCS codes are placed **statically** on the chargemaster. Whenever a given line item entry is invoked, the statically placed code will appear on the UB-04. This often occurs in radiology, laboratory, ER, physical therapy (PT), and similar areas. In other cases, particularly surgery, the codes are developed **dynamically** by professional coding staff. In this case the chargemaster contains no code; the coding personnel develop the code that then appears on the UB-04. In a hybrid situation, a **default code** is statically placed in the chargemaster and may later be overridden by coding staff. Great care should be taken to ensure that if coding staff overrides a code, it is also overridden on the UB-04 or 1500 claim forms. Health information management (HIM) staff may also be called upon to develop modifiers on a dynamic basis. Care should be taken to ensure that these modifiers, along with statically placed modifiers, appear on the claim form correctly.

Drugs and self-administrable drugs

Self-administrable drugs in an outpatient setting under the Medicare program are non-covered items and must be billed to patients; other drugs must also be specially billed. Certain chemotherapy drugs require the use of RCC 0636 with a J code. Likewise LOCMs (low osmolar contrast materials) often require the use of Q codes with RCC 0636.

Non-covered items and services

A number of items are considered non-covered, for example, take-home supplies such as Therabands and Theraputty from the PT and occupational therapy (OT) areas. In the inpatient area, questions arise about coding for the convenience packs given to patients. They typically include items such as tissues, hand lotion, slippers that are certainly non-covered. The self-administrable concept can be further extended for items that should not appear on the chargemaster. Under Medicare, for example, the application of hot and/or cold packs in PT and OT are typically provided as part of another service and can (generally) be self-administered. Thus

CPT code 97010 should not be used because the packs are part of a bundled service. In other words, charges for these packs are bundled into charges for other services and should not be billed at all.*

Special payment system requirements

The chargemaster is routinely altered to meet special demands of third-party payers. One third-party payer may accept a particular revenue code while another wants a different code. Some third-party payers are not fully up-to-date with CPT and HCPCS and may require different coding for the same service. Different services and supplies may be subject to special bundling rules. The variations are too numerous to delineate. In each case, the chargemaster coordinator must be sensitive to compliance considerations when making special alterations to the chargemaster.

An example of this can be seen in the CMS requirement relative to RC 0623. The 062X series is an extension of the 027X series for supplies. Over the years, CMS issued guidance that has mutated with the implementation of APCs. Currently, the 0623 code can be used with certain take-home surgical supplies using mainly A codes and then are then paid through a fee schedule.† This shows how a special requirement from a single third-party payer can significantly alter the chargemaster and create significant problems with claims that must meet certain requirements.

Charging interface

The chargemaster may be correctly developed with all line-items properly aligned and up to date. However, this does little good if the personnel inputting charges have not been fully trained in their areas about how the chargemaster works and what happens when they input a charge. Inputting multiple supplies and the proper use of units can be challenging. In areas such as PT, OT, and ST, 15-minute increments can be used as units to make it easier for charge entry personnel to understand what the units mean. Similarly, some modifiers may be implemented through the chargemaster, and personnel inputting charges must be trained to input the correct line item that applies the modifier.

APG and APC considerations

The advent of payment reform in the hospital outpatient area in the form of APGs (ambulatory patient groups) or a CMS variant designated APCs (ambulatory payment classifications), means that a number of compliance areas of concern for the chargemaster continue to evolve. For APGs and APCs, supplies and drugs are generally bundled. The exceptions are chemotherapy drugs and expensive radiopharmaceuticals.‡ Thus supply items for APCs are very much like supply items under DRGs; that is, most supplies are bundled for payment purposes. Because no separate payment is involved, it would seem that fewer compliance concerns should surround categorization of supplies. Unfortunately, this is not the case and supply categorization for the chargemaster continues to be a significant compliance problem.

APGs and APCs both reimburse based upon CPT and HCPCS coding, making coding interface for the chargemaster critical. No single best way to code and generate appropriate claims exists. Coding may be static (through the chargemaster) or may be developed dynamically outside the chargemaster.

Key learning area: Proper use of the chargemaster is a complex challenge for CBR compliance personnel. It is the focus of direct concern relative to organization, assignment of revenue codes, and pricing. Adding to the complexity are numerous interfaces to areas such as cost report, coding, billing, and charge capture processes.

OIG resources

Some of the richest sources of information pertaining to compliance problems and opportunities lie with the Office of the Inspector General (OIG). Four of the main types of documents that should be routinely reviewed by CBR compliance personnel are:

1. Fraud alerts
2. Annual work plans
3. Advisory opinions
4. Special reports

All these documents are available at no charge on the OIG website. Additionally, the OIG issues compliance guidance through the *Federal Register*. CBR compliance personnel are urged to routinely review the last

---

* Obviously they should be billed to third-party payers that recognize this CPT code and are willing to pay for these services. For Medicare, see the Physician Payment Reform or RBRVS *Federal Register*, usually issued every November. CPT 97010 is listed as a Status B (bundled).

† Check current rules and regulations in specific area. This scenario is provided only as an example of the confusion that can arise with special third-party payer requirements.

‡ These are the drugs requiring a J code with RCC 0636.

five years of the OIG's work plans in order to follow developments. See the appendix for Internet addresses and instructions for obtaining these and other documents.

Cost reports

Medicare cost reports are targets of direct compliance audits and reviews by Medicare auditors. Note that these documents are also used by state Medicaid programs in various ways. Depending on the payment system, a cost report can be a significant mechanism for reimbursement. For instance, critical access hospitals (CAHs) are cost-based reimbursed for many of their services as are rural health centers (RHCs) and federally qualified health centers (FQHCs).

A cost report is also a critical element for establishing cost-to-charge ratios (CCRs) used by Medicare to translate hospital charges back into hospital costs. These calculated costs from all hospitals are then used as a foundation for complex statistical processes that determine the relative weights for the DRG and APC categories.

Developing cost reports is a detailed and arduous process. Large hospitals and/or IDSs may well have their own personnel develop such reports. Smaller hospitals tend to have outside firms prepare their cost reports. However such reports are developed, many decisions must be made and supported by judiciously selected supporting documentation. Hospital staff should always be prepared to provide all information required or requested by cost report personnel. Generally, the higher the level of detail in the cost report, the better will be the report.

Several types of mistakes can make a report incorrect. The most fundamental issue is inappropriate cost, i.e., reporting a cost that is not reasonable. Note also that the chargemaster and the assignment of revenue codes may influence a cost report. Consider for example Schedule C on which various cost-to-charge ratios (CCRs) are listed by department. It is an interesting exercise to see whether the CCRs make sense. A cost report may show, for example, a CCR of 1.20 for therapy services, a figure that indicates that the department's costs are 20 percent higher than its charges. Does this make sense? What could explain the ratio or cause what is clearly an aberration?

Another aspect of the CCRs can create overpayment concerns. The cost reporting process usually lags several years behind because the report must be filed and eventually approved through Medicare. This produces a time lag in updating the CCRs. One calculation in which the CCRs are used is for cost outlier payments under both DRGs and APCs. If a hospital increases pricing over several years, a current CCR may be lower than one from several years ago. If the old CCR is in use, it may generate an incorrect cost outlier payment.

Case study 3-18. Cost-to-charge ratio. Apex Medical Center imposed no price increases for a number of years, then began raising prices. Over the past three years, the total increase in charges averaged 30 percent. The CCR from three years ago was 0.60. Assuming that costs have remained steady and that we do not compound the increases, the center's current CCR should really be 0.46. This indicates a significant change in the CCR over a three-year period, and this type of difference would certainly skew cost outlier payments.

Another simple cost report issue is what is or is not included. If a hospital employs non-physician practitioners (NPPs) such as PAs, NPs, CNSs, and the like, their salaries may or may not have to be included on the cost report. If the NPPs have their own NPIs or provider numbers and bill for on 1500s, their salaries should be omitted from the hospital's cost report. However, if the NPPs are simply employees and reimbursement for their services is achieved through the technical or facilities components on UB-04 claims, their salaries should be included.

The cost report is also very sensitive to the way in which certain activities are structured. For instance, hospitals often own or develop clinics that may be operated as independent structures. The physicians may or may not be employed; employees may be on the payroll, contractual, or leased. Facilities may be owned or leased, and joint ventures may be involved. All these factors can influence the way in which a cost report is developed.

A thorough discussion of the cost reporting process and potential areas of concern is beyond the scope of this book. It is sufficient to stress that cost reporting personnel must be apprised of all activities of the hospital or IDS. Additionally, it would also be desirable if they were involved in planning processes. In many cases, the impacts of planning and organizational changes should be assessed before final decisions are made. Cost reporting personnel should be proactively involved in planning and not relegated to a reactive mode after the fact.

Key learning area: The cost report is a complex and detailed document. Cost reporting personnel must have full information about the organization and should be proactively involved in planning process. Numerous cost report compliance issues must be carefully navigated.

Organizational structuring

The organization of a healthcare delivery system is a major area of ongoing compliance concern. The relationships of physicians to hospitals, clinics to hospitals, joint venturing arrangements, employment contracts, service contracts, management service organizations, physician–hospital organizations, integrated delivery systems, hospital mergers, hospital acquisitions of clinics, free-standing entities versus provider-based entities, residency programs, and a host of other arrangements must be considered from a compliance perspective. Virtually all of these arrangements impact the coding, billing, documentation, and reimbursement processes. CBR functions are often not considered until after an arrangement is negotiated and in place. Great care must be taken to analyze relationships of all types.

As noted, the healthcare industry faces many organizational structuring issues. This section will consider (1) provider-based clinics and (2) physician–hospital joint ventures.

The area of provider- or hospital-based clinics has become increasingly contentious as hospitals continue to explore ways to optimize reimbursement. A hospital-owned clinic may be organized as a free-standing or provider-based entity. From a CBR perspective, the easiest way to distinguish the two organization types is that a free-standing clinic files only 1500 forms (or CMS-1500 forms for Medicare). A provider- or hospital-based clinic files **both** UB-04 (CMS-1450) and 1500 (CMS-1500) claims.

Notes

1. *Free-standing* is used in an organizational sense. A clinic may be free-standing (physically separate) or may exist within a hospital complex.
2. Billing and claims filing implications are significant, particularly with respect to the place of service (POS) cited on a 1500 claim form.
3. A hospital's cost report may also be affected, depending upon which organization form is chosen.
4. Rural health clinics (RHCs) are special organizational forms and are subject to specific rules.
5. NPPs may be treated differently, depending on organizational structure. In a free-standing clinic, certain NPPs (PAs, NPs, CNSs) can be billed as "incident-to" the services of a physician.
6. When both UB-04 and 1500 claims are filed under the Medicare program (RBRVS), reductions in payment may apply to certain physician services. This is known as site-of-service differential. See the current RBRVS *Federal Register* for affected codes and amounts of reductions. The difference in payment is reflected in facility versus non-facility RVU differences.

Comparison of organizational structures

One of the major reasons for organizing a clinic as a provider-based entity is to increase reimbursements. As a result, this structure has become more popular in recent years even in light of the Medicare site-of-service differential and structuring has become a compliance issue after CMS promulgated rules and regulations relative to qualification as a provider-based clinic.[*] Hospitals involved with provider-based clinics should carefully conform to CMS criteria for organizing in this fashion.

The basic thrust of the criteria is that a clinic is truly a part of a hospital as evidenced by a number of factors. Common accreditation, geographic proximity, common management, common ownership, and similar factors are required. In the CBR area, probably the two biggest areas of concern are (1) the medical record-keeping system and (2) the billing system.

If a provider-based clinic is indeed to be a part of a hospital, it makes sense for the two administrative systems to have some degree of commonality. The immediate question is: "What constitutes an appropriate degree of commonality and/or integration?" Obviously, if both the medical records and billing systems are truly centralized at the hospital, this criterion is met. In most cases, the clinic—provider-based in this case—will have its own patient recordkeeping system and may well have its own specialized billing system. What must be done to make them common? Is a cross reference system back to the hospital medical record-keeping system enough? Is common management of the computer system required and/or must the computer systems be networked? These are the types of questions that must be addressed and resolved with respect to organizational structuring. CBR compliance personnel and corporate compliance personnel must pay close attention to these and similar criteria.

Note also that such provider-based clinics may provide other types of services such as PT and OT. If the clinic is a part of a hospital outpatient department, these PT and OT services can be billed just as they would be if they provided in the hospital. However, if the clinic is free-standing (organizationally) and PT and OT services are provided there, due consideration must be given to how the PT and OT are to be billed. As with the clinic, the PT and OT services could be billed as free-standing (1500) claims or the PT and OT operations could be organized as part of the hospital, with

---

[*] See provider-based rule (PBR), 42 CFR §413.65.

services claimed via the UB-04. If the PT and OT operations are organized to be provider-based, the facility would have a split use, that is, partially free-standing (i.e., the clinic) and partially provider-based (i.e., the PT/OT services). Split utilization brings additional cost reporting implications to consider. See Chapter 12 for further discussion of the provider-based rule as a special regulatory area.

The physician–hospital joint venture is an equally complex area. Whenever physicians become involved in ownership or partial ownership situations, they face the potential for the self-referral or Stark laws to come into play, as illustrated by this simple case study.

> **Case study 3-19. Hospital–physician joint ASC.** A group of physicians in a joint venture with a hospital decides to establish a free-standing ambulatory surgery center (ASC). Capitalization of the ASC is evenly divided between the hospital and group of physicians. The property upon which the ASC is built is leased from the hospital. ASC personnel are leased by the hospital with the exception of the administrator who is independently employed by the ASC. CRNA services are contracted separately from the hospital. Billing for services is via 1500 for both technical and professional components. A separate computer billing system has been purchased for use by the ASC. However, the ASC medical record-keeping system is integrated into the hospital's medical recordkeeping system.

The facts in any case will vary and analyzing these types of joint ventures under both Stark and the more general fraud and abuse laws requires great care and possibly the expertise of legal counsel. See Chapter 12 for a further discussion of the ever-expanding Stark regulations.

CBR compliance personnel are urged to think about possible organizational structuring. For instance, what if the hospital in Case study 3-19 contracted with the ASC to provide hospital outpatient services? The basic idea is that these services as billed by the hospital could receive higher reimbursement than that received by the ASC under the ASC's payment process. Could this process present some coding, billing, and reimbursement compliance concerns?

> **Key learning area: The organizational structuring of healthcare service providers must be carefully considered. CBR compliance personnel should be proactively involved in planning considerations and determine how to properly code, bill, and document services provided.**

Operational considerations

Most arrangements listed in the preceding section represent external organizations and deal with ownership, control, and associated payment system issues. Internal structuring and operations also play an important role in CBR compliance. While many operational aspects including patient flow, support personnel, documentation development and others are relevant, only two will be addressed in this section (1) the organization of the coding process and (2) the use of computer billing systems. A careful study of analysis process and alternative approaches in this area is essential. Every healthcare provider that develops and files claims will have to consider variations requiring separate analyses.

Consider the coding process or function within a hospital.* For an example, assume that the fictitious Apex Medical Center has a normal array of hospital service areas. Coding in this case covers all types including inpatient ICD-9-CM diagnosis and procedures coding for DRGs and diagnosis and CPT procedure coding for various outpatient and ancillary services. Some key questions provide a focus: When is coding done? Where? And by whom?

The typical model for inpatient DRG coding is to centralize this function in a health information management (HIM), or equivalent department by having completed medical records reviewed and coded by coding staff. Thus the coding is performed after the episode of care in the HIM department by professional coding staff. This centralized model often forms the basis for all hospital coding considerations. The outpatient coding process discussed in more detail below tends to challenge this centralized process. Even for inpatient coding, the centralized model may be augmented by concurrent coding—performed concurrently with the provision of care. In this process, the coding staff goes to the acute care floors, interacts with physicians and other providers, reviews the medical record as it is developed, and codes the case as it develops.

From a compliance perspective, the concurrent process is generally superior† because the coding staff can collect better information while on site and can also request physicians to document in a manner that ensures the medical record meets various coding guidelines. Thus, coding staff do not have to guess or request additional information well after the fact.

---

* The analog for this analysis exists for all types healthcare providers including clinics, home health, skilled nursing, etc. The documentation, abstracting, and coding processes vary by setting.

† It is also superior from a reimbursement perspective.

Moving from inpatient to outpatient coding entails subtle but important changes. The greatest change is that outpatient services are encounter-driven rather than considered on the basis of length of stay or episode of care. While this seems obvious, the ramifications are not. Many cases require a change in the way we think about the whole process of providing care. Since outpatient coding is encounter-driven, the timeliness factor comes into play for both documentation and coding. Delaying the coding process for days after a service is performed under a centralized organizational model is not really acceptable. Moreover, having a medical or patient record physically tied up in a coding area for days can create havoc with patient care because the record may be required for additional encounters.

Access to records is another problem. In many large hospitals and IDSs, the medical recordkeeping system may be decentralized or dispersed at different locations.* The access problem, the trend toward some form of record decentralization, and the need for records to be near areas where care is provided causes the coding function to become decentralized or dispersed. As with concurrent inpatient coding, the closer the coding staff is to the physicians and other clinical providers, the more likely better documentation will be developed and that the subsequent coding will be correct. This in turn leads to a greater probability of compliance.

Case study 3-20. Dedicated ED coding staff.
Apex Medical Center has finally decided to have two coding staff members dedicated to coding for the ED. These two individuals will handle all E/M codes, surgical codes, and diagnosis coding. An office near the ED has been established to house this dedicated function. The two staff members are still officially a part of the HIM department but also report to the physician who serves as medical director of the ED.

The result of this process of decentralization is immediacy in the feedback loop to and with provider staff from those who code and/or review the documentation. One weakness of the centralized model is the limited opportunity for coding staff to interact with providers when or shortly after the services are provided.

The strengths of centralized coding include consistency, common training, uniform adherence to coding policies and guidelines, and opportunities to interact with other coding staff when dealing with complex coding issues. Centralized coding is advantageous from a compliance perspective. For this reason, it is

---

* Record access may represent a compliance problem for provider-based entities.

generally recommended that management of such functions remain centralized in a decentralized coding operation. Thus a matrix organization in which the director of HIM continues to be the line manager while coding staff may report on a functional basis to other service areas of the hospital is recommended. Note that the matrix organization can be superior to the classic hierarchical organization, but it requires additional skills in management.

Another major issue for CBR compliance personnel is a computer billing system. For purposes of this discussion, computer billing includes the billing and claims generation software and the databases of information generated from CBR activities. It may also mean dealing with several different systems if multiple types of services are provided. For example, hospitals with provider-based clinics will sometimes have a clinic or physician billing system for 1500 or CMS-1500 claims while utilizing the main hospital system for UB-04 or CMS-1450 claims. Likewise, skilled nursing and home health may also have dedicated systems.

In today's healthcare environment, computer billing systems are essential. They perform tasks that would be nearly impossible to perform manually. However, the complexity that provides the advantage can also create compliance problems. If the billing system does not generate appropriate statements, clean claims, secondary claims, and bills while meeting special third-party payer requirements, compliance can be compromised. Moreover, if compliance problems for coding and billing already exist, computer systems tend to magnify them. On the other hand, computer systems can provide significant assistance in checking, cross checking, analyzing, and reporting potential CBR compliance problems. Four brief case studies illustrate some of the issues that can arise from using—or misusing—healthcare billing systems.

Case study 3-21. Code overrides.
Apex Medical Center is studying the coding and billing process in its ED. Currently, the physician professional claims on the 1500 are generated through the chargemaster. The physicians check off appropriate E/M levels and then check off any surgical procedures performed. A billing clerk in the ED inputs charges that drive through the chargemaster to pick up the correct codes from which the claim is generated. To test and study this process, two HIM coding staff members review the coding performed by the physicians. The reason for this test is that audits of samples of ER physician claims showed that E/M coding documentation guidelines were not always followed for

items checked off, especially with respect to code level.

Over a two month period, the HIM coding staff members reviewed the documentation, sometimes moving the level of E/M codes down and, in a few cases, moving the levels up. They also discovered that in a surprising number of cases, procedures were performed but not checked off. Coding staff made the changes through their abstracting system. Training sessions with the ED physicians and staff were conducted to reduce the incidence of coding errors. While everyone was pleased with this new process, several months someone discovered that the codes input by the coding staff did not override the E/M codes generated through the chargemaster. This billing system glitch exacerbated the problems caused by under-coding and failure to check off procedures. As a result, incorrect claims were submitted and revenues were lost. A formal audit was conducted and Apex began to consider using dedicated coding staff instead of coding through the chargemaster.

Case study 3-22. Secondary payer claims. Apex Medical Center learned that while its computer system was proficient at generating primary claims, in some instances, it could not generate secondary claims. Most cases in which this technical error occurred were considered minor, and the hospital simply wrote off the balances because no secondary claims were being filed. However, during a routine review of the computer billing system, the determination was made that such write-offs, when measured against Medicare Fraud, Abuse, and Anti-Kickback Law standards, might be construed as inducements.

Case study 3-23. CMS-1500 Claim form diagnosis coding. One major feature that distinguishes 1500 and UB-04 claims is that a diagnosis code on the 1500 can be correlated back to a line item. This is done by numbering the diagnosis codes 1 through 4, and then placing a 1 and/or 2 and/or 3 and/or 4 to the right of the line item. Acme Medical Clinic started noticing a number of claim rejections and requests for additional information after starting to use a new computer system. An investigation revealed that only a 1 appeared on each claim and for each line item. Thus line items that were billed in conjunction with other diagnosis codes were rejected as medically unnecessary because of improper correlation. It was also dis-

covered that some third-party payer claims went through adjudication even though the diagnostic justification was inappropriate. After significant discussion with the computer vendor, the system was modified to prevent the discrepancies.

Case study 3-24. Type of bill (TOB) on UB-04. During an audit of claims for various outpatient services, Apex Medical Center discovered an inconsistency in computer-generated TOBs. This was particularly evident in connection with TOBs 831 and 131. The former were subject to the ASC payment limitation; the latter were not. While it was not known whether reimbursement was affected for compliance purposes, an investigation was launched to determine how the computer system generated TOBs. Surprisingly, the function that would allow the computer system to generate TOBs had been turned off! TOB were generated by admitting clerks at registration. After the TOB-generating function was turned on, the algorithm for generating TOBs in conjunction with other information was reviewed and the problem was resolved.

Numerous other examples related to computer interfaces and/or department operations can be cited, but one important but sometimes overlooked fact is that in many instances a computer works properly. The way in which the computer is used can create compliance problems. For this reason, it is imperative to review and monitor all operational systems that affect the coding, billing, documentation, and reimbursement processes.

Key learning area: All operational systems affecting the CBR process must be carefully reviewed and monitored on an ongoing basis. Problem areas can often be identified by tracing the end products, statements, and claims back through the overall system.

Coding and payment system demands

With the advent of the HIPAA Transaction Standard/Standard Code Set (TSC) rule, the same claim for a service should be filed to each third-party payer. Using a standard code set on a standard claim form should produce the same claim regardless of the third-party payer involved. While this is certainly a goal of the TSC, achieving it is many years away. The demands made by the various coding systems and the associated payment systems are continuing sources of compliance problems and mechanisms for information development. The main coding systems fall into two categories:

1. Procedure coding that identifies the procedure or service provided
2. Diagnosis coding that identifies the condition, illness, disease, sign, or symptom related to provision of service

These two types of systems involve the use of detailed and sometimes confusing rules, regulations, and guidelines. Conflicts about use of coding systems sometimes arise between billing office* and coding† personnel. The billing office's primary objective is to file claims to obtain reimbursement. Coding personnel follow specific guidelines sometimes designed for global data production and statistical analysis. These two objectives sometimes conflict with each other. From a compliance perspective, it is extremely important to resolve such conflicts.

Key learning area: Conflicts sometimes arise between the billing and coding functions. These differences often pose compliance issues relative to claims filing and should be appropriately resolved to satisfy compliance constraints. The resolution of such situations should result in written policies and procedures.

Procedure coding

This section discusses two general procedure coding systems used by healthcare providers. The first is Current Procedural Terminology (CPT), developed by the American Medical Association. The current system is CPT-4; CPT-5 will upgrade it in the near future. CPT is widely used in connection with services provided by physicians. NPPs such as therapists, psychologists, and nursing staff can also use some of its codes within prescribed limitations. The format for these codes is always five digits.‡ The CPT system is updated annually with hundreds of changes, and the system continues to grow and be refined. One particularly interesting feature is how the codes are used in various combinations. One example shows how three codes might be used for an ER encounter:

- 99283-25—Level 3 ER encounter
- 12002-59-51—Simple laceration repair
- 12032—Intermediate laceration repair

As this example also shows, a number of modifiers must be used in conjunction with this coding system. The -25 modifier indicates that the Level 3 encounter (an E/M code) is separate from the surgical procedures performed (without the modifier, the E/M service would not be paid). The -59 modifier indicates that the two surgical procedures are distinct (without the modifier it is possible that both surgical procedures would not be paid). The -51 modifier signifies multiple procedures, in this case multiple surgeries. This modifier is generally informational and used by physicians. However, the use of this modifier for a given adjudication system could result in a reduced payment.

Note: Another modifier that might be required for ER physicians is the -54 (intraoperative only) modifier used to indicate that post-operative services will be transferred to another physician. For example, a patient may be directed to see his or her own primary care physician to have sutures removed after a laceration repair.

An adjunct to CPT is a special coding system developed by CMS, namely the Healthcare Common Procedure Coding System (HCPCS).§ This system is applied in a number of special areas including supplies, DME, dental, pharmaceuticals, and the like. Unfortunately, HCPCS was developed on an ad hoc basis over the years, so it is not a well organized coding system. The HCPCS may be referred to as Level II National Codes. Theoretically, Level I is reserved for CPT. In the past, Level III or local codes were also used, but HIPAA TSC did away with Level III codes.¶

The national codes are recognized across the U.S. even by some non-Medicare third-party payers. The codes are updated annually around the time the CPT is updated. Unlike the five-digit CPT codes, a typical HCPCS code starts with a letter followed by four digits.

HCPCSs have more than two hundred modifiers generally consisting of two alphabetic characters. Both the HCPCS codes and the various modifiers can

---

* "Billing office" is used generically to describe a department or area with a particular function. The organizational entity may also be called patient accounting, patient financial accounting, accounts receivable, and the like.

† The coding function within a healthcare organization varies widely. Typical department designations are health information management (HIM), medical records, abstracting, and the like.

‡ Note that the format for CPT is the same as for the postal service zip codes. Because the CPT codes are copyrighted by the AMA, some interesting questions arise when a CPT code is identical to a zip code.

§ HCPCS were originally developed when CMS was still HCFA and HCPCS meant HCFA's Common Procedure Coding System.

¶ Even at this late date you may still find HCPCS codes starting with X, W, Y, or Z—the initial letters in Level III codes.

be used in highly different ways by different types of healthcare providers. Two simple examples are:

- E0785—Implantable intraspinal (epidural/intrathecal) catheter used with implantable infusion pump, replacement
- A4614—Peak expiratory flow rate meter, hand held

Modifiers for Level II codes generally have two alphabetic characters, for example: -GN, indicating service delivered under outpatient speech–language pathology plan of care.

Another general procedure coding system is Volume 3 of ICD-9-CM, due to be replaced by ICD-10-PCS (Procedure Coding System). This system is currently used in connection with the DRG for inpatient services. The format for these codes is the same as for the diagnosis coding described below.

All the procedure coding systems involve extensive guidelines, some embedded in the systems and some developed externally. Because different payment systems and third-party payers may make unusual demands relative to coding and/or combinations of codes, written policies and procedures are necessary to support decisions about how to use these coding systems, when to use modifiers, when not to use certain code combinations, etc.

> **Case study 3-25. PT Fabrication of splint in ED.** Occasionally, an ED physician will request that a physical therapist (or occupational therapist) come to the ED to fabricate and apply a special splint. On these occasions, the physical therapist returns to his or her department and checks off the appropriate charge that drives through the chargemaster and generates the proper splinting code. However, an outside auditor noted that a code included a –GP (service delivered under outpatient physical therapy plan of care) modifier. Because this service was not provided under a physician-generated physical therapy plan of care, the auditor maintains that no modifier should have been included and payment for the service under Medicare should have been claimed under APCs (no modifier) as opposed to the Medicare Physician Fee Schedule (MPFS) that would have been driven by the modifier. In this case, improper payment was made.

This case study illustrates the distinction between therapy-only codes and not-therapy-only codes. Certain codes, including splinting, can fall into either category. The differentiation lies in the use or non-use of the -GP (or -GO for an occupational therapist) modifier. Because of ambiguities in this area, it is wise to consult the most current CMS guidance for the specific type of case.*

Diagnosis coding

The coding system for diagnoses is well established and continues to be refined. ICD-9-CM (Clinical Modification) is being replaced by a much more detailed system, ICD-10-CM. An ICD-9-CM code can consist of three, four, or five digits. Typically, a period follows the third digit if a code requires additional digits. Coding personnel strive for the greatest level of specificity allowed within a coding subsection.

Note: Inside computer systems, the period in an ICD-9 code is omitted. Thus, a five-digit ICD-9 code will look exactly like a CPT code. It is critical to understand the context of the data to be certain of the kinds of codes represented. Also note the present-on-admission (POA) indicator may also require a trailing character added to the diagnosis code on the UB-04.

ICD-10-CM represents a significant departure from ICD-9-CM. The format has been increased to seven alphanumeric characters. Generally, the first character is alphabetic. This system is much more detailed and its implementation will require significant changes to computer systems and claim forms and extensive retraining of coding personnel. As with procedure coding, many guidelines, rules, and regulations must be followed with diagnostic coding. Some of these guidelines are embedded into the system and others were developed relative to their use with different payment systems.

Key learning area: Healthcare coding systems are complex. For compliance purposes it is important that qualified staff be trained (and retrained) to perform coding functions properly. Acquiring a thorough knowledge of CPT, HCPCS, and ICD-9 codes and the associated processes is a lifetime endeavor.

Note: Throughout this book, you will find references and expanded discussions of these major coding systems that have now been standardized under the HIPAA TSC rules.

---

* See CMS Publication 100-04, Medicare Claims Processing Manual, Chapter 5, §20.

Revenue codes

Revenue codes (RCs) are somewhat loosely organized. They are used on UB-04s and are typically coded into chargemasters. Revenue codes can also influence the way cost reports are developed. This system is expanded and modified on an irregular basis through the National Uniform Billing Committee (NUBC) which is hosted by the American Hospital Association. These codes and other UB-04 information are generally provided through state hospital associations that sponsor state level uniform billing committees. A national level UB-04 manual is available from the NUBC.

This system developed on an as-needed basis and is therefore not always logically organized. Similarly, the descriptions of the revenue code uses can be cryptic and open to interpretation. To further complicate the issue, third-party payers tend to interpret and/or require the use of different RCs for various purposes. As discussed in the chargemaster section, the proper use of RCs is a compliance issue as is their correlation with the CPT/HCPCS codes.

> **Case study 3-26. Revenue code assignment.** Sylvia, the Chargemaster Coordinator at Apex Medical Center is in a quandary. The hospital's managed care contracting team indicated that several contracts pay more for RC 0278 (other implants) than they pay for RC 0272 (sterile supplies). Sylvia is encouraged to classify expensive catheters and balloons for angioplasties (items that have HCPCS C-codes) as 0278 to increase reimbursements. Is this proper?

Payment systems

Selected payment systems will be discussed in more detail elsewhere in this book. A brief list includes:

- LCC—Lesser of charges or costs
- DRGs—Diagnosis-related groups
- APCs—Ambulatory payment classifications
- RBRVS—Resource-based relative value system
- RUGs-III—Resource utilization groups

Payment systems also have variations. One variation of DRGs is the AP-DRG (all-patient DRG)* APCs are specific implementations of the more general APGs (ambulatory patient groups). Considering the various managed care and capitated payment systems, the number and variety of payment systems are significant. Each payment system and its specific implementation imposes slightly or significantly different requirements for filing claims. The interplay between the coding systems and associated documentation and the payment systems creates a number of compliance concerns, the major one relating to filing false claims. Compliance can concern:

1. Services or items not supplied
2. Incorrect procedure codes
3. Incorrect modifiers
4. Incorrect or incomplete diagnosis codes
5. Medical necessities not indicated
6. Documentation incomplete or too ambiguous

It is important to note that diagnosis codes are used to provide medical necessity justification. If questions arise, the documentation can be further studied and amended to show medical necessity if required. A detailed bill or itemized statement is considered part of a claim for auditing purposes. It is not submitted with a claim, but auditors will request this information when conducting formal audits.

All these systems impose specific claims filing requirements on both 1500s and UB-04s. The capabilities of billing computer systems to generate correct claims represent great challenges of all healthcare providers. Equally important are the needs to keep coding and billing staff up to date and provide access to current accurate information. It is also imperative to find a way to ensure that third-party payers, who often have their own unique requirements, provide timely and accurate answers to compliance-related questions.

> **Key learning area: Coding and payment systems represent one of the most complex areas for CBR compliance. The most common compliance problem is false claims arising from a variety of mistakes. Healthcare providers must take extra precautions to prevent mistakes by hiring and retaining competent professional staff and by developing coding and billing policies and procedures.**

Safe harbors

Additional information for identifying potential compliance problem or opportunity areas can be found by reviewing the safe harbors established in connection with various laws. The following safe harbors (exceptions) are listed in the Code of Federal Regulations (CFR) Section 1001.952:

---

* As this book was written, CMS was in the process of significantly changing DRGs through the implementation of MS-DRGs (Medicare severity DRGs).

- Investment interests
- Space rentals
- Equipment rentals
- Personal services and management contracts
- Sale of practice
- Referral services
- Warranties
- Discounts
- Employees
- Group purchasing organizations
- Waivers of beneficiary coinsurance and deductible amounts
- Increased coverage, reduced cost-sharing amounts, or reduced premium amounts offered by health plans

See also the following *Federal Register* entries that provide more background information about these safe harbors:

- 57 FR 3330, January 29, 1992
- 57 FR 52729, November 5, 1992
- 57 FR 2135, January 25, 1996

Note that a healthcare organization may be involved in an arrangement that does not meet every condition of a safe harbor. This does not necessarily mean that the arrangement is in violation of a law. It simply means that no protection or safe harbor is afforded. Note as well that the OIG under the Balanced Budget Act (BBA) of 1997 solicits suggestions for possible new safe harbors. See the CD accompanying this book for additional resources.

Key learning area: CBR compliance personnel should be familiar with the various safe harbors, monitor developments in this area, and be able to research and obtain appropriate information and/or supportive citations from the *Federal Register* and the *Code of Federal Regulations*.

Statistical and benchmark utilization

Developing and monitoring various statistics can help identify possible compliance concerns. In the CBR area, statistics typically result from various aspects of the payment system. While some statistics are fairly complex, most involve simple frequency analysis and various ratios.

DRGs, APGs, and CMS's APCs have case-mix indexes. For APGs and APCs, they are generally called service-mix indexes or encounter-mix indexes. These index numbers, if monitored over time, provide a means of tracking changes. For example, a sudden increase (or decrease) in a DRG case mix over the course of a year may raise concerns. A specific case can easily illustrate this situation.

Case study 3-27. Index change. Apex Medical Center noticed that the DRG CMI over the course of a year increased from 1.0120 to 1.2001. This increase was significant and will produce substantially higher payments. The movement of this index must be investigated, even though it may be legitimate. For example, the number of certain types of complex surgeries may have increased, a new inpatient program may have been developed, or the hospital may have switched to concurrent coding instead of after-the-fact coding.

Whatever the reason, the difference between these index numbers over time is an indicator of change. For compliance purposes, it is wiser to investigate than assume compliance.

Case study 3-28. DRG CMI Analysis. Samuel, the chief financial officer of Apex Medical Center has been contacted by an outside consulting firm. Apex's DRG CMI has been slowly but surely dropping over the past three years. The outside company suggests a special study to determine why Apex coding personnel are not correctly coding inpatient cases. What should Samuel do?

Significant changes in the DRG CMI should be investigated. However, the presumption in the case study is that a coding problem exists. This may or may not be the issue; other factors may influence the DRG CMI.

The index numbers for APGs and APCs can be used in the same way. Because of the more complex grouping process for APCs, different indexes can be developed. For instance, an overall-encounter or service-mix index may lump together all the APCs generated or a case-mix index may calculate APCs within each case before averaging.

Ratios of codes and/or groups can also be monitored. One of the major concerns with the DRG-type payment systems is the classification of cases within a severity-refined group. CMS DRGs basically specify two groups for certain types of cases (1) those with complication or comorbidity (CC) and (2) those without complication of comorbidity. More refined DRG systems may have three categories, for example, a base DRG, a DRG with a CC, and a DRG with a MCC (major complication or comorbidity). Ongoing concern surrounds CMS's DRG system related to proper categorization of severity levels. Consider the following pairs:

1. DRG 89 (simple pneumonia) versus DRG 79 (bacterial lung infection)
2. DRG 297 (nutritional and miscellaneous metabolic disorders without complicating conditions) versus DRG 296 (nutritional and miscellaneous metabolic disorders with complicating conditions)
3. DRG 293 (other endocrine, common nutritional and metabolic OR procedures without complicating conditions) versus DRG 292 (other endocrine, common nutritional and metabolic OR procedures with complicating conditions)

A quick check of the CMS-DRG weights will indicate that payment levels for these three pairs of codes varies significantly based on the presence of a CC. The new MS-DRG system expands the severity levels by also having an MCC (major complication or comorbidity). While general ratios have been established for these pairs under the old CMS-DRG system, there is no history relative to the new MS-DRGs. Thus, hospitals will need to monitor frequencies within different sets of the MS-DRGs. Because the numbering system for MS-DRGs is completely different, CBR compliance personnel will need to translate the old norms into new norms for conducting special problem DRG audits.

Simple frequencies can be used in a number of areas. Consider physician coding, more specifically E/M (evaluation and management) coding. For a physician practice, consider using the new patient sequence of CPT 99201 through 99205. Statistics can be developed about the use of these codes and relative frequencies will vary according to specialty. For simplicity, we will classify the physicians as primary care or "specialist."

Figure 3.1 shows a comparative bar chart of the E/M percentage distribution for Acme Medical Clinic. The frequency of the use of the codes varies significantly between the two groups of physicians. Note also that specialists will probably not use the new patient codes as much as they will use the consultation codes.

Once again, if codes of an individual physician vary from either the established norm at the hospital or from established state or national norms, CBR compliance personnel should investigate to make certain that codes are used properly and that documentation standards are met. This same type of frequency analysis can be used for hospital technical component E/M coding as well.

Also, within the E/M coding system in CPT, average times that can be associated with each level are provided. The frequencies of code use can thus also be

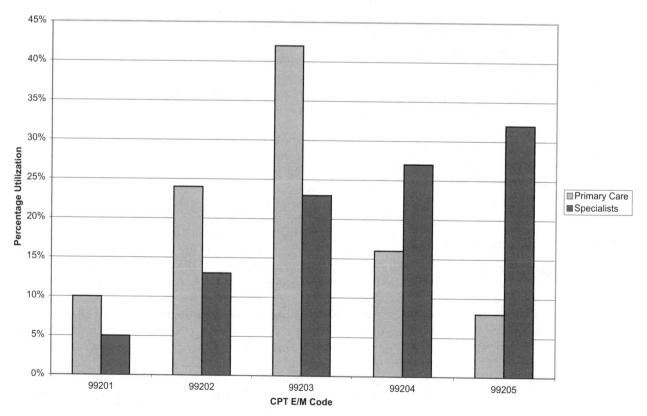

Figure 3.1 Comparative E/M percentage by physician classification.

converted to overall times. While the time provided at E/M level is not supposed to be used this way, auditors may opt to do so.

Case study 3-29. Total time for E/M services. At Acme Medical Clinic, a single day of a primary care physician is analyzed. The following sequence of E/M code utilization occurs:

E/M Code	Number	Average Time (minutes)	Total Time (minutes)
CPT 99201	1	10	10
CPT 99202	5	20	100
CPT 99203	2	30	60
CPT 99212	8	10	160
CPT 99213	10	15	150
CPT 99214	8	25	200
CPT 99215	2	40	80
CPT 99222	3	50	150
CPT 99232	6	25	150
Total			1060

The total time spent based on these CPT averages (1060 minutes) a little over 17 hours!

In a single day, this physician saw 45 patients (including 36 in clinic), admitted 2 patients to observation, admitted 3 patients to inpatient, and visited 6 patients on hospital rounds. While this analysis does not show it, the physician also performed several minor surgeries in the clinic. This scenario could certainly occur and every entry may be correct, properly documented, and medically justified. However, from an auditing view, this situation would be suspect, particularly because the physician was only in the clinic for 7 hours and at the hospital for 2 hours.

Note that CPT cites no average times for ER E/M levels of service. In an area such as ER along with other types of physician services, quantitative monitoring generally uses a relative value system such as CMS's RBRVS (Resource Based Relative Value System). RVUs are routinely updated yearly and published in the PPR (Physician Payment Reform) *Federal Register* issued every November or December. These same relative values can be used for productivity measurement and even for calculating productivity bonuses for physicians.

Key learning area: CBR compliance personnel must be conversant with various benchmarking and statistical analysis techniques for use with quantitative aspects of different payment systems.

Summary

For CBR, numerous situations can be considered compliance issues. The variations and nuances stemming from various laws, rules, and regulations seem endless. CBR compliance personnel can use a two-pronged approach to identify potential problem areas. One is external, e.g., reviewing OIG advisory opinions, OIG compliance work plans, legal cases, newsletters, and the like. The other approach is internal and involves examining and analyzing various aspects of coding, documentation, statistics, sampling audits, organizational structuring, provider relationships, baseline compliance audit comparisons, and the like.

Key learning area: Hospitals, clinics, IDSs, and other healthcare providers generally have little trouble identifying compliance problems. It is generally a matter of prioritizing areas that need to be addressed with the resources available. Ongoing monitoring is also essential to make certain that no aspects of the CBR process are inappropriately skewed.

---

four

Investigation and problem solving

Introduction

The *systems approach* is a very powerful tool for CBR compliance personnel. It is an organized, step-by-step approach that, if used correctly, covers all important issues and helps compliance personnel make certain that nothing is overlooked and that analyses are reasonably complete. This is not to say that the systems approach is perfect. It is only as good as the personnel performing investigations and solving problems. As noted in the preceding chapter, every healthcare provider faces no small number of real and potential healthcare compliance problems. Often, identifying a problem or opportunity area is easy; identifying the underlying cause may be more difficult. Just as often, a provider may have a lurking concern that a process is performed incorrectly, but no one is really sure how. Thus the ability to probe for problems is also important.

Note that associated techniques derived from the fundamental systems approach may be used in the compliance area. Business process reengineering and benchmarking are two disciplines or approaches typically used for quality or performance improvement. Six Sigma encompasses many quality improvement techniques developed over the past 20 years. These and other techniques can also be used to address various aspects of investigating compliance issues. Note also that the OIG has indicated that one benefit derived from compliance programs is increased performance and quality improvement through the thoughtful application of these techniques.

Key learning area: Full statutory and contractual compliance promotes quality improvement and excellence. While compliance may be viewed as a burden or process that must be accomplished to avoid penalties, it should really be viewed as a positive process that promotes qualify improvement.

Systems approach

The systems approach is the single most powerful tool that CBR compliance personnel have at their disposal. This approach provides a means of thinking about and developing solutions to problems. A seven-step process (Figure 4.1) is suggested:

Step 1—Problem/opportunity identification
Step 2—Problem/opportunity analysis
Step 3—Solution design, external
Step 4—Solution design, internal
Step 5—Solution development
Step 6—Solution implementation
Step 7—Situation monitoring and remediation

No facet of the seven steps is inherently magical nor are the steps magical or even absolute. Those using the systems approach may need to modify the steps, depending on circumstances. One of the great strengths of the systems approach is that it is flexible. Let us consider each step in terms of CBR compliance.

Problem/opportunity identification

Real or potential compliance problems can be identified through a number of different sources, for example:

- OIG fraud alerts
- OIG work plans
- Current litigation activities
- Lists of potential compliance problems
- Corporate integrity agreements (CIAs)
- Experiences of others (requires networking)
- Routine audits and reviews
- Baseline benchmark audits and reviews
- Employee reports and suggestions
- Hotline information
- Fiscal intermediary and carrier cease-and-desist letters
- Fiscal intermediary and carrier inquiries
- Third-party payer audits
- External audits
- Claim denials and reduced payments
- Cost report challenges
- Patient complaints

The list does not include every source. The simple fact is that in today's healthcare fields, regardless of the type of services provided, hundreds of potential compliance issues must be considered. You do not have to look for them. They will come to you whether you want them to or not.

The OIG issues periodic fraud alerts citing significant problems. The OIG annual work plans provide information about areas currently under investigation.

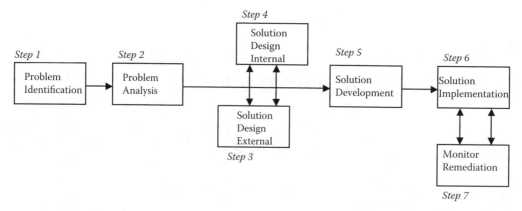

Figure 4.1 Seven-step systems approach.

The increasing length of work plans and the number of areas they address are clear indications of the scope of potential problems. Current litigation and CIAs can provide insights about problems experienced by other healthcare providers. CBR compliance personnel can also learn much by reading general and specialized news reports. Another good source of updates on current activities is networking with others in healthcare, particularly on a person-to-person basis via contacts made through workshops and professional organizations. Other good sources are e-mail lists or listservs. Routine audits and reviews (and general baseline audits) are excellent tools for identifying problems and investigating potential problem areas. These processes are discussed in Chapters 8 and 9.

Employees who perform work daily can also recognize potential problem areas. This is true for those providing services and entering charges and those who process the charges, maintain the chargemaster, and generate claims. Whether potential issues are reported on a regular employee-to-manager basis or anonymously through a compliance hotline, the information revealed may be extremely valuable. Team reviews and/or flowcharting processes and activities can also stimulate employees to question certain activities or end results. Likewise, during training sessions, whether specific to compliance or other topics, issues and concerns may be uncovered.

Medicare administrative contractors (MACs)* and other third-party payers are also sources of information. These entities adjudicate claims and often pick up certain patterns or unusual claims activities that may result in denials or reduced payments. Third-party payers may also perform periodic audits. A healthcare

provider may also retain external consultants to perform audits.

Pay attention to patient complaints and questions, particularly in the coding and billing area. Most patients do not understand their bills or the ways third-party payers do or do not pay the claims. While many of the questions and concerns can be addressed without much difficulty by anyone who understands the process, there are certainly cases where even the healthcare provider cannot decipher exactly what is happening.

Note: Visits and special audits performed by the MACs and the OIG are often generated from patient complaints. As much as possible, CBR compliance personnel should be sensitive to patient questions and reactions about billing.

While many compliance problem areas are well known, and some are even well publicized, there is almost always an element of discovery associated with the process of problem identification. A general problem area may be known, but recognizing the specific problem within that area may be difficult. Probably the greatest challenge in recognizing compliance problems is identifying areas that are likely to be under investigation in the years to come. Obviously, if we know something will be a problem three or four years from now, we can take steps to make certain that appropriate preventive steps are taken today. Conversely, one of the more difficult tasks for CBR compliance personnel is going back in time to address issues from the past that have created problems in the present.

Key learning area: While numerous compliance problem areas require attention, the experience and knowledge base of CBR compliance personnel must come into play to identify and recognize potential compliance problems or opportunities.

---
* This book generally cites *Medicare administrative contractors,* but also mentions fiscal intermediaries, intermediates, carriers, and specialized regional carriers (e.g., durable medical equipment regional carriers (DMERCs)).

Problem/opportunity analysis

Because compliance problems appear in many types and forms, problem analysis is diverse and complex. Every possible tool should be brought into play if there is a possibility that a compliance situation exists. Investigation may involve interviewing personnel, reviewing processes, diagramming events, and checking computer system processing. It may also mean reviewing samples of claims, medical records, and/or bills, having an outside consultant assess the situation, reconsidering personnel competency and training levels, checking coding and billing resources, and other activities. Four simple case studies from the fictitious Acme Medical Clinic and Apex Medical Center discuss potential problems and how CBR compliance personnel approach them.

Case study 4-1. E/M Level inconsistencies. Billing personnel express concern because of the five physicians at the Acme Medical Clinic, two consistently have high levels of E/M codes, even though all five doctors work about the same amount of time and see similar types of patients. One approach in investigating a situation like this may involve first a review of overall frequencies and/or percentages of E/M code utilization and then comparing them to national norms for the specialty. Another approach would be to review a sampling of claims and associated documentation to see whether they conform to current standards.

Case study 4-2. Claims payment irregularities. A claims specialist at Acme Medical Clinic notices that certain physician claims are not being paid. While the claims have not been denied, it appears that the services were bundled, even though the documentation shows that separate and distinct services were provided. The problem may relate to the use of modifiers and/or the physician's understanding of what can be billed. One approach to resolving this concern is to review such claims with coding personnel to see whether the coding is correct and/or appropriate modifiers are used.

Case study 4-3. Injection/Infusion charge capture. Nursing staffs on the medical–surgical floors of Apex Medical Center are concerned about charges. While injections and infusions are clinically documented, the nursing staff does not know when a patient is in observation. As a result the nurses do not know when to enter charges for injections and infusion services. A simple probe audit and analysis of observation flow may help determine the extent of this problem.

Case study 4-4. Self-administrable drugs in ED. Apex's ED has received a number of complaints about self-administrable drugs. For Medicare, the drug charges are billed to the patients as non-covered. According to the patients, some of the charges are high, and some patients consider the charges excessive and fraudulent. Investigation of this situation requires examining the charge-master, charging structures, and the overall billing process.

These simple examples are realistic. Other issues may be exceedingly complex and require more thorough examinations. Note that the results of problem analysis may not always lead to identification of a compliance situation. In Case studies 4-2 and 4-3, the main problem is likely reimbursement and not compliance. However, failing to code and bill appropriately and thus not receiving appropriate reimbursement constitute both compliance and financial issues.

Key learning area: Identification and analysis of compliance problems in the CBR area often reveal a reimbursement problem. Full compliance often means increased reimbursement.

After the real problem has been identified and analyzed, the next step is to design a solution. This is a two-part process: external solution design and internal solution design. In some cases the distinction is trivial but it can be significant. For instance, service area personnel may not be fastidious about correctly assigning supply items from a dispensing machine to proper patient accounts. The solution is relatively simple: instruct the employees to make certain all items are properly assigned. On the more complicated side would be a solution requiring a change of the logic inside the billing system. Separating external and internal designs may be useful in complicated situations.

External solution design

External design is simply the way the changed system will look to those who use it. The concentration is on the desired final output or outcome. For example, modifiers on both 1500 and UB-04 claims are sometimes required. While this may be viewed only as a compliance requirement (coding and billing correctly), it is also a reimbursement issue. From an external design perspective two important points should be considered:

1. The final outcome: correct modifiers associated with proper CPT HCPCS designations on claim forms

2. The supporting information and documentation needed to justify the use and generation of modifiers: A way to verify that the modifiers selected (and what they relate to) are appropriate and correct

We concentrate on the final product first, then address the necessary inputs, namely the documentation and/or other information required to generate and/or justify the outputs. Note that the order is important. Review the outputs of the process and then trace back to the necessary input information. You may see or hear the term *black box* in connection with this activity. With a black box process, we know the inputs and outputs, but do not know the internal processes used to convert the inputs into outputs. In some cases, particularly with third-party payer adjudication systems, black box audits may be kept secret.*

Thus the external design concentrates on the *what*, i.e., what the solution should look like, how it should act, what will be the outcomes, etc. The *why* question also needs consideration, for example, a full understanding of why a requirement exists. Modifiers are generally required for two possibly overlapping reasons. Some modifiers are informational; they simply provide additional information for statistical monitoring. Others are payment modifiers; they may allow payment to be made and/or increase the amount of the payment. Armed with the proper external design information (the *what* and the *why*), CBR compliance personnel can begin to address the *how* component of the solution that serves as the core or internal design solution.

Internal solution design

Internal design concentrates on how to develop or implement the external design. The external design may be easy if you know what is to be accomplished and why without much probing. The *how* question may not be so easy to answer. Continuing our example of modifiers on claim forms, consider how these modifiers are added to claim forms, for example, the UB-04. While several service areas may be involved in using modifiers, the following general breakdown accommodates our brief discussions:

- Outpatient surgery
- Laboratory
- Diagnostic radiology
- Therapy services
- Cardiovascular interventional radiology
- Other

These areas differ and development of internal solution designs that meet the external design parameters will probably vary.

The first real consideration is what computer capabilities are available through the billing system generating the claim forms. Whatever the answer to this question, the computer capabilities will affect the design. For each of the above service areas the main question is the same: "Is there a logical point in the overall service-documenting-coding-claims generation process where the modifiers can be developed?" From a compliance perspective, the objective is really to find that point in the process in which a knowledgeable decision, based upon the existence of proper documentation, can be made concerning modifier utilization.

For outpatient surgery, the relatively logical answer is that outpatient surgical cases are typically coded by HIM professional coding staff.† Thus a logical point for modifier development is HIM coding personnel. Obviously, resources such as personnel, computer editing, reference books, etc. must be available. The solution should also provide a means of external feedback. For instance, when two surgeries are performed, it is possible that payment may be bundled unless the -59 (distinct services) modifier is used. Since many thousands of edits appear in this area, modifier use may be missed. However, having a feedback loop—at an editing point or later in the process—to identify cases where payments are bundled can help address this situation.

For the laboratory and diagnostic radiology, the general answer to the question of where modifiers can be developed and input into the coding and billing cycle is only at the very front end, i.e., at order entry. The coding for radiological services is typically driven through the chargemaster with no human intervention. Thus the chargemaster must be set up in conjunction with the order entry system to capture the appropriate modifier or modifiers when the services are entered into the computer system.

For physical therapy and occupational therapy, the need for modifiers is limited. The -GO (occupational therapy) and -GP (physical therapy) modifiers can be entered in the chargemaster and then automatically generated through charge entry. However, claims in this area sometimes need a -59 (separate procedure) modifier and developing this modifier is a challenge. Someone must review the need for it as charges are entered

---

* The opposite of a black box is the white box in which the internals of a subsystem process are visible and known. For instance, the CMS CCI (correct coding initiative) edits are fully known so that users know how the editing will take place during claims adjudication.

† Professional coding staff may be located in areas other than HIM.

or an edit may be invoked during the claims generation process, indicating the need to consider a modifier.

Cardiovascular interventional radiology is one of the most difficult coding areas for outpatient services. A careful examination of the overall coding and billing flow must be made to determine how the many modifiers in this area should appear on claim forms. The other areas can similarly be considered. The important thing to note is that the first step is to identify the *what* and the *why* (external design) and the *how* (internal design).

Key learning area: The design phase of the systems approach is divided into internal and external designs. For complex situations, both aspects are useful; for simple situations the two may be merged.

Solution development

After a solution has been designed, it may be necessary to further develop it. Our modifier example may make it necessary to acquire and/or program editing tables into the computer to check for modifier utilization. The chargemaster or fee schedule may have to be altered relative to finalizing the solution. A training program may need to be developed to meet compliance criteria. A new documentation system for physicians and other providers may assist in meeting documentation criteria. Keep in mind that a solution may address a compliance standard and also improve reimbursement cycles.

In some cases, the distinction between design and development may be minor. At the very least, it is usually necessary to develop policies and procedures along with training materials and/or other documentation.

Solution implementation

Solution implementation can range from minor to major effort. Our modifier example for the surgical situation involved a combination of implementation by HIM personnel of new coding policies and procedures along with possible computer system changes. Training will probably be necessary so that coding personnel have a good knowledge of modifier development. Keep in mind simply knowing the rules is not enough. Solution implementation also depends on a basic understanding of the process and requirements. For modifiers, it is useful to understand those required for informational purposes and those that affect payment.

For the diagnostic radiology situation, after the chargemaster and order entry interface have been set up, implementation of the solution revolves around proper training of the personnel who input the services through order entry. It is also critical to ensure that appropriate documentation is in place to provide the necessary information for modifier choices.

Any implementation may involve considerations beyond the control of the organization and these may affect the change. In implementing a solution relative to post-operative observation status, for example, it is imperative that the surgeons be involved because they must provide the necessary documentation to support medical necessity and clinical pathway data for observation services. Similar situations exist for most types of healthcare providers. Physicians in a clinic situation may enter their own E/M codes, but if their documentation does not adequately support the level chosen, a problem ensues. Implementing a system correctly means ensuring that the correct level of coding is used.

Whenever possible, automated solutions via computer technology should be employed. It may be necessary to implement a temporary manual solution prior to developing and implementing a computer-based solution.

Solution monitoring and remediation

The final stages are the post-implementation monitoring and remediation. In the CBR area, this involves checking documentation, claims and statements on routine and random bases. A hospital may have taken significant steps to prevent up-coding relative to DRG assignment. Since specific DRGs are typically involved, it is appropriate to simply pull a sampling of the records and associated claims and review the documentation to ensure that the appropriate major complications and/or comorbidities along with regular complications and/or comorbidities are documented to justify the DRG assignment. Similarly, if a system is in place to ensure that pre-admission services are bundled into the DRG billing, the process can be checked by pulling a sampling of cases for review. Checks should also be made for proper present-on-admission (POA) indicators because the DRG assignment can be affected.

Graphic tools

Input–output modeling is frequently used to diagram processes and as an aid for thinking through situations. See Figure 4.2. A second and somewhat newer method is the object–action approach. It is more general and allows a greater degree of non-linear thinking. See Figure 4.3.

The input–output model is used in flowcharting processes and activities. Often, the emphasis is on the process or activity, with less emphasis on the data or

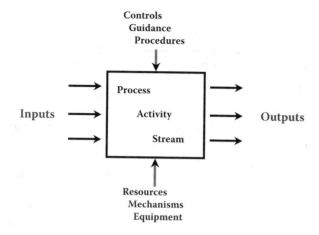

Figure 4.2   Input–output diagram.

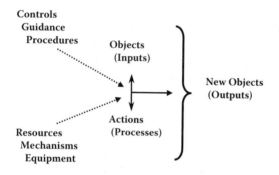

Figure 4.3   Object–action diagram.

items processed. This approach derives directly from the mathematical study of functions. It is widely used in associated disciplines such as Six Sigma, Total Quality Management (TQM), Activity-Based Costing (ABC), and Business Process Reengineering (BPR).

The object–action approach is newer and will probably be less familiar. It also derives from a mathematical discipline called category theory.* It provides a more general approach that gives equal weight to both the actions or activities and the data or items acted upon. This approach is currently receiving wide recognition in information systems development in the form of object-oriented design and programming.

A number of other graphic tools can aid in modeling and analyzing complex processes or flows. The most useful and easiest to use come from TQM. (See the bibliography for further information.) For problems that appear totally disorganized, a very general and useful technique called mind mapping is available.† See Figure 4.4. This is a free-form approach that allows

ideas to be placed on a diagram as they come to mind. After the ideas are recorded, they can be reorganized through this charting technique.

Consider a CBR compliance officer trying to analyze a diverse situation such as observation services. The analysis may seem overwhelming because so many different issues must be considered. Developing a mind or semantic map involves noting a central idea or area in the middle of a sheet of paper and noting various associated ideas as lines radiating from the center. Figure 4.4 shows an initial map for observation. Simply noting every idea or facet of the observation issue produced this map.‡ Additional information was inserted for some of the branches.

Key learning area: CBR compliance personnel should become conversant with various graphic tools that can help with creativity and organizing thoughts and information. The reimbursement cycle is heavily involved with processes and thus process analysis and improvement are important.

Multiple perspectives

The CBR process typically involves a number of departments or areas. Participants at the beginning of the process are the service areas and providers. The documentation process follows provision of services. The next steps are coding, billing and claims generation, quality assurance, and utilization review. Thus different people with different objectives, backgrounds, and concerns are involved.

Looking at a situation from different angles is essential. In addition, interfaces among the personnel involved in the CBR process can create some very real problems. For instance, coding personnel may have certain guidelines that conflict with the ability of the billing personnel to achieve full reimbursement. Another example concerns the need for provider personnel to fully document services both for quality of care purposes and also to meet coding and reimbursement guidelines.

Whenever you investigate a compliance problem area or design a solution to resolve a compliance problem, it is important to analyze the situation and/or solution from all applicable perspectives: service area, coding, billing, chargemaster, utilization review, etc. This concept is so important that several metaphors apply. For example, we need a "new set of eyes" to look

---

* The author's Ph.D. dissertation is in the area of category theory.

† This graphic technique has many names. Computer software is available to develop these charts.

‡ This mind or semantic map was generated by MindManager® Pro7.

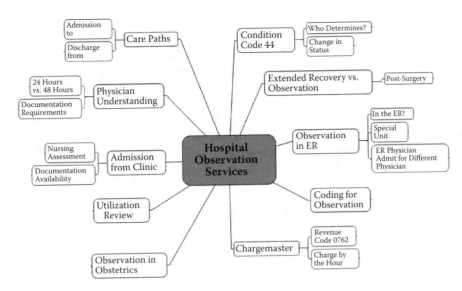

Figure 4.4 Mind/semantic map of observation services.

at a problem or must "walk in another person's shoes" to understand that person's perspective.

Raised perspective

A systematic or step-wise approach and view from different perspectives may not be enough. In some cases, it is necessary to elevate the perspective and thus broaden the horizon for associated interfaces and subsystems. For instance, a billing compliance problem such as dispensing self-administrable drugs in an outpatient setting may easily be resolved through a computer change.

One solution may be to make all such drugs for all patients non-covered and bill them as such. CBR compliance personnel may be fully satisfied with this analysis of the problem and the solution. Service area personnel, providers, coding staff, and billing employees may all agree with the specifics of the solution. However, it may be best to raise the perspective and broaden the scope of consideration to include patients, third-party payers, and public relations personnel. While the solution may be workable, patients may have to be informed of it in advance. Some third-party payers may not consider self-administrable drugs to be non-covered so their billing will have to be different. Public relations personnel like to know about changes that might impact patient concerns and complaints.

Key learning area: The systems approach is a powerful tool for CBR compliance personnel. A stepped or phased approach that accommodates multiple perspectives and adjusting the scope of consideration can often help solve difficult and complex problems.

Designing audits

Audits are potent tools for CBR compliance personnel. They can be used to identify problem areas and monitor adherence to a solution intended to maintain compliance. The highest level of auditing is the baseline compliance type discussed in Chapter 9. This special type of auditing has its own design parameters. For CBR compliance purposes, audits fall into formal and informal categories.

CBR compliance personnel frequently use informal audits. The simple process of pulling a cross-section of claims for review can be enlightening. More information can be gained by examining the associated itemized statements and documentation. Informal audits still need to be designed, and it is always important to understand audit form and function. What is the purpose or objective of the audit? Is the audit episodic or part of a cycle? Who is to be involved? What guidelines are to be used for the audit review? What type of post-audit report will be issued?*

A formal audit is more likely to be used by external consultants or auditors. One of the major differences between the two types of audits lies in the choice of sample. The size of the sample and the selection method are very important. Questions about confidence levels relative to sample size and selection must be analyzed and documented. This process requires knowledge of statistical concepts related to choosing sample sizes and selection processes. Formal audits are typical tools for external auditors including government auditors. If, for example, government auditors take a sample,

---

* It is important to document all activities and the results thereof. Even informal audits should be documented by a report or memorandum.

analyze it, and detect overpayment, the total amount of the overpayment will be calculated. The calculation process involves extrapolating the sample findings to the total universe of cases. Consider the following simplified example.

> **Case study 4-5. E/M Utilization audit.** Government auditors are at the Acme Medical Clinic performing a sample audit of office visits relative to proper documentation supporting a certain level of service. For the period under consideration, the audit determines that overpayment (code level not supported by documentation) occurred 10 percent of the time. This 10 percent is then applied to the total set of encounters over the same period. The extrapolation process depends on the applicability of the findings in the sample to the entire population.

One way to prepare for such audits is to conduct them internally before the external auditors arrive. A hospital or clinic can actually design an audit and use selection techniques similar to those used by the OIG and other government entities. A hospital might conduct such an E/M audit for the ED using current guidelines for technical component E/M coding. Internal or mock audits can use the same techniques used by CMS or OIG auditors. In fact, OIG's software package for case selection is freely available on the Internet. (See the CD accompanying this book.) The auditing process is further discussed in Chapters 8 and 9.

Key learning area: The process of designing an audit and then performing it effectively is a challenging but critically important tool for CBR compliance.

Fact gathering and interviewing techniques

Data and information can be gathered in a variety of ways. CBR compliance may have to document specific systematic components of the CBR process. The steps involved, the computer systems used, the interfaces between and among computer systems, personnel involvement, fee schedules, chargemasters, and the like can all be analyzed and documented. From such documentation, problems and opportunities can be identified. Flowcharting or other diagramming techniques can be used to gather information related to the various processes.

Interviewing techniques can also be effective. Talking with personnel involved in a process (individually or as a group) can yield significant data about problems and/or frustrations with the way a system does or

does not work. Interpersonal communication skills are extremely valuable in interviewing and eliciting information by talking with people. CBR issues may appear to involve technical processes that can be addressed quantitatively without undue human interaction, but many compliance issues involve significant human interaction and behavior modification issues.

Note: A word of caution for interviewing personnel involved in processes targeted for audits: such interviews may raise sensitive issues. In a hospital setting, categorization of supplies is a compliance issue. While a simple reclassification of certain supplies may be appropriate from a compliance perspective, such a change may impact the revenue generation for a department which, in turn, will affect its budgeting process. Any issue affecting a department budget is certainly going to be sensitive!

Team approach

An interdisciplinary and/or interdepartmental team in the CBR area is essential. Problem situations can often be identified and resolved by such a team. The team approach is an application of the multiple perspectives discussed above relative to the systems approach. The following example shows the advantages of a team approach.

An ED E/M compliance problem has been uncovered. Generated claims indicate higher levels of E/M services than those provided or, at least, documented. Coding personnel are amazed because they review the documentation and input codes into the abstracting system. The chargemaster coordinator quickly recognizes that the CPT E/M code appearing on the claim is the chargemaster code driven by charge entry. The information systems person in attendance can resolve the problem by making a change in computer system parameters or, if necessary, making a programming change. The change will allow the E/M level developed by coding personnel to override a default code in the chargemaster.

Information analysis

Data and information gathered via the techniques described must be carefully analyzed before it is used to design any type of solution involving changes. Since the whole area of coding, billing, and reimbursement constitutes a process, it is natural to flowchart the various steps and interactions of the process. This, of course, is only the beginning. Other areas will have to be analyzed, by graphic means or via a systematic process such as root cause analysis.

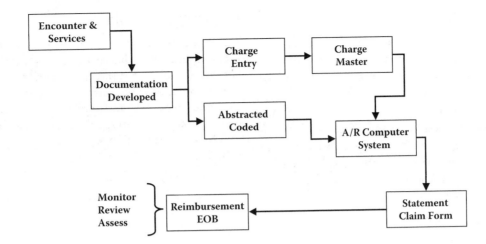

Figure 4.5 Extended input–process–output diagram.

Figure 4.5 illustrates the generalized process using a simplified input–process–output diagram. The chart is bifurcated (split into two branches) and the final box in the sequence contains additional annotation. The diagram could contain more detail by including the additional information provided in Figure 4.2, i.e., by including controls, guidance, methodologies, resources, equipment, manpower, etc. The diagram can also be developed and/or translated into an object–action diagram using the newer object-oriented techniques as illustrated in Figure 4.3.

A number of graphic or charting techniques can be used. The objective is to organize the information and then systematically analyze it. Because process flow involves so many different types of situations and variations, the techniques used may vary. As indicated above, the most generic technique is the mind or semantic map. The ideas, processes, or key points of a situation are noted on the diagram; relationships of ideas, processes, or points can then be developed and the chart can be revised. Flowcharts emphasize processes or activities while object–action diagrams encompass processes and their components.

Investigation of observation services provides a simple example. Assume that information has been gathered from various service areas and the chargemaster, and a claims review to determine where services are provided has been performed. The findings indicate the following locations are involved:

- Emergency department
- Obstetrics
- Outpatient surgery
- Acute care
- Physician's office (direct admit)

Interviews with personnel in these areas about providing observation services yielded interesting information after the following questions were asked:

- How does a patient get to observation status?
- Who is involved?
- How is care provided?
- What documentation is developed?
- What are the criteria for admission and/or discharge?
- How is this service coded and billed?

Figure 4.4 shows a preliminary mind map of the observation situation. Subsequent analysis may then yield a simplified input–process–output analysis of the type shown in Figure 4.5. The various flows required by provision of observation services can also be developed as a flowchart.

The results of this information gathering and analysis reveal that no physician involvement occurred in obstetrics so true observation did not occur. The solution here is to reclassify this service differently, e.g., obstetric holding, and bill it accordingly. Likewise, the analysis reveals that ER service did not constitute a true observation situation either. However, the ER physicians could have provided observation services and documented them.

In information analysis, the skill and experience of CBR personnel are of the greatest importance. While many techniques can aid CBR staff in organizing and analyzing data, creativity and ingenuity are critical.

Key learning area: Information analysis and decoding complex processes can seem overwhelming. A variety of tools can be effectively used to facilitate an understanding of these processes.

Root cause analysis

It is important to fully investigate situations in the CBR compliance area. The basic idea of root cause analysis is that the investigation and questioning of a situation should proceed to the point where the real problem is identified, and not the symptoms. This typically involves posing successful levels of questions. The process relies on digging until the real problem or its root cause is identified. (See the bibliography for additional references for this technique.)

Statistical basics and graphic representation

Many different statistical techniques and graphic presentation techniques have been designed to manage analyzed data. The best approach is simplicity. One of the most common errors with statistical or quantified data is to read too much into the data and fail to fully identify the context from which the data was taken. By changing the context statistics can be manipulated to mean almost anything.

Data and relative data arrays

Identified data elements are usually presented in table format in ascending or descending order. The following example shows arrays of frequency of two triples of DRGs in ascending order.

Respiratory infections and inflammations
DRG 177 with MCC →	50
DRG 178 with CC →	60
DRG 179 without CC/MCC →	100

Pneumonia and asthma
DRG 196 with MCC →	40
DRG 197 with CC →	25
DRG 198 without CC/MCC →	120

This type of data array allows easy analysis and comparison. After such an array has been developed, for example, ask yourself what the relative percentages within these two triples should be. Then ask what the relationship between the two triples should be. The relative frequency of utilization for certain DRG combinations is a significant compliance issue requiring careful attention. While the DRG pairs, triples, and/or quadruples may vary over time, CMS and other third-party payers using DRGs are concerned about up-coding and resulting overpayments.

Frequency distribution

The frequency distribution is a form of data array. Relative and cumulative frequency distributions are common. They are typically shown in graphic format although the base data must be displayed as well. The example below covers frequency distribution of E/M code utilization by an FP physician; distribution is limited to Medicare patients.

99212 → 45
99213 → 113
99214 → 115
99215 → 57

Graphs and charts are discussed below.

Percentages, percentiles, and proportions

Percentages are well understood and do not need to be redefined here. Percentiles are used to split arrayed data points (ascending or descending) into 100 groups. For example, the 25th percentile is a value that divides the array into one fourth versus three fourths. Note that the 25th percentile may not be a data point. Proportions are similar to percentages and can be used in areas such as choosing a sampling. For instance, it may be desirable to develop a sampling that will find errors within a proportion of 0.05 (or 5 percent) with a confidence of 90 percent.

Measures of central tendency

The **arithmetic mean** is determined by adding the data points and dividing the sum by the number of data points. The **geometric mean** is found by multiplying data points, then calculating the nth root of the product where n is the number of data points. As an exercise, calculate the arithmetic and geometric means for the following data points:

4, 7, 7, 9, 10, 26

To arrive at the arithmetic mean, add the numbers to obtain 63. Divide 63 (total) by 6 (number of data points) to obtain an arithmetic mean of 10.50. To calculate the geometric mean, multiply the numbers to obtain 458,640. Then find the 6th (number of data points) root to obtain 8.78.*

Note that the geometric mean is a better measure of central tendency when outlier data such as the 26 in the above set of data points is present.

---

* The geometric mean is often calculated using logarithms equivalent to this formula. A special calculator or electronic spreadsheet such as MS Excel is needed for these calculations.

Median—Basically the middle point or the average of the two middle points. For the above six data points the median is the average of the two middle points, i.e., the average of 7 and 9, which is 8.

Mode—The most common value. It may not exist and may not be unique. The most common value for the above six data points is 7. Note that for a sampling as small as this, the mode has little meaning.

Outlier—Unusually high or low data points relative to the central tendency. For the above six data points, 26 is an outlier.

Note: Outlier data is common in the healthcare field. Consider average charges across all hospitals for the same service. Hospital pricing is significantly different for many reasons and thus charges for the same service can differ enormously and create outliers.

Index numbers

Index numbers represent a special class: they are not expressed in units. They are used for comparative purposes, usually geographically or over time. They are commonly used in healthcare, particularly with prospective payment systems. Examples are:

- APG/APC Weights
- DRG Case Mix Index
- RBRVS Relative Values
- APC Service Mix Index
- Consumer Price Index
- Wage Index

Graphic examples

One of the best ways to represent quantitative data is with a chart or graph. Many types can be used. This section contains two simple examples. (See the bibliography for additional information.) Note that graphing techniques help organize data so that it can be visualized and then further assessed.

A quick look at the percentage frequency distribution of new patient E/M codes for two physicians easily shows a significant disparity in the relative use of levels (Figure 4.6). This may be a significant aberration if both are primary care physicians and see the same types of patients. However, if one is primary care (Physician A) and the other is a specialist (Physician B), the distribution may be inappropriate.

Figure 4.7 illustrates two different triples of DRGs within the MS-DRG system. DRG triple 177–179 covers respiratory infections and inflammations. DRG triple 196–198 indicates pneumonia and asthma. Hospitals must be careful to compare their distributions within these triples relative to national norms.

Probability and distributions

A discussion of probability and distributions is beyond the scope of this section. CBR compliance personnel should have a basic knowledge of these subjects, particularly relative to normal distributions and standard deviations, so that they understand the process of choosing sample sizes for auditing purposes. (See the bibliography for basic references on these topics.)

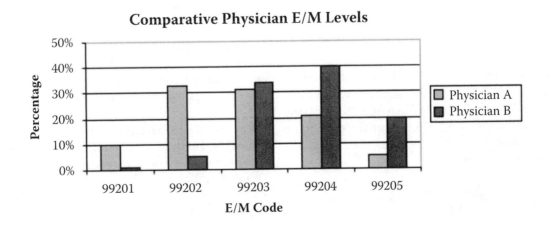

Figure 4.6 Frequency distribution of new patient E/M codes.

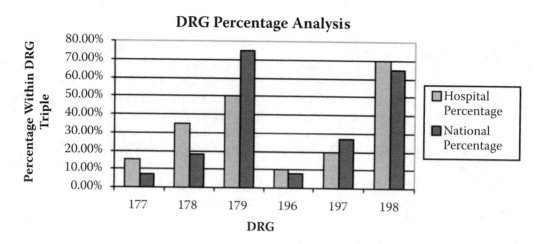

Figure 4.7 Frequency percentage by DRG severity triple category.

Sample sizes and confidence intervals

These important aspects of compliance issues involve statistical inference—a sample size for an audit is generally chosen so that we can statistically infer that certain criteria are met. It is best to pick a sample size for an audit that will assure with a probability of 95 percent that we are within 0.05 of the proportion of actual errors based on population size. A simple formula typically used is

$$n = \frac{z^2 \pi (1-\pi)}{E^2}$$

This will give us the number of cases needed; then we fill in the variables. E = 0.05 (stated proportion relative to errors). z = 1.960 (95 percent confidence level; see Table 4.1). π = 0.5 (worst case; see Table 4.2). The calculation then becomes

$$n = \frac{3.84 * 0.25}{0.0025} = 384$$

A few simple calculations will indicate that the number (n) of cases to be reviewed is sensitive to the three parameters. Consider that E = 0.025 (within 0.025 of true proportion of errors). z = 2.575 (99 percent confidence level; see Table 4.1). π = 0.5 (worst case; see Table 4.2). The calculation becomes

$$n = \frac{6.63 * 0.25}{0.000625} = 2,652$$

This represents a significant increase. Using this formula is easier using Table 4.1.

Table 4.1 Value of z for Given Confidence Level.

	99%	98%	95%	90%	80%	50%
z =	2.575	2.330	1.960	1.6450	1.280	0.675

If other values of z are required, i.e., for a confidence level not shown in Table 4.1, consult the Standard Normal Curve Table to be found in one of the statistics references. The table can provide precise values.

The value of π should represent the estimated proportion of errors in the population. For most work in the CBR area, this estimate is unknown. A small sampling of, say, 30* cases could be taken to better determine this estimate. If some information is known, the starting point for π can be better determined. Consider Table 4.2.

Table 4.2 Value of Proportion (π) for Initial Choice

π =	0.1	0.2	0.3	0.4	0.5	0.6	0.7	0.8	0.9
π(1 − π) =	0.09	0.16	0.21	0.24	0.25	0.24	0.21	0.16	0.9

Note that the value of π(1 − π) is both maximized and symmetrical about π = 0.5. Thus, in the absence of better information, the worst case can be assumed and the value of the estimated proportion set at 0.5.

Key learning area: Knowledge of basic statistics for CBR compliance personnel is a prerequisite to using sample size formulas to conduct a formal compliance audit.

---

* The 30 has special significant in statistics. It is considered the minimum number for any sampling to have meaning.

See Chapter 8 for a further discussion of audit design and see the bibliography for additional sources of information. The CD accompanying this book contains information about the OIG's RAT-STATS program for choosing sample sizes and selecting random samples. Note that this is a highly technical area and appropriate research and understanding are required to use these methods correctly. Extensive documentation with the RAT-STATS program explains the more advanced statistical formulas used.

Business process reengineering

Business process reengineering (BPR) has a number of different forms and can be utilized at different levels. Many fine techniques have evolved from BPR. The emphasis is on processes. One of the underlying philosophies is the process is broken; the people performing the process are not. While this philosophy can be debated, it does allow for focusing on processes which, if improved, can produce better performance, increased effectiveness, greater efficiency, and *improved compliance.*

For CBR compliance considerations, the BPR techniques can be applied at different levels:

- Individual process reengineering
- Department reengineering
- Corporate reengineering
- Enterprise reengineering

These levels simply represent the use of the raised perspective of the systems approach. With BPR, only the level and focus of consideration change. As an example, consider the number of different types of coding and levels involved in a complete analysis of a significant project or system:

- Individual coding
- Overall department coding
- Hospital-wide coding
- IDS coding*

Questions surrounding the individual coding process involve the personnel performing the coding, computer encoder availability, documentation available to coding personnel, coding guidelines, and other reference materials. The objective is to have both coding staff and the process generate correct codes.

At the department level, questions surrounding the infrastructure and organization of the process and personnel come into play. The coding process may involve specialization. Some coding personnel may be dedicated to inpatient coding, some to outpatient surgery, and some to clinic and/or ED coding.

At the hospital level, questions that arise related to centralized versus decentralized coding. A hospital, for example, may have embarked upon a strategy of decentralizing the coding staff to the various service areas on a functional basis while line management still resides within the health information management department.† Another hospital level coding issue involves the chargemaster and whether coding takes place through the chargemaster from charge entry. Static coding involves placing the codes in the chargemaster and having the charge entry drive the coding. Dynamic coding involves developing the codes outside the chargemaster, generally by professional coding staff.

At IDS level, the reengineering process may concentrate on uniformity and consistency of the end result of coding. Often this involves the development and application of enterprise-wide coding policies, procedures, and guidelines to ensure that personnel code in the same way and the outcomes of the coding process are uniformly accurate and consistent.

Quality improvement

Quality improvement techniques for healthcare often involve the following disciplines:

- Six Sigma
- Continuous Quality Improvement (CQI)
- Total Quality Management (TQM)
- Quality Circles
- Quality Function Deployment (QFD)

All these disciplines use a number of techniques that can assist CBR compliance personnel to gather information and perform analysis. Six Sigma is the culmination of many years of quality improvement methodologies. Its six different levels of capabilities are embodied in a progression roughly analogous to the system used in karate, for example, green belts progress to black belts who, in turn, progress to master black belts.

It is advantageous to review and study the other techniques as well. The Quality Circle technique is one of the oldest and is still used. In simplest terms, the team approach to improving the quality of processes relative to coding, billing, and reimbursement is really an application of the systems approach at an organizational level. CQI, TQM, and QFD provide a range of tools, techniques, and approaches that can assist in problem identification, analysis, and solution development.

---

* For this example we will assume that the hospital in question is part of an IDS.

† Matrix organization.

Healthcare is generally a service industry. These quality improvement tools must sometimes be translated from a product development view to a service orientation.

Benchmarking

Benchmarking can be a highly formalized process that can be utilized in a number of different ways. Consider the following activities*

- Performance benchmarking
- Process benchmarking
- Strategic benchmarking
- Internal benchmarking
- Competitive benchmarking
- Functional benchmarking
- Generic benchmarking

Benchmarking is typically used to improve quality and can be applied to compliance-related issues. This is particularly of the baseline compliance audit that is really an internal benchmarking process and may be called a benchmark compliance audit. This process is discussed more fully in Chapter 9. Note that an important part of CBR compliance concerns the use of normative or benchmark data from external sources. This technique is used in many different areas of CBR compliance, if for example, the relative percentages of DRGs 177, 178, and 179 along with the 196, 197, and 198 triple can be tracked over time to determine identifiable changes or trends. It can also be useful if a comparison of the frequency of ED physician utilization of CPT E/M codes for ED visits raises questions, or for evaluating the relative frequency of the use of consultation codes by physicians at a clinic. In the latter two cases, hospital or clinic information can be compared against other normative data.

---

* See Andersen, *Benchmarking Handbook: A Step-By-Step Process.*

> **Key learning area: Disciplines such as Six Sigma, Business Process Reengineering (BPR), Total Quality Management (TQM), and Benchmarking should all be reviewed for applicability to CBR compliance programs.**

Summary and conclusion

The process of investigating, analyzing, and developing solutions to CBR compliance problems can be facilitated by a number of techniques. Information can be gathered from a variety of sources and activities including record reviews, process studies, and interviews of personnel. Some investigations in the CBR area may be relatively simple; others may be complex and interlaced with many facets and considerations. CBR compliance personnel must be familiar with a variety of qualitative and quantitative tools. Skills in interpersonal communication and persuasive techniques are also important. Since many aspects of coding, billing, and reimbursement involve process analysis, a functional approach to analysis is often used.

The systems approach is invaluable. Utilizing this systematic, step-by-step approach enables and empowers the thinking process in complex situations. Such a process also helps ensure that all aspects of a situation are addressed. As a part of the systems approach, it is helpful to consider multiple perspectives and elevate the perspectives as appropriate. Looking at a situation through the eyes of different people from different areas can add depth and scope to a problem. In some situations, it is essential to look at the bigger picture—that is, to look at the forest as well as at the individual trees.

Tools used in disciplines such as Six Sigma, TQM, benchmarking, root cause analysis, and BPR can also be used to deal with compliance issues. While such tools can provide significant assistance, the real asset is the ability of personnel to logically analyze complex situations and then utilize the tools and techniques appropriate to a situation.

five

Development of CBR policies and procedures

Introduction

Among the most powerful tools for CBR compliance personnel are the written policies and procedures developed as part of a compliance program. These typically cover the coding, billing, and chargemaster areas can also extend to documentation, utilization review, and quality assurance. Developing and writing policies and procedures requires careful craftsmanship. A number of interfaces must be considered within the overall view of the final product. In addition, the rate of change in the CBR area for all healthcare providers is significant. Thus, this intricate process also requires ongoing monitoring and revision. The approval and implementation processes are equally important. Some policies and procedures will be simple and easy to manage; their approval and implementation may be straightforward. At the other end of the spectrum, an attorney may have to consider potential legal ramifications before a policy can be developed and procedures set in motion.

Developing and writing policies and procedures

A major part a CBR compliance program involves identifying and solving compliance challenges. The solutions designed and implemented result in the development of various policies and procedures. The scope and volume of the policies and procedures correlate directly to the size and complexity of the healthcare organization and associated services. A small free-standing physician clinic in a rural area will require fewer policies and procedures than an urban hospital providing a wide range of services. *However, the need for well-crafted policies and procedures remains exactly the same.* A single manual with several chapters may suffice. In some cases, separate policy and procedure manuals devoted to areas such as:

- Coding
- Billing
- Chargemaster
- CBR compliance review and auditing
- Utilization review
- Quality assurance and outcome management

Because a part of the solution of many CBR compliance problems is the development of policies and procedures, careful analysis must be applied. For example, a conflict may arise concerning the assignment of a date of service. Such a situation might occur if a patient presents to a hospital late in the evening and is an outpatient for several hours before admission as an inpatient after midnight. The episode of care started on the original date of presentation, but for billing purposes, the following day may be used for the inpatient services on the bill. To complicate matters, health information management personnel may decide that for coding purposes the date of service commenced on the first date the patient was seen which corresponds to the episode of care. Note that something as simple as this question may require careful investigation of rules and regulations involved and a consensus of those involved.

The solution to such an interface problem is to have representatives from health information management work with the billing or claims transaction office. Note that external guidelines and/or requirements may be involved. Health information management may have an abstracting policy in place relative to the episode of care. Billing personnel may be under specific requirements from a third-party payer relative to the date of service. This simplified example may require revision of health information management's abstracting policy and development of a new overall policy to address this situation. One way to approach this might be to abstract the episode of care as two encounters, outpatient and inpatient. Regarding the issue of specific payment systems directives, a critical access hospital would code and bill the services separately. A hospital under the Medicare DRG system would have to consider the three-day DRG pre-admission window. The development of the needed policies and procedures in this area can serve as the mechanism to change the coding and billing processes so that correct and compliant bills and claims are generated.*

Keep in mind that the overall objective and anticipated outcome of developing and utilizing policies and procedures is to perform processes correctly and

---

* In some cases external national guidelines for billing and/or coding may conflict with both reimbursement and compliance.

within compliance guidelines. Also, the policies and procedures show auditors that compliance considerations have been made, documented, and put into place. While a policy or procedure may not be correct in every detail, the fact that a genuine effort with careful investigation was made can help a healthcare provider avoid penalties. The development of policies and procedures is thus a significant line of defense as well as a mechanism to increase efficiency and improve reimbursement.

Key learning area: The processes of developing and writing CBR compliance polices and procedures constitute an important part of the systematic process of recognizing and solving CBR compliance problems.

Form, format, and organization of policies and procedures

A healthcare organization of any significant size will already have a number of policies and procedures in place. The form, format, layout, and processes involved will have already been determined. A hospital will most likely have a standing committee (such as a forms committee) to deal with these organizational considerations.

This section addresses the basic elements required for written policies and procedures to cover coding, billing, and reimbursement. The specific format is not critical; follow whatever format is dictated by your healthcare organization. Below is an outline of the typical items to cover in an individual policy or procedure:

- Subject
- Date
- Previous Issuance Date
- Policy Number
- Effective Date
- Affected Areas/Processes
- Approving Authorities
- Policy Statement
- Distribution
- Cross Referenced Policies and Procedures
- Revision Sequence
- Notes and Discussion

You may also want to include meta data items such as keywords or indexing information. For example, a CPT or HCPCS coding system may include references indexed to specific coding policies and procedures based upon individual codes or code combinations. For larger healthcare organizations, the process of organizing and accessing the hundreds of policies and procedures can be a real challenge. While the policies

and procedures may be in paper format, most large healthcare organizations now use electronic formats that make dissemination much easier and also allow convenient updating. This is discussed in more detail at the end of the chapter. We will now examine a simple CBR policy and procedure from Apex Medical Center.

**Apex Medical Center
Billing Policy and Procedure Statement**

Subject: Billing for Observation Services

Date: February 15, 2008

Previous Issuance Dates: June 1, 1998; October 1, 2004

Policy Number: CBR01002152008

Effective Date: March 1, 2008

Affected Areas/Processes: Billing Process, Chargemaster, Outpatient Service Areas, Utilization Review, Quality Assurance

Approving Authorities: [Insert appropriate titles, e.g., Director of Finance.]

Policy Statement: Observation services can be charged and subsequently billed only if the following criteria are met:

1. A written physician order was issued.
2. Documentation from the physician meets the appropriate level for use of E/M codes 99218, 99219, 99220 or 99234, 99235, 99236 and must include indicated levels of the following elements:
   a. History
   b. Examination
   c. Medical decision making
3. The documentation provided by the physician requesting admission to observation status must indicate appropriate medical necessity for the provision of such services.
4. Services must be provided for a minimum of 8 hours.
5. Services will be billed on an hourly basis.
6. For Medicare, observation services can be provided for up to 48 hours. For all other providers, observation can be provided for up to 24 hours.
7. Before the first 24-hour period is reached, Utilization Review will assess the observation services and confer with the attending physician concerning proper disposition of the patient.

Distribution: Director, Health Information Management; Director, Patient Accounts; Director of Finance; Chargemaster Coordinator; Director, UR/QA; Director, Information Systems

Cross Referenced Policies and Procedures:

Revision Sequence: Original December 1, 1997; Updated June 1, 1998; Updated March 1, 1999; Updated June 2000; Updated January 2003

Notes and Discussion:

1. See current *AMA CPT Manual* for definition of documentation requirement relative to observation coding.
2. Observation services are outpatient services that generally arise from three different types of cases:
   a. Admission to observation status from the ER after administration of services. An ER or attending physician may make the admission.
   b. Admission to observation status directly from a clinic. This requires assurance that documentation is on file from the physician relative to meeting the record and medical necessity requirements.
   c. Admission to observation status in a post-outpatient surgery situation. The patient is generally admitted to observation status from the recovery room or extended recovery status. Care must be taken to distinguish between observation and extended recovery relative to documentation and medical necessity criteria.
3. Note that the documentation requirements for admission to observation status are essentially the same as for admission to inpatient status. However, the medical necessity criteria are not as stringent.
4. For Medicare, observation is an area of significant compliance concern, particularly in post-outpatient surgery situations. Medicare has indicated that observation services are not always justified through medical necessity. Claims showing revenue code 0710 (recovery room) and revenue code 0762 (observation services) raise the possibility that documentation justifying the provision of observation services may be requested.

Note that this policy and procedure statement is overly simplified and is intended to serve only as a general guideline for developing a policy and procedure statement. Most of the entries in this sample are self-explanatory. Some of the more important areas are discussed below. Every healthcare organization may have its own standards and format for written policies and procedures. This sample policy is oversimplified

because observation services is a large and intricate area. Multiple policies and procedures are needed to address the many facets of observation services. For instance, the use of Condition Code 44 is extremely complex because Medicare has adopted a definition that is different from the one used by the National Uniform Billing Committee (NUBC).

Indexing and numbering

Care should be given to the indexing structure of policies and procedures. The complexity of the process will vary widely for different healthcare providers. Small organizations may find it necessary only to index by title of the policy or procedure. Larger organizations will need to categorize policies and procedures into different areas such as coding, billing, chargemaster, cost report, etc. Within the various categories, a numbering system can be developed based on further categorization or on a numbering scheme including the date.

Dates

Issuance date, effective date, and a full history of revision dates should be included. It is important to show that each policy has been regularly reviewed and revised. Dating serves as a useful indicator to external auditors that an organization keeps abreast of compliance issues. Save copies of all previous policies and procedures for archival purposes.

Approval process

The approval process is very important because policies and procedures usually affect a number of departments. Every affected area should review and approve a policy and procedure statement. Consider each of the following departments that might be involved:

- Health Information Management for coding aspects
- Patient Financial Accounting for claims filing and transaction data
- Chargemaster Coordinator for chargemaster operations
- Utilization Review for review criteria
- Medical Staff for provider recognition

Depending on the organization, more departments or entities may need to participate in approval or at least participate in the review phase. Developing what appears a logical and appropriate policy and procedure may later produce unintended impacts on the organization. While the review and approval process may be more difficult if multiple reviewers are involved, the dividends accrued in a high quality and acceptable policy and procedure are worth the effort.

Distribution list

As with most aspects of developing CBR policies and procedures, distribution is important. Note that different departments and/or service areas will have interrelated policies and procedures. Thus some policies and procedures are distributed for implementation by a department while in others may be provided for informational purposes only. Thus a distribution list may include departments in addition to affected areas.

The most typical distribution method is on paper. However, as discussed below, alternative formats such as e-mail, networks, and intranets are available. Policies and procedures should also be stored at a centralized location. Historical archival documents relative to the policies and procedures should also be retained at the central location. For most healthcare organizations, archives of old policies and procedures may be maintained in a computer system. The information systems personnel can best advise on this process and on alternative mechanisms for distribution.

Cross-referenced policies and procedures

The sample policy and procedure related to observation services cites a number of cross-referenced policies and procedures. For instance, observation services involve an extensive set of care paths or clinical pathways relative to:

1. Medical necessity criteria for admission to observation status
2. Medical necessity criteria for keeping a patient in observation status beyond 24 hours
3. Medical necessity criteria for discharging a patient from observation status to home or lower level of care
4. Medical necessity criteria for moving a patient from observation status to hospital inpatient status
5. Medical judgment relative to changing from inpatient status to observation status using Condition Code 44

The coding for observation services follows from the general E/M coding documentation guidelines that are probably embodied in a general E/M coding policy and modus operandi for the coding staff. Similarly, the chargemaster has most likely been established on a time basis, typically by the hour with differentiated charges based upon the type of observation service provided. For example, a patient may be in observation status in the ER, in an acute care bed, in the telemetry unit, and/or in a special observation (cardiac or pediatric) unit. Different costs are incurred and thus pricing will be gradated.

Utilization review personnel will usually be subject to established guidelines when reviewing observation services that should be part of the applicable policies and procedures. Guidelines typically involve post-surgical observation services and proper determination of observation versus inpatient status.

General compliance policies and procedures may also cover periodic auditing and the inclusion of these types of services in the baseline compliance auditing process. All of these cross-references should be noted in a policy and procedure so that anyone reviewing it can acquire a complete picture of a situation.

Notes and discussion

The notes and discussion section provides an opportunity to explain why a policy and procedure has been established. This section also provides the means to provide more detail. Personnel required to meet a policy and procedure may be much more amenable if they understand why the policy and procedure are required. The notes should indicate the compliance area addressed, i.e., medical necessity, false claims, Medicare fraud, abuse, and anti-kickback issues, patient dumping, etc.

Additional information concerning the legal citations, rules, and regulations can also be cited in this section or in a separate section created specifically to serve that purpose. Note that some CBR compliance policies and procedures will be established relative to the interpretation of legal matters. In cases where Medicare, third-party payers, and/or professional organizations have not established specific guidelines related to coding and billing issues, your organization may have to make interpretations and act accordingly.

Meta data

Meta data is simply information about data, in this case, applicable to policy and procedure statements and directives. Thus, relevant meta data will involve index information, keyword information, cross reference entries, and other reference tools that may be used to navigate the various policies and procedures. One reason policy and procedure statements are so complex is that the same issue may be addressed from different perspectives. These different perspectives (e.g., coding versus billing versus chargemaster) must be properly correlated so that the overall system works smoothly.

Key learning area: CBR policy and procedure development and implementation are formal processes requiring careful consideration and documentation. Policies and procedures form the foundation of a healthcare organization's commitment to compliance in the CBR area.

Areas of concern

Dozens, if not hundreds, of CBR-related policies and procedures may have to be developed and implemented because of the numerous areas of concern, many of which are discussed in this book and illustrated in case studies. Although the numbers, types, and levels of compliance issues are significant, prioritizing them depends on the organization. Certainly a primary impetus for developing CBR policies and procedures arises from internal or external identification of specific compliance concerns. The sample presented in this chapter is only one example. Another might relate to the relationship of a hospital that owns a medical clinic and must therefore address pre-admission or post-admission bundling rules. The list of potential issues changes constantly. Several simple case studies illustrate the problem-solving process in relation to the need for formal, written policies and procedures.

Case study 5-1. Clinic gastroenterology: Endoscopic control of bleeding. At a gastrointestinal specialty clinic, the physicians go to one of several hospitals and an ASC. They note information about services performed on 3 × 5 cards, for example, colonoscopy performed, two polyps removed, biopsy taken, and bleeding controlled. Coding staff then codes cases based on this information and inputs charges into the billing system that then checks for the CCI (correct coding initiative), edits, and flags the biopsy and control-of-bleeding codes as needing a -59 (separate procedure) modifier. Clinic coding staff have simply added -59 whenever the edits occurred. A recent audit revealed that some uses of this modifier are inappropriate and that incorrect claims have been filed.

Control of bleeding and biopsies form the bases for a number of CCI edits. The basic logic is that if an endoscopy is performed to control existing bleeding, the control-of-bleeding codes should be used (with -59 modifier attached as appropriate). However, bleeding caused by the endoscopic procedure is considered a normal complication of the procedure and the control-of-bleeding codes should not be used (no -59 modifier).

A similar logical argument concerns biopsies. Sending a tissue sample to pathology is fairly typical for GI endoscopic services. However, the tissue sample sent may simply be a polyp removed by the snare technique. Thus, the intent of the procedure was not to take a biopsy; the tissue sample was incidental to another procedure. If the biopsy was the main procedure, the biopsy code and a -59 modifier should be used as appropriate. If the biopsy was incidental, the biopsy code should not be used or at least the -59 modifier should not be used.

For Case study 5-1, a policy and procedure should be developed to make certain that the -59 modifier and associated coding are used correctly. That means training physicians to use correct coding or giving coding staff ready access to documentation related to the services provided.

Case study 5-2. Hospital gastroenterology: Endoscopic control of bleeding. At Apex Medical Center, the coding for both upper and lower GI colonoscopies is performed by charge entry through the chargemaster. When service area personnel input the charges, a reminder pop-up screen appears in case they need to add modifiers. Over the past several years, billing personnel have provided feedback on the need for the -59 modifier. GI service area personnel have learned when to use the -59 modifier to skirt CCI edits. A recent external audit found that the modifier is used incorrectly for biopsies and control-of-bleeding claims.

Case study 5-2 extends the concepts discussed in Case study 5-1. It applies to a hospital setting where compliance issues become more complex. The chargemaster and billing personnel may claim that a charge is required because control of bleeding was performed. This is based on the premise that coding is performed to reflect resource utilization on the hospital outpatient side. The hospital may have a need to capture the charge that would normally drive the development of a CPT code. It may decide to drop the code and retain the charge, a decision that will deal with a simple set of circumstances. The -59 modifier should not be used, but if it is not used, the editing system will kick out the claim. The mechanics of implementing a solution will require careful analysis of billing logic. Moreover, a written policy and procedure describing and substantiating this rationale will be essential for compliance purposes.

Case study 5-3. Injections and infusions. Apex Medical Center is struggling with the new CPT codes for injections and infusions that were fully implemented in 2007. The problems include charge capture for observation services and a number of questions involving the use of multiple codes. While procedural issues must be address, the hospital also has a clear need to develop a comprehensive policy and procedure covering the chargemaster, coding, and subsequent billing. Because service area personnel, particular nursing staff, must capture charges and thus code through the chargemaster, a large number of employees must understand the coding and billing logic associated with hydration, injections, and infusions. (*Note:* Chemotherapy is not usually as much of an issue because specialized nursing staff is dedicated to providing these services.)

A complete policy and procedure related to infusions and injections might fill a small book. While coding logic (primary versus secondary versus concurrent logic) must be delineated, so must coding conventions of hierarchical sequencing (explaining which codes to use if two or more services can be considered primary). An extensive number of examples should be included for training and education purposes. The following list of concerns and examples that should explain how coding is to be performed.

- Medical necessity
- Written order
- Drugs charged separately
- IV solution charging
- Start/stop times
- 15-minute rule—IV injection versus IV infusion therapy
- Half-time unit rule ← see separate hospital-wide policy and procedure
- First hour plus each additional hour logic
- Keep-vein-open (KVO) circumstances
- Multiple drugs
  - Injections—mixing of drugs
  - IV Therapy—concurrent concept
- Multiple sites
- Vein failure
- Separate encounters
- Discontinue/reestablish
- Routine, integral part ← see separate hospital-wide policy and procedure
- Multiple injections of same drug
- General injection, hydration, infusion therapy logic
  - Primary/initial versus secondary/subsequent
  - Concurrent

- Add-on code utilization
- CPT guidance

A number of chargemaster and associated billing policies and procedures will be needed because the coding and charge capture process may be distinctly different across service areas. A brief list of service areas in which specific charge capture and flow processes must be considered follows:

- Emergency department
- Medical/surgical floors (observation)
- Pre- and post-surgery areas
- Outpatient service areas
- Provider-based clinics

To summarize, the coding, billing, and claims filing process for injections and infusions requires careful analysis and development of policies and procedures along with appropriate training.

Case study 5-4. Half-time unit rule. The half-time unit rule has its origin in the Medicare program. Simply stated, when multiple time units are reported, the last subsequent time unit cannot be billed unless at least half of that time unit is provided. In some cases this is quite straightforward; in other cases, it becomes a little involved. Apex has made a policy decision that the half-time unit rule is to be applied to all circumstances in which time units are used.

Time units may be generated from the coding structure or via structuring of the chargemaster. A representative sampling includes:

- Physical therapy and occupational therapy—15-minute units
- Infusions and chemotherapy—1-hour units
- Critical care—1-hour units
- Anesthesia, professional—15-minute units
- Behavioral assessment—15-minute units
- Medical nutrition therapy—15- or 30-minute units
- Observation services—1-hour units
- Recovery—1-hour units (chargemaster decision)
- Surgery—5-minute units (chargemaster decision)
- Anesthesia, technical—15-minute units (chargemaster decision)

The policy decision in Case study 5-4 is reasonable, particularly in light of Medicare's concern about charging for a proper number of units. The development of a policy and procedure is straightforward and should be supplemented with appropriate training materials.

Time units are difficult to apply in physical therapy and occupational therapy. The difficulty stems from the fact that several treatment modalities provided may all use time units. Physical and occupational therapy use 15-minute time units. Thus, to count the last subsequent time unit, at least 7.5 minutes (rounded up to 8 minutes) must be used. Consider the following sequence of three different modalities:

Modality A	23 minutes → 2 units
	(15 minutes + 8 minutes)
Modality B	38 minutes → 3 units
	(30 minutes + 8 minutes)
Modality C	23 minutes → 2 units
	(15 minutes + 8 minutes)
Totals	84 minutes, 7 units

These numbers were manipulated to make the point that dividing the total time (84 minutes) by 15 minutes, yields 5.6, rounded up to 6 units. This is distinctly different from the 7 units generated. Thus, the policies and procedures for the half-time unit rule should include examples of this type to illustrate the way the half-time unit rule is to be applied.

Case study 5-5. Critical access hospital CCI edits.

Coding and billing staff at a rural critical access hospital (CAH) recognize that CCI edits and use of the -59 modifier do not apply to them. However, the need to code correctly is of concern and a policy decision has been made to obtain a CCI editor and check claims for any CCI edit violations and adjust coding accordingly. This policy decision is based on the need for complete, accurate, quality coding.

CAHs, under Medicare, are cost-based reimbursed. Thus, surgical coding does not directly drive the payment process. Charges are required and adjudicable claims must be generated through a non-OPPS claims editor. Correct coding is still an issue because auditors may review cases and assert that the claims were incorrect, even though no payment increase was involved.

Case study 5-6. Utilization review use of Condition Code 44.

Apex Medical Center has difficulties with one-day inpatient stays. Patients are frequently admitted in the late morning or early afternoon and then discharged the next morning. A review indicates many of these patients should have been treated as observation cases because of the short duration of services. A policy decision was made to have utilization review see any patient admitted to the hospital by the end of the morning of the second day of service. Thus a procedure is established whereby a UR nurse will assess patients before discharge to determine whether their cases should be switched to observation using Condition Code 44.

Case study 5-6 illustrates that policies and procedures may be required in associated areas such as utilization review and/or quality assurance. The policies and procedures can then be dovetailed and/or cross-referenced to any associated coding, billing, and chargemaster policies and procedures. Our final case study in this section illustrates developing policies and procedures for the coding, billing, and reimbursement compliance areas.

Case study 5-7. Routine CBR audit and review listing.

Apex Medical Center is developing a list of routine periodic audits and reviews that should be conducted. Some of these will be internal projects and others will use outside consultants from an independent review organization (IRO). Due consideration is being given to annual inpatient and outpatient coding reviews concentrating on Medicare DRGs and APCs, respectively. Several ongoing issues from recent OIG work plans are also under consideration including those addressing one-day inpatient stays, three-day stays prior to skilled nursing facility admissions, observation stays, and emergency department coding and billing.

Obviously, the discussion in Case study 5-7 may be extended to other audits and reviews. The challenge in CBR auditing is paring down the list of all possible issues and/or potential problem areas. Most healthcare organizations do not have the budgets or resources to review every possible compliance concern. However, projects that are chosen, particularly those that are performed periodically, should be established as written policies and procedures. The results of these types of audits should be carefully documented to establish the organizational intent to monitor compliance issues.

Key learning area : A number of different areas require policy and procedure development as part of a CBR compliance program. They include:

Coding
Billing
Chargemaster
CBR compliance review and auditing
Utilization review
Quality assurance and outcome management

Developing CBR compliance manuals

A significant part management of CBR compliance manuals relates to development, maintenance, and implementation of policies and procedures. CBR compliance includes other activities such as:

- Infrastructure for CBR compliance process
- Auditing processes and methodologies for different areas of concern
- Prospective compliance checking and analysis including computer-based tools
- Retrospective compliance checking and analysis including computer-based tools
- Baseline compliance auditing activities
- Documentation of CBR-related activities including training, education, audit activity results, policy, and procedure development
- Patient complaints, employee reporting, and/or compliance hotline activities including resolution
- Disciplinary and/or remedial actions taken relative to CBR compliance issues

CBR compliance manuals should carefully document handling of CBR compliance activities. In a healthcare organization such as a small hospital or clinic, the CBR compliance activities will probably be addressed by a single individual and thus continuity and consistency lie in the hands of that individual. Likewise, the interface of the CBR compliance program with the corporate compliance program is typically straightforward because the CBR compliance person may well serve as the corporate compliance person. The same applies if corporate compliance personnel and CBR compliance personnel form a close-knit team.

Large healthcare organizations such as systems of hospitals and IDSs require distinct organizational structures in which several designated individuals address different areas. In these situations, the structure and the job functions involved must be carefully documented. The documentation must include details about reporting relationships, credentials and qualifications, and more. The relationship of the CBR compliance program to the corporate compliance program must also be clearly defined. In most larger settings, the chief compliance officer will not be a CBR expert. In such cases, the reporting relationships and the ways in which individuals and departments communicate become important.

As suggested, teams may be required to handle various compliance projects. Information about these teams (or in some cases committees) must be documented and minutes of meetings should be prepared and retained. Documentation of problems resolved, actions taken, training provided, and policies and

procedures developed should also be maintained. Because of potential legal issues that can impact CBR compliance issues, documentation should be suitable for presentation to a judge.

Computer technology presents challenges and serves as an aid for CBR compliance personnel. On the one hand, the computer billing system or network of systems often creates compliance problems through the claims generation process. However, computer technology can provide a significant means of monitoring and checking various CBR issues and how they are addressed. The best way to make certain that a claim is correct and meets compliance criteria is to be proactive and check it before it is sent. Proactively addressing the vast number of issues involved in CBR compliance can lead to programming changes and/or prompt the adoption and use of front-end and back-end computer systems to aid the main accounts receivable system.

Retrospective reviews using information and special reports from the billing system can also be of significant value. Carefully constructed reports can be invaluable in determining a sample population to audit or review a particular situation. Most CBR compliance personnel are not versed in reporting or report generation. Thus, a good working relationship with information system personnel is of real value.

If you want to review emergency department services that involved fracture care, you can probably generate a report to look for CPT codes covering fracture care, but how will you look for a patient who had a fracture if the record contains no CPT code indicating fracture care? The answer is to generate a report based on diagnosis of fractures but includes no fracture care CPT code. This is only preliminary because a patient may have been diagnosed with a fracture but only a temporary measure such as splint or strapping may have been provided. However, using this type of logical construct that plays diagnosis codes against procedure codes can generate interesting sample populations for review.

Key learning area: Computer technology is a valuable tool for implementation of solutions, both prospective and retrospective. The use of computer systems should be carefully documented and included as part of the CBR compliance program.

The development of policies and procedures intertwines with baseline compliance audit activities that can be covered as a separate section within a CBR compliance manual or constitute part of a larger baseline compliance audit process. (See Chapter 9 for further discussion of baseline compliance audits.) Whatever the case, it is important to document the activities, problems identified, and actions taken, including development of CBR policies and procedures.

Patient complaints can lead to concerns in the CBR compliance area. While many complaints stem from a lack of understanding of the CBR process, patient concerns and complaints must be given proper attention because they can trigger audits if they are made to the Medicare FI or carrier or even the OIG. Thus policies and procedures that cover investigation and resolution of such complaints should be included in the CBR compliance manual or contained in a separate manual for the patient accounting area.

Activities and processes detailed in a corporate compliance program will also filter into CBR compliance activities, for example, a hotline number for employees to report concerns anonymously and mechanisms for employees to voice concerns and/or make suggestions about improving compliance. While these mechanisms are usually handled at corporate level, the CBR compliance apparatus should document all fact-based problems and complaints along with changes that address or resolve them. In addition, any disciplinary action taken relative to CBR compliance problems should be documented.

Special publishing of policies and procedures

The basic format for developing CBR policies and procedures is in writing. Distribution, however, can be accomplished in a number of ways, typically in connection with special training and educational activities. Policies and procedures necessary for implementation of CBR compliance solutions should be retained as a formal part of documentation of the organization. This is particularly true for establishing evidence of an organization's good faith endeavors to address compliance concerns, both proactively and reactively. Because policies and procedures may be updated frequently, an organization must establish a system to ensure timeliness relative to updating and implementation processes.

For compliance purposes, old policies and procedures should be kept on file so that the change process can be documented historically. Investigations by the OIG or federal attorneys may relate to cases and situations that arose seven to ten years earlier. An organization may be in compliance today, but was it in compliance six years ago? Can you regenerate claims produced six years ago? Does your organization archive the chargemaster on a monthly basis? Do you have access to fee or charge structures from the past seven to ten years?

With the growth of healthcare provider organizations and the commensurate rapid rate of change in the coding, billing, reimbursement, and documentation areas, it is appropriate to use all available technology for publishing and distributing these documents. Simple reproduction, facsimile, and/or electronic mail can transmit basic documents. Other electronic formats allow retrieval, even from remote locations.

Because healthcare organizations are increasingly integrated and geographically dispersed, some form of networking for information dissemination and retrieval is appropriate. For many organizations, the solution to the dissemination challenge is to use what is known as an intranet, a process of using standard Internet technologies [browsers,* file transfer protocol (FTP), or transmission control program/internet protocol (TCP/IP) to set up a network on a controlled basis]. Only those authorized or physically connected to the network can access documents that can be retrieved, reviewed, and/or printed as needed. As appropriate, electronic mail can be used to alert selected personnel as policies or procedures are issued or updated.

A number of decisions must be made as to how the documents will be formatted and made available on an organization's intranet. The main formats are:

- Standard word processing
- HTML (hypertext markup language)
- PDF (portable document format)
- XML (extensible markup language)
- SGML (standard generalized markup language)

These documents can also be formatted in the most standard generic format available: plain ASCII† text. The standard word processing approach is probably the easiest if an organization has an internal standard for word processing and other office-based software. HTML allows personnel to retrieve the documents from the intranet and then simply print them through the browser. PDF is an increasingly popular format for document interchange. PDF documents require the use of the Adobe Acrobat Reader or an equivalent for reading and printing documents. PDF is the format of choice increasingly used by government agencies to distribute documents such as the *Federal Register*, OIG fraud alerts, and OIG advisory opinions. One disadvantage of the PDF format is that making changes to documents is difficult unless you go back to the base document and regenerate the base document as a new PDF file.

---

* The dominant browser in the Windows environment is Microsoft Internet Explorer although there are alternatives.
† ASCII = American Standard Code Information Interchange.

XML and SGML are advanced formats typically used in large organizations that employ dedicated personnel to develop and maintain archives of information. See your information processing personnel if you need information or guidance about these techniques. Regardless of the technology used to store and disseminate policies and procedures, remember that the urgency is getting the right information to the right people at the right time.

Key learning area: Computer technology provides innovative ways to publish and distribute documents, including policies and procedures for CBR compliance. Use any technology that enhances the dissemination and access to CBR policies and procedures.

Summary and conclusion

A significant amount of time and effort will surround the development of written policies and procedures and a CBR compliance manual or manuals. While the form, format, and process for development and implementation of CBR policies and procedures will vary based on the type and size of the healthcare organization, the function of these policies and procedures is to effect changes in the CBR process and to show that the organization is committed to and has taken the necessary steps to ensure compliance. A compliance manual and/or associated policies and procedures will also vary depending on the interface of the compliance program to the corporate compliance program.

six

Implementing changes

Introduction

The implementation stage within the overall systems process is the culmination of a great deal of work and preparation. Changes made to the organization structure and within the organization can be minor or extensive. Regardless of the extent of change, careful consideration must be given to how change will be implemented and what impacts it may impose on affected areas. As with many aspects of organizational change, how the change is made is often more important than the change itself. Be prepared for unexpected impacts, particularly if a complicated process or procedure is the subject of the change. While we tend to concentrate on the technical issues within the solution design, human and behavioral elements also must be considered.

Analyzing change impact

A careful analysis should be made of how the change will affect an organization's structures, processes, personnel attitudes, computer systems, and so forth. The number of potential impacts can be significant. A relatively simple example easily illustrates this point.

Case study 6-1. Simple chargemaster code change. Under the Medicare program, the classification of a CPT code was changed from active to "bundled." Apex Medical Center decided to remove this code from the chargemaster for Medicare but retain the code and associated charge for other third-party payers. Apex CBR personnel had to examine the interface between the chargemaster and billing system to ensure that the line item associated with this charge (primary or secondary) would indeed be billed only for non-Medicare patients. This meant that the impact on the billing computer system including possible programming changes had to be carefully assessed.

The service area to which the code applied was contacted and a meeting was held to discuss the situation, the change required, and the reason for the change. The department manager was concerned that this change would decrease revenue generation and thus affect the department's budget. Under normal circumstances, the charge for the deleted item would be prorated among other services in the department. Because the code was eliminated for only one third-party payer, the decision was made to adjust the budget. The financial department was contacted to see how the budget for the department could be adjusted so that the impact of change would be minimal. The financial department agreed to perform an analysis of how revenue generation (charges) would be affected and to make an internal adjustment to the budgeting process.

The next thing to be discussed was the question of changing charge slips. Because this code would be used for most third-party payers, no change of the form was needed. The charge would continue to be checked off, but the billing system would simply not include it on itemized statement or on UB-04s. Because charge entry procedures did not change, no special training was required for personnel.

Even a simple change such as the one described in this example will affect a number of different interfaces. Consider the list of those mentioned in Case study 6-1:

1. Chargemaster
2. Billing system
3. Budget generation
4. Charging interface

Case study 6-2. Clinic billing system. Apex Medical Center purchased the Acme Medical Clinic two years ago. No significant changes were made other than having the clinic administered by hospital personnel and bringing Acme employees under the hospital's umbrella. Organizationally, Acme was left as a free-standing clinic filing claims only on 1500 forms. Acme's billing system had not been changed since it was developed and was optimized for physician billing, use of modifiers, and proper generation of reports.

Apex Medical Center decided to reorganize the clinic so that it would become provider-based. Because the clinic's billing system had to be significantly updated and better meet the need for an integrated billing system between the hospital and the clinic for compliance purposes, the decision was made to move the clinic billing process onto the hospital's mainframe billing system via remote terminals and printers at the clinic.

The hospital's information technology department was directed to conduct an analysis of the required changes for the mainframe computer system to accommodate the integration. They also noted anticipated software changes and a need to set up the remote devices and/or appropriate network.

Meetings were held with clinic personnel concerning the changes. While the changes were to be as transparent as possible, they would involve new software and hardware. Safeguards would be included to ensure that the new system would generate the physicians' 1500 claims properly, that all current reports could be replicated on the new system, and no degradation would occur in service or response time. Another decision was to electronically transfer all current data (fee schedules, reimbursement schedules, appointment scheduling, and historical data for two years) to the new system. Due to the sensitive nature of the clinic's computer system, the two systems were to run in parallel for at least one month and possibly two to ensure a smooth transition. Training preceding the conversion was scheduled for clinical personnel.

During discussions relative to transferring the physicians' fee schedule to the hospital's mainframe, it was realized that the fee schedule would now become a part of the chargemaster, and the chargemaster coordinator was consulted about the proposed changes. She expressed concern that the fee schedule might need to be changed to correlate with other employed physicians' fee schedules. Because the clinic would now be provider-based, a new fee schedule for facility charges would also have to be developed. Additionally, clinic personnel would now be entering charges for both professional and technical components and the reimbursement schedules required modification at least for Medicare because its site-of-service differential reduction would affect certain codes.

The HIPAA security and transaction standard requirements also had to be addressed. The clinic's billing system was not previously networked with the hospital's mainframe. The changes would require significant networking and remote access from the clinic to the hospital's mainframe computer. Thus, a number of changes would be necessary to ensure compliance with HIPAA concerns.

The discussion related to the numerous issues described in Case study 6-2 could continue at some length. The process of assessing impacts and developing project plans for changes of this type can become quite involved; in many cases, they will mushroom as more changes and associated impacts are recognized.

Case study 6-3. Emergency department coding and billing. Due to an increasing number of denials for services provided in its emergency room, Apex Medical Center decided to institute a three-tiered system for coding and billing for services:

- True emergencies
- Urgent care
- Clinic level services

Recognizing that all patients presenting to the emergency room would receive a medical screening for EMTALA purposes, the emergency physicians made a commitment to go ahead and care for all of the patients presenting, regardless of the reasons—whether true emergencies or not.

The chargemaster must be completely revised to accommodate the three different levels of technical, facilities and professional physician charges. Thus, six different chargemaster sections must be developed, and new revenue codes such as 0451 (EMTALA emergency medical screening services), 0452 (ER beyond EMTALA screening), and 0456 (urgent care) must be put into place. During the design of the chargemaster sections, a number of questions concerning coding and use of modifiers arise. As a result, representatives from health information management and patient accounting are called to form a team to analyze the situation, assess the changes required, and revise the necessary flows.

It is also obvious that encounter forms for professional services and charge slips for technical services will be significantly affected. To offset the impact, three sets of forms and slips and one pair of encounter forms and charge slips will be developed for each of the three levels of services. A color-coding scheme is developed. The new encounter form and charge slip designs will be reviewed by a team composed of personnel from the emergency department, health information management, patient accounting, and information systems.

Patient accounting and the chief financial officer are concerned about potential financial impacts. An analysis of impacts relative to the major third-party payers has been conducted. Surprisingly, because of the high rate of denial (particularly for facility charges), it is projected that revenues will actually rise with the new system in place.

Another important aspect of implementation is training all personnel involved in the change. The CBR compliance personnel have already developed a number of policy statements related to the change, along with certain other policies and procedures suggested by the emergency room physicians and staff. These policies and procedures prompted modifications to emergency room care paths since non-emergency services including observation will now be provided by the emergency department. All these policies, procedures, and modifications form the bases for the training materials that will address the interface of those providing services and those handling billing and coding processes.

Another important concern is the need for patient education. To minimize the concern, brochures are to be developed for distribution to the community, letting prospective patients know about the expanded services provided at Apex Medical Center. Additionally, joint sessions are scheduled for Apex medical staff and community physicians who should be apprised of the changes.

Note: Theoretically, Case study 6-3 may be construed as a series of proactive actions by the hospital as it delineates three different types of services in the emergency department. In practice, this process is typically reactive and involves a series of steps taken to meet specific third-party payer demands relative to levels of care in the emergency department. This case study is not intended to establish any policy recommendation.

The main compliance issues addressed in this example are medical necessity and the need to eliminate false claims. Note that the number of impact areas and the activities required to address them can be extensive. This case study involved these areas and activities:

- Chargemaster
- Coding—health information management
- Charging interface—patient accounting
- Computer changes—information systems
- Emergency department physicians and personnel
- Training and education
- Quality assurance and utilization review—care paths

- Medical staff—education
- Patients—education
- Third-party payers—announcement

A careful analysis of impacts involves review of all possible interfaces throughout the entire coding, billing, and reimbursement cycle. Some aspects of this analysis are computer-based. Others involve manual systems and interfaces between subsystems and/or computer systems. Careful analysis can help prevent problems. The systematic steps suggested to address various CBR compliance problems separates the external design (what a system should look like) from the internal design (how it will work). (See Chapter 4.) These steps and the distinctions in design facilitate development of the implementation plan and the associated implementation process.

Designing implementation plan

Implementation can be a difficult process. Even with careful preparation, good design, and a thorough impact assessment, problems may still arise. In planning for implementation, the CBR compliance personnel must dynamically adjust to difficult and unanticipated situations.

While the billing system for a healthcare organization may not warrant the highest priority (this honor generally goes to the payroll system), it is near the top of the list. Thus, when making changes to the overall coding, billing, and reimbursement system, the CBR team must exercise great care in deciding what to change and how to change it. An item that appears to be a small change can suddenly develop into a major problem that results in claim rejections, denials, or reduced payments that lead to problems with accounts receivable. Large receivables or sudden growth in receivables will attract attention because of cash flow impacts. Thus, the potential impact of implementation of even the smallest changes cannot be overemphasized.

Consider the simple chargemaster change illustrated in Case study 6-1. Modify this simple example to a situation that includes changes to certain revenue codes. Such a change, for instance, may result from a decision by a certain third-party payer that the use of RCC 0490 (other ambulatory surgery) is no longer acceptable relative to interventional radiology. The third-party payer then indicates that RCC 0761 (treatment room) is not acceptable, and that RCC 0329 should be used because charges for interventional radiology are now to appear under radiology as the services are provided in radiological suites.

Note: The type of situation described in the example is often accompanied by a mandate to use revenue codes ending with 9 that designate generic "other" services. Generally, a revenue code ending with 9 should only be used when specifically requested by a third-party payer. As noted in the discussion concerning the revenue code set, this is a somewhat irregular coding requirement and is not always well defined. A simple solution would be to simply change all the facility billing for interventional radiology surgery to this revenue code. However, this may lead to rejections of claims by other third-party payers. Additionally, the interface to the cost reporting process will now also change as surgical charges are directed into a radiological area via the revenue code.

As these examples show, implementing changes can be risky. To lower the potential for risk and unanticipated problems, the implementation process should be divided into (1) pre-implementation preparation, (2) implementation, and (3) post-implementation monitoring.

Pre-implementation preparation

This stage of implementation involves activities such as documentation, computer changes, training, changes in forms, changes in order entry, and the like. Typically, those engaged in this part of the implementation planning process have the luxury of time and should use that time to perform certain aspects correctly. Training is a key element of change implementation and personnel sometimes tend to be resistant. Even those who do not resist the change may need time to understand and/or adjust to it. The time spent training personnel can provide significant benefits in the longer term.

Information system personnel have long known that organizations must devote the necessary resources to development and testing before implementation. This concept should be adopted by everyone involved in pre-implementation planning and beyond.

Implementation

Implementing solutions for the wide variety of CBR issues can vary significantly from organization to organization and even within organizations. Some changes allow little latitude in the timing of implementation. This is often the case if a healthcare organization is out of compliance and must adjust its systems and processes immediately. In extreme cases, it may even be necessary to suspend billing for certain services until the compliance issue is resolved. But even in these situations, it is important to take the time to consider which implementation strategy to use. This section describes four different approaches to implementation:

- Experimental or trial run
- Phased or sequential
- Parallel operation
- Full implementation

The experimental or trial run approach is often used when making very specific and limited changes to a billing system, e.g., changes to the chargemaster. If time and circumstances permit, this approach has significant merit since potential problems can be identified and resolved quickly and efficiently, without creating chaos in other areas. The basic idea in the claims processing area is to simply submit some claims with the changes and then monitor the results.

In more complex situations, the phased or sequential approach can be used. In some cases, this may be the only way to implement a change. Consider as an example the implementation of bundling for a window such as DRG pre-admission. This should really be done through a computer system change, possibly involving the networking of the hospital billing system with other computer systems that bill for the services from owned or operated entities.* As a starting point, it may be necessary to manually compare services from an owned or operated entity to admissions to the hospital. In time, the system can be automated so that the computer systems can check whether diagnostic or non-diagnostic services related to the principal diagnosis for admission were provided.

A parallel operation is, in a sense, an extension of the experimental or trial run, except that it is performed during a longer predetermined timeframe. Running systems in parallel is often not possible for remedying CBR compliance problems, but it works well in some situations. In Case study 6-2, for example, the new computer system for generating 1500s was run in parallel with the old system. The desired change in this example was to meet organizational requirements relative to provider-based status. Parallel operations are often used with sensitive conversions of computer systems.

The full and immediate implementation is the so-called "cold turkey" approach. The change is simply put into place. For severe compliance problems, this may be the only approach. In some cases, billing for certain services may have to be halted while a change is implemented. Billing can be resumed after implementation. A simple example of when such a process might occur during a routine claims review is the discovery of double charging. This might be the case, for instance, if an endoscopic room charge and a surgery room charge are entered for certain gastroenterology endoscopic

---

* The trigger for the DRG pre-admission window to apply for outpatient services is provision of the services by an organization owned or operated by the hospital.

procedures. This can occur if the endoscopy center cannot accommodate a case and it is moved to a surgical suite. The problem arises when both the endoscopic and surgical personnel make facility charges. In a case of this type, billing can be suspended while an internal billing arrangement is made so that the surgical personnel can charge the endoscopic center for use of the surgical suite. The endosocopic center can then bill normally and both departments maintain their revenue status.

Post-implementation monitoring

Monitoring via reviews and audits is a typical process for CBR compliance personnel, and post-implementation monitoring of a specific change or series of changes should be immediate and focused. Depending on the extent of impacts and the number of interfaces, significant monitoring can be required. In some cases, the process of assessing proper implementation will be easy. Personnel involved in the change will report problems as they occur. In other cases, it may be necessary to probe and review the changes. Whatever the case, a logical process for ensuring proper implementation should be created.

Key learning area: The implementation of CBR compliance changes can involve significant impacts and must be treated with great care. While various approaches can be chosen, pre-implementation preparation and post-implementation monitoring must be included in every implementation.

Facilitation and organizational buy-in

As discussed in the case studies above, the implementation of changes to meet various CBR compliance issues can be complex and may involve many departments. Two important functions for CBR compliance personnel are encouraging and facilitating implementation. Part of the facilitator role means using persuasive techniques. This does not mean that management at all levels should not be involved; it simply means that accomplishing goals quickly and with minimum turbulence is often easier and more effective when an informal approach is used to deal with resistance that can potentially sabotage change endeavors. Obtaining organizational buy-in can be considered at the levels of (1) administration, (2) management, and (3) workers.

The approach at each level may vary; your organization may require additional levels, particularly if it has an integrated delivery system. At administrative level, the process of compliance resides totally in the corporate compliance plan. Thus the details of various CBR compliance implementation issues will not normally be of concern. However, if significant financial or operational impacts will occur, administrative personnel may well become involved. At this level it is best to be proactive. This means alerting administrative staff in advance of situations that might cause mid-level management to react at an operational level.

It is best to include management level personnel or their direct representatives in team activities related to solution development and implementation. Whenever possible (and as much as possible), staff should be involved in team activities. However, it is not always practical to involve too many people in such activities. If the number of people becomes a concern, CBR compliance personnel in their capacity as team leaders should encourage team members to meet with their own staff or operations personnel to assess necessary changes, impacts, training requirements, and resistance concerns.

Teams come in all sizes, shapes and fulfill a variety of purposes. Some teams have designated leaders while others are self-directed. Despite these differences, all organizational teams have common characteristics, most of which reflect the organizations in which they work. The two most important aspects of the team process are the anatomy of the team and the knowledge, skills, abilities, and personal characteristics (KSAPCs) of team leaders. These concepts are addressed below.

Membership—Teams should generally be as small as possible, utilizing only the participants needed to achieve the overall purpose and objective of a project. For CBR activities, this almost always means including representatives from the departments involved in coding, billing, documentation, and reimbursement. If an organization has latitude in choosing participants, those who work best together should be selected.

Project objective—The CBR area may already have an existing team that tackles compliance-related projects as an ongoing function. This core team will probably remain fairly constant (represents of HIM, IS/IT, patient accounting, and CBR compliance) and can be integrated with other participants on an as-needed basis (e.g., laboratory personnel for addressing a laboratory compliance problem).

Organizational context—For any team to succeed in meeting project objectives, it must be committed to the team process and have organizational support. If some members of a team (particularly members in management) send substitutes to meetings instead of attending, they send a message that other projects take priority over team activities. If this occurs often enough, teamwork and team morale are compromised.

Focus—A team arrangement should focus on achieving results and working together to achieve common goals.

Systems relationships—CBR compliance can involve a number of systems and processes all the way up to the organizational level. Thus it is important to recognize all the interfaces and organizational sensitivities that exist.

Management support—As noted above, management support is critical to team success. This involves participating in meetings as needed and having an administrative mission statement that applies to the project the team is working on.

Formally or informally, CBR compliance personnel will be thrust into leadership roles, and thus must consider their capabilities as leaders, communicators, and facilitators. Consider the following list of skills and abilities that might be called upon.

Leadership—Leadership can take different forms, even from the same person, within the context of a team. In some cases, a leader must be authoritative while in others, more facilitative. Authority can mean directing (organizational authority), informing (technical authority), or confronting (consultative authority). On the facilitative side, leadership may require eliciting (drawing out thoughts), supporting (appreciating member thoughts), and releasing (creating excitement or releasing emotions).

Planning and task coordination—This is the technical aspect of team activity. As mentioned below, computer software can be helpful in this area but it cannot replace hard thought and sequencing of activities.

Goal and objective setting—If a team's goal or objective is clearly stated, the team process becomes much easier. In some instances, the objective of the team's work might change, but the goal will usually remain constant. If a goal is clearly in sight, it is much easier to reach.

Operation—This relates to the ability to effectively and efficiently run team activities. Simple ideas such as setting written agendas prior to meetings, setting time limits, distributing appropriate materials in advance, forewarning team members what they need to do before meetings, and the like are examples of good operational techniques.

Interpersonal communications—This is probably one of the most important skill areas for team leaders. The ability to effectively and patiently listen is critical. Team leaders should always remember that not only the words but also non-verbal communications and interactions play roles in communications.

Note that this brief discussion addresses the *effective individual*, but that the characteristics applied to this person can and should be translated into *effective team performance*. This translation process can be extended to the *overall enterprise*, the *integrated enterprise* (integrated healthcare delivery system), and finally, in today's world, the *internetworked organization* (see the Internet). The bibliography and CD accompanying this book contain references concerning teams, small groups, and organizational development.

Key learning area: Implementing CBR compliance solutions often requires CBR personnel to act as facilitators at different levels within an organization. A well designed team can assist with facilitation and achieving organizational acceptance of solutions.

Computer technology

In many organizations, various aspects of the coding, documentation, billing, and reimbursement process have been automated through computer technology. In some cases, the implementation of CBR compliance solutions will depend on changes to computer systems. Usually, these changes will apply to software, and most will be minor (such as revising the chargemaster to accommodate certain modifiers). Other changes will be more significant and may require programming changes.

Because of the trend toward automation, CBR compliance personnel must be familiar with all computer systems used for any work in which compliance issues or concerns exist, and must be particularly familiar with changes made to those systems. While this familiarity will primarily be at the user level—that is, changes in parameter files that drive the features of the system currently in use—but compliance personnel may also have to work closely with information technology personnel and even programming staff whenever changes are considered or implemented.

A complicating factor is a computer system may be internally maintained by a programming staff that modifies or maintains the system, but may be worked on just as often by an external vendor that develops or modifies functions or installs new ones as requested. Work with an external vendor requires a vendor support interface, typically through a healthcare organization's information system personnel. If a vendor makes changes or modifications, it is extremely important for the organization and the vendor to establish liaison relationships of people who work together to effectively address the necessary system changes.

Note that computer-based billing systems may involve other interfaces such as computer-based medical records, decision support, and various front- and back-end systems. Both the capabilities of these systems and the ways in which they interface with the main billing system must be well understood.

Key learning area: CBR compliance personnel must learn all the capabilities of the various computer billing systems and become familiar with all interface systems. Additionally, appropriate liaisons with information systems personnel must be developed and maintained.

Project planning skills and software

CBR compliance personnel often address complex situations that require a great deal of thought and careful planning, and computers are directly affected by and also affect various CBR compliance situations. Computers can also be extremely useful tools for planning and monitoring implementation processes. For larger projects, the need to carefully map and track who is doing what, when it should be done, how to know when it is done along with the resources utilized is imperative. Computer software can keep such data organized and manageable. It can also help in the planning process where a particularly implementation may involve multiple phases.

For all these reasons, an investment in project planning software is most appropriate. Keep in mind that the actual cost of the software and its implementation representation only a fraction of the real cost that often takes the form of personal commitments required on the part of users to learn all the ins and outs of the software, how to print charts, and how to keep the system updated as the project implementation proceeds.

Consultants

Implementation of some solutions to CBR compliance problems may require the use of outside resources. At the implementation level, resources most often are consultants rather than legal counsel. Legal counsel will generally be involved in formulating solutions, not in their implementation.

Many areas of an organization can benefit from the expertise a consultant can provide and a healthcare organization may choose to consult someone outside for a number of reasons, one of which is employee resistance to change. Because the implementation of CBR compliance solutions may be questioned or actively resisted by employees and others directly involved, it may simply be easier and less inflammatory if the bearer of what is perceived as bad news is someone outside the organization. This is not much different from the strategy of using consultants to gain organizational leverage for organizational buy-in with respect to recognizing problems and properly addressing them.

Note also that training is a key element in the implementation of many CBR compliance solutions. In many instances, CBR compliance personnel, with assistance from the training and education department can effectively address training, but in some cases, a skilled and knowledgeable instructor from another organization, i.e., a consultant, may be more effective. A consultant can often help develop training materials and provide the training. He or she might even develop multimedia or videotape training for use throughout the organization and thus eliminate the need for a trainer.

Organization information flows

CBR compliance solution implementation should always include careful consideration of the ways information flows through an organization. Assuming that healthcare personnel are honest and that false claims are caused by mistakes rather than deliberate fraud, a problem might be traced easily to not having the right information at the right time in the right place. Because errors are often caused by information gaps, it is critical that the organizational information flow path be accessible to people who need it. This path should be easy to follow, but sophisticated enough to store, update, and disseminate information of varying complexity and depth. It should also have interface capabilities that allow cross-departmental access if and when needed.

Case study 6-3 above shows that in making major changes in the way in which emergency department charges are managed, one critical element is the ability to distinguish the different levels of services (true emergencies versus urgent care versus clinic care). This process is subjective, but over time, the system can be refined by information gleaned from internal reviews, external reviews, and/or reimbursement denials. As the process is refined, it is critical to have informational feedback mechanisms to inform those involved about what is being learned. This may even involve additional training sessions or discussion groups addressing special cases.

Key learning area: No implementation of a CBR compliance solution is static. Ongoing dynamics require feedback loops and information flows to keep all those involved updated about changes and progress made toward addressing any situation that may arise.

Summary and conclusion

The implementation of CBR compliance solutions can range from simple and mundane tasks to major projects involving significant parts of an organization.

No matter how small or big, the key word is *change*. Whenever change is introduced into an organization or its processes, reactions will occur. Thus the planning of any implementation must assess the impacts: who will be affected, what processes will be affected, and whether a change is only internal or will create external effects as well. The process for implementation must also be considered. Certain critical behaviors must change immediately; others can be phased in over time. The need to plan the overall implementation may require the use of teams and/or external consultants. For complex implementations, project management software may also be appropriate.

seven

Developing effective training

Introduction

Training is a key element in the development and implementation of CBR compliance initiatives and it can be delivered in a number of ways with a number of techniques. Various levels of personnel must be trained, and multiple languages may need to be employed. Specially educated training personnel can serve as valuable resources in developing and presenting effective training programs. CBR compliance personnel should consult training personnel at their healthcare organizations for further guidance.

Learning modalities

Training personnel recognize that people learn in a variety of ways. The most common learning styles are (1) visual, (2) auditory, and (3) kinesthetic.* Visual learners must see material presented; they respond well to charts, graphs, pictures, and a host of other visual materials and techniques (television, multi-media, etc.). Auditory learners must hear the material. They respond well to the spoken word and audio tapes. Kinesthetic learners need to feel what is presented. The kinesthetic learning mode is challenging to trainers on two levels: how can trainees learn by feeling and how can I teach kinesthetically when most of the information relative to compliance has no physical form? One way to reach kinesthetic learners is to have them write material presented in oral form. The delivery is auditory (the students must listen), but writing is a tactile activity and becomes a form of kinesthetic learning.

It is important to note here that most people learn best when instructors use all three approaches: If people see it and hear it and feel it, they are more likely to learn it. These three modalities can be appreciated in the following statement attributed to Confucius:

What I hear, I forget.
What I see, I remember.
What I do, I understand.

Silberman, in his book *Active Learning: 101 Strategies to Teach Any Subject*,† extended this principle:

What I hear and see, I remember a little.
What I hear, see, and ask questions about or discuss with someone else, I begin to understand.
What I hear, see, discuss, and do, I acquire knowledge and skill.
What I teach to another, I master.

Both statements emphasize the three learning modalities: Visual, auditory, and kinesthetic. Silberman's statement also reveals an interesting aspect of the learning and teaching relationship—that one of the very best ways to learn is to teach. An instructor who can develop materials (visual), present them (auditory), and involve participants (kinesthetics) will learn new things about the material taught and will also learn how to be a better teacher.

Another way to approach training is to separate knowledge development from skills development. Much of the work in compliance relies on knowledge development. The way various coding systems are used requires extensive knowledge of the development and proper use of coding systems. It may also be necessary to train personnel to use a computer system effectively. That, in turn, affects the compliance stance of a healthcare organization. While knowledge development may depend more on the visual and auditory, skills development almost always requires a degree of kinesthetic involvement. CBR compliance personnel should take every opportunity to use a multimodality approach in compliance training.

Key learning area: CBR compliance training personnel should carefully design training materials to meet the needs of a variety of learning styles with emphasis on the three main learning modalities: visual, auditory, and kinesthetic.

Training techniques and modes of delivery

Training can vary from a very simple meeting to a full-blown training curriculum involving facilitators using

---

* Two other sensory systems, olfactory (smell) and gustatory (taste), can be involved in training and education or interpersonal communication in general. Because they are atypical and seldom used in this context, these modalities are not included in our discussions.

† See bibliography.

multimedia materials in multiple locations. Several different techniques will be discussed. The choice of a given technique or even combination of techniques depends on various criteria including cost and effectiveness.

Technology

A wide range of technology can be used for training and education. A simple lecture without notes, visuals, or other materials is probably the oldest approach, but it takes no advantage of available technology. No matter what kind of training is presented, written material should always be distributed. This allows participants to read and see the materials as they are presented. Having participants take notes may further enhance the learning process.

Visual technology includes overhead projectors, slide projectors, and laptop computers with special projectors. Using a sequential set of visuals is a relatively inexpensive approach and can be very effective. Multimedia approaches include various combinations of videotapes, audiotapes, written materials, and computer-based animation. Computer-based materials make it possible to provide an ongoing stream of information through the Internet or an intranet.

Self-paced, self-study materials can be provided in a variety of formats, from reading materials with questions and answers to audiotapes and videotapes to Internet sources that can be easily accessed through a Web browser.

Lecture–recitation

This is a very basic technique that instructors can enhance by using overhead transparencies, slides, and other technology. If a lecture is part of a self-paced training component or directed at remote learners beyond a traditional classroom setting, presenters or facilitators may find video teleconferencing extremely effective.

Developing training materials

The materials and the modes of presentation are the basics of a training program. Some programs, depending on whether the training is general or highly specific relating to a given problem, may also be integrated into an overall curriculum. A good example of specific training is having technicians explain whether a radiological examination requires an anatomical modifier when the service is logged into an order entry system. A general training need is the OIG compliance suggestion that healthcare organizations provide general ethics training relative to compliance.

Key learning area: No matter what modes or techniques are used for compliance training, it should always include hand-outs, a workbook, and/or other documentation. Attendees should always receive written materials.

The process for developing the training program can be divided into several different factors using a modified form of the systems approach. Keep in mind that the overall objective of training is to change behavior: Personnel need to change the way they work or a process in which they are engaged must be changed. The recommended breakdown of factors includes:

- Need
- Behavior
- Content
- Method

A simple example of how these four steps translate into a training sequence is presented below:

- Need → Have proper modifiers placed on radiology CPT codes.
- Behavior → Order entry personnel must determine anatomic site and whether a specific modifier applies.
- Content → Policies, rules, and regulations require the use of modifiers along with the technical skills for inputting information into the computer along with the chargemaster and documentation interfaces.
- Method → Real-time training sessions with a lecture portion, hands-on computer demonstration, and practice using actual sample cases.

The training materials should be appropriate for the content. A general training session on ethics and ethical behavior may, for example, involve viewing a videotape with case studies and then having a facilitator lead a discussion on the material viewed and its implications for training participants. Specific billing training may be much more focused on processes and changes in processing and thus may involve practicing at a computer terminal or understanding a charge capture change through the chargemaster.

Most formal educational programs require lesson plans, stated objectives, explanations of methods of presentation, and so forth. The most basic tenets to follow in CBR compliance training are:

- *Tell* the participants what you are going to *tell* them.
- *Tell* them.
- *Tell* them what you *told* them!

This may sound redundant (and it is), but part of the teaching process is to make certain that required material is learned, and this can rarely happen if material is presented only once. The real challenge in conforming to this important tenet is to find a way to repeat things without being boring. One way to do this is to approach a concept from different perspectives. Teaching involves the ability to make certain that a principle or technique is learned and that behavior will change. This occurs through repetition but only if the learners remain involved and engaged.

Training materials may be highly detailed or loosely structured in outline form that may be supplemented with supporting detailed material. When presenting complex material, it may be appropriate to have participants take notes or make drawings to reinforce what is learned kinesthetically. If the material taught involves computers and/or keyboards, participants should perform the required steps rather than take notes as someone else performs the action. This again reinforces the kinesthetic aspect of the learning process.

Developing and assessing training for specific audiences

The old adage "know your audience" may have arisen from compliance training. The objective is to achieve a particular outcome or behavior, and achieving this objective means a trainer must know his or her target audience, what the target audience needs to know, and how the target audience learns best.

Healthcare organizations employ a broad spectrum of personnel who must be trained in different areas of compliance. Additionally, these people may be widely dispersed, and this may require different modes of training such as on-site lecture/recitation or self-paced individual studies through the Internet.

Personnel types do not fall into simple or clear-cut learning categories. Each group must be considered individually. The best approach is to analyze the target audience relative to the three modalities of learning discussed above. Keep in mind that any person can and will learn in all three modalities but a group may learn best in a primary learning mode. For example, physicians as a group tend to be highly visual. Thus the material used for presentations to physicians should include color charts, graphs, pictures, and the like. Other staff members may learn better by listening or doing.

Logistics

The logistics associated with training and education activities may be neglected. The overall ambiance of a training location is important. Some compliance training and education can be provided in a classroom setting. Other training may need to be accomplished in a work setting, particularly if it involves the use of computer-based systems and/or software. Training personnel should be sensitive to the environment. Proper space, appropriate privacy level, freedom from interruptions, food and beverages, lighting, temperature, and ventilation are all important environmental and comfort factors that can make a session run smoothly and aid learning.

CBR compliance training for the most part is technical. In some cases, particularly with coding activities, trainees will have a need to spread out and peruse reference manuals and guidelines and even use laptop computers. Some training will involve the use of a computer system, thus requiring a computer lab. If at all possible, the training should take place away from the normal work environment to reduce interruptions. Pagers and cellular phones should be turned off or left at the door!

Attention span is another factor to consider. Long training sessions, even with breaks, may prove ineffective. Because compliance training is so critical, it may be best to have several short sessions rather than a single long session.

Note also that most healthcare organizations have staff that work various shifts every day of the week. To accommodate these individuals and their schedules, special off-hour sessions and even week-end sessions may have to be scheduled.

Note: Some of the training provided in conjunction with CBR compliance may involve personnel who are not employees such as physicians who are on the medical staff but not otherwise associated with a hospital. Providing training and associated amenities such as food and snacks with no charge to participants should be reviewed for compliance appropriateness.

Keep in mind that most compliance training is mandatory. For this reason alone, every training program should be a rewarding experience for participants. Where possible, consider the possibility of making CBR compliance training part of a continuing education package and having training sessions qualify for continuing education units (CEUs).

Training at different levels and in different languages

Compliance training in the coding, billing, documentation, and reimbursement area is likely to involve personnel with varied backgrounds, education levels, professional and technical credentials, and learning styles. Some may speak multiple languages; others will have varying levels of English language proficiency. All these factors must be taken into account when designing compliance training. Care must be taken to craft policies and procedures in a language format appropriate to the level of participants' education and language skills. Depending on the geographic location and demographics of the organization, it may be necessary to provide the training in different languages.

Training trainers

Much of this chapter provides guidance on how to train. This section addresses an often neglected part of the training process—how to learn to train. While it would be wonderful to have a professional trainer provide the training (and in some cases this may be the best answer), the level of technical knowledge necessary to provide training may limit or preclude the use of professional trainers. Thus it is necessary for CBR compliance personnel to learn presentation techniques and also learn how to design training sessions. Obviously, a complete discussion of this process lies well outside the scope of this book, but a few important points must be made.

Training personnel are accustomed to the dual nature of training. One major component of this purpose is transmitting factual information on procedures, processes, policies, and the like. A smaller, but perhaps equally important component, is behavior modification. This process involves taking training a step further by integrating the information with actions and activities performed by the individuals involved. This transition from theory to practice is one reason for emphasizing the three main modalities of learning (visual, auditory, and kinesthetic). Achieving behavior modification depends on truly integrating the information on the processes and procedures with what participants do.

Those providing training must be fully cognizant that the words spoken in verbal communications are often one dimensional. Intraverbal and non-verbal communications are often more powerful than words. Intraverbal communication involves volume, tonality, and pace. Non-verbal communication involves gestures, facial expressions, and movements. Training personnel must be attuned to these communication modes as they can enhance or diminish a presentation and also influence attitudes about the importance of a training session.

A trainer's credibility can also be an issue. Credibility derives from his or her expertise or knowledge base. Sometimes, credibility is related to authority, especially if the trainer is an outside facilitator and is not a member of the organizational authority hierarchy.

At other times, a trainer may be someone who would ordinarily be viewed as a "lesser mortal" in the health-care personnel hierarchy. To be effective, trainers must establish credibility with the participants. Sometimes this is a question of nuance—letting participants know in a subtle way who is in charge. While it is important to keep presentations interesting and informative, it may be best in some cases to skip light introductory comments and go directly to the core information to be presented.

Consider the process of training physicians who may be employees of the organization or simply may be associated with the organization through the medical staff. It is vital to establish credibility very quickly with physicians and other highly trained professionals by going directly into the training material. As previously noted, physicians tend to be visually oriented. Thus graphs, pictures, and charts are appropriate. Moreover, most physicians have been trained to make decisions quickly so establishing credibility must be a priority: The sooner they see that the trainer is credible, the better their responses to the trainer and the training will be.

Note: On the specific issue of a hospital's ability to direct physicians who are simply on the medical staff is interesting from CMS's view. In the April 7, 2000 *Federal Register* CMS indicated that hospitals were responsible for correct coding by physicians of the place of service (POS) entries on 1500 claim forms relative to provider-based clinics. This hospital responsibility was established from CMS's perspective on the basis that a physician is on the medical staff of a hospital (65 FR 18519).

Learning objectives

The training objective relative to coding, billing, documentation, and reimbursement compliance issues is to change behavior. This addresses what is called ***behavioral learning*** and involves the development of knowledge and competencies relative to procedures, operations, methods, techniques, processes, and the like. Although this is the main objective, trainers also need to address attitudes, feelings, emotions, and values. This is referred to as ***affective learning***. While some affective training (such as ethics training) is designed for the corporate compliance level, affective learning components should also be included in CBR compliance training. While the training may emphasize behavior modification, it should also include materials and techniques that communicate appropriate values and attitudes. Case studies and/or scenarios can be very useful teaching tools in this area.

Cognitive learning involves the acquisition of concepts and information to the point where cognition occurs and the information can be used to analyze organizational situations and processes in a work setting. Healthcare organizations often face complex coding, billing, and reimbursement issues, both directly with the relevant processes and also with the organizational structuring of healthcare provision. For example, it is not enough to train personnel to accept the fact the hospitals cannot provide free rent to physicians or bill Medicare for self-administrable drugs. Personnel must also understand the Medicare Fraud, Abuse, and Anti-Kickback Laws and the concepts of non-covered services, drugs, and supplies. They must then be able to apply this fully understood information to related situations.

Meta learning takes the concept of cognitive learning a step further by providing personnel with the tools needed to more effectively apply what is learned cognitively. For example, effective development of and participation in team efforts is very important. Since the various CBR processes typically cross departmental boundaries, the use of teams becomes essential for fully analyzing the processes. Problem-solving techniques and creativity in general should also be tied to meta training. These areas are often addressed in management training and should be carefully extended to more specialized CBR compliance training.

Tips for effective training

This section will focus on some of the most important training techniques and provide a few pointers. As previously noted, CBR compliance personnel are often not trained as trainers; they are often chosen to train because they have the technical knowledge bases to teach others about CBR processes and associated compliance issues.

Team teaching

Unless you have skilled training personnel, it is best to have several presenters or use a single presenter who can draw on experts in specific fields or departments to supplement the material presented, answer complex questions, or simply provide relief if a session is especially long and arduous.* Additionally, it is wise to have someone observe the training and/or record questions and associated discussions.

---

* Appropriate physical conditioning and proper pacing are requirements for long and arduous training sessions.

Preparation

It is important to be well prepared with hand-out materials, visual aids, a good opening, and key points that emphasize the most important content of the presentation. In an organizational setting, timing can be important. While some tangential issues may be pertinent or amusing, keep on track and cover the materials that correspond to the overall objectives of the training session.

Interpersonal communications

The attitude of an instructor is fully communicated by non-verbal behavior or body language. An instructor must use intraverbal communication that is suitable for the material taught and for the target audience. Voice tone, quality, and pitch are important. Similarly, eye contact with the audience and reading the audience to see whether material is understood and absorbed are essential. Watch for resistance or lack of comprehension. Stance and movement are also forceful communication devices. Non-verbal and intraverbal communications during training sessions are as important as verbal and/or written communications. The best material can quickly be eroded by an instructor who treats the training process as busy work.

Audiovisual aids

Few things are more frustrating for trainers and trainees than attending a session where audiovisual aids are ineffective. Training personnel must take the time to learn how to use audiovisual aids effectively. Flip charts and white boards are easy to use. More advanced audiovisual aids include overhead projectors, slide projectors, and/or computer projectors. Sophisticated aids include fiberoptic and satellite network productions. Even for a seasoned trainer, some of the new technology can be somewhat overwhelming. Thus training personnel should take the time to master audiovisual technology before using it.

Note that participants should always receive copies of visual aids used in a presentation. No matter how much planning takes place, it is always possible that some of the participants may not be able to see and/or hear all the material presented. Providing written materials ensures that all participants have back-up information.

Facilitating learning

CBR compliance personnel involved in providing training must go beyond teaching or explaining. Some concepts or modified processes may require what is sometimes called *explication*. This means that a trainer must move beyond teaching raw material and instill the concepts and/or procedures into the students' knowledge and behavior patterns. Simply repeating the material may not achieve this goal. Use metaphors, change the context, and look at material from a different perspective. Have the students explain what they learn in their own words.

Addressing resistance

CBR compliance training is typically mandatory. Participants must attend, learn, and certify that they have been trained and understand the processes, procedures, and principles involved. CBR compliance training tends to be specific and addresses complex billing, coding, and documentation issues. Like other students, healthcare personnel may not be eager to attend mandatory classes and often need incentives to participate in spirit, not by simply attending.

Training very often provides no guarantee of advancement in the organization and in most cases does not qualify for CEU credits. Thus, a trainer needs to find another way to motivate trainees to participate. The most typical way is to remind them of the serious nature of the training. Review the need for compliance relative to specific cases in which significant fines were levied and/or hospital personnel and/or physicians went to jail. Show the participants that if a certain procedure or process is not changed, claims might be considered fraudulent and civil monetary penalties (CMPs) of $5,000 to $10,000* per claim can be imposed. Examples of potential impacts can go a long way to help motivate employees to learn to perform correctly.

Note that negative motivation should be balanced with positive motivation. Participants should be told that changes that enhance the compliance stance of a healthcare organization often improve and increase revenue generation. Overall increases in revenue can strengthen an organization and thus enhance job security.

The best approach is to use both the stick (potential penalties) and the carrot (increased revenues) to help motivate employees to meet various compliance challenges through training.

Prerequisites for participants

One seemingly obvious point is often overlooked in training programs even though it may be the most critical component of training success. It is important to make certain that the students trained have the proper background, training, and experience to understand the material presented. At the very least, an instructor should be fully knowledgeable about the backgrounds

and abilities of the participants. Whenever possible, personnel to be trained should be separated into groups with similar backgrounds and abilities. These groupings may make the training process more effective, but this technique does place an additional burden on training personnel who must make certain that the training is consistent and that the proper objectives are achieved for every group.

Unlearning

It would be wonderful to simply walk into a training session and train personnel on the proper way to handle various CBR compliance issues. Unfortunately, the process sometimes requires a preliminary step—"unteaching" old procedures and habits that have become ingrained. This means addressing both the short-term or working memories and also the long-term memories of the personnel being trained. It also means understanding that unlearning is often more difficult than learning. The process involves repetitive techniques and approaching subjects from different perspectives.

One of the best methods for ensuring that information and behavior are unlearned is to make certain that participants know and understand why certain changes are required. If they are simply told that certain changes must take place and not given a reason, the unlearning–relearning process will take longer and be less effective. If students are told, for instance, that they must change the way modifiers are used without knowing the reason for the change, they may resist unlearning. If they are told, however, that the incorrect use of modifiers is rampant in both physician coding (1500) and facility coding (UB-04) and that this is both a compliance issue or requirement and also a reimbursement (revenue enhancing) issue, they are more likely to comply with the desired unlearning–relearning process.

Key learning area: A number of tips and tricks can be effective for training. CBR compliance personnel should carefully prepare for and think about the way in which training is to be provided.

See the bibliography for additional source material about the training process and the various techniques.

Coordinating internal and external training

Much of the discussion in this chapter has concentrated on in-house or organization-based training, but

---

* CMPs can vary, depending upon the specific law, rule, and/or regulation violated.

an organization may have a pressing need for personnel to attend external training sessions and/or conferences or to bring external training personnel into the organization. Obviously, external, off-site training for large numbers of people is prohibitively expensive. If specialized training is necessary for a significant number of people, an external trainer should be retained and brought on site.

Part of a CBR compliance training program should be directed toward CBR compliance personnel. Much of the training will need to be external in terms of workshops, conferences, and related professional activities. In some cases, these people can act as scouts by going outside the organization, obtaining the necessary information, and bringing it back to the organization for use. Activities similar to benchmarking may be appropriate and can be accomplished by having CBR compliance personnel visit other organizations to review their compliance systems, training approaches, and even training programs.

Key learning area: CBR compliance personnel along with other specialists in the coding, billing, and reimbursement areas require special training that typically can be obtained only externally through special workshops. A carefully coordinated plan should be developed to balance the internal and external training processes.

Recordkeeping

Because compliance training is an important part of both corporate compliance and more specific CBR compliance programs, it is important to maintain accurate records of all training activities, noting who attended, what was covered, and who provided the training. Copies of training materials should be catalogued and archived. It is best to have participants sign in so that attendance can be verified. Self-study and self-paced computer-based training requires an administration system and appraisal mechanisms that determine appropriate completion of a program. Sign-in sheets and a facilitator to monitor and direct activities should also be used for video conference and/or teleconference presentations.

Summary and conclusion

Training and education are critical elements for implementation of compliance programs in general, and are of even greater importance for the highly complex and detailed coding, billing, documentation, and reimbursement area. Developing training materials and presentations and conducting the training warrant high priority. Effective training is a challenge. CBR compliance personnel, because of the technicalities involved will often be thrust into training roles. Non-trainers who will have to provide training should consult the pertinent references in the bibliography. Seeking advice from other healthcare training personnel is also recommended.

eight

Monitoring and corrective action

Introduction

Monitoring CBR compliance processes involves reviews and audits. Corrective action feeds back through the systems approach to the problem identification and problem solution processes. Reviews and audits for coding, billing, documentation, and reimbursement functions can be formally designed with tight objectives and outcomes. At the other end of the spectrum are CBR review and audit activities that are informal in nature and smaller in scale. These reviews and audits involve small samplings for audits and/or informal reviews of specific situations. Monitoring activities are intended to ensure that changes put into place through compliance policies and procedures are indeed working and look for current or developing problem areas.

Note: This chapter concentrates on the mechanics of monitoring and taking corrective action. Specific review and audit areas are discussed throughout this book. See Chapters 12 through 15 for a discussion of special areas of healthcare compliance concern.

Designing reviews and audits

Expertise in designing and conducting reviews and audits is important for CBR compliance personnel. Reviewing and auditing are highly technical areas and due consideration must be given to the service area being audited or reviewed. Because of the different areas and different types of compliance concerns, CBR compliance personnel go beyond the standard approaches used by engineers. In some cases, recognizing the need for and performing an audit or review are almost art forms and require special insights.

For our purposes, the processes related to reviewing and auditing are separated into two parts, similar to the two parts of the design phase within the systems approach. The first part is the review design that addresses the *what* question; the audit design then addresses the *how* question. Note that much of the differentiation in this area relates to whether an approach is formal or informal. Formal reviews and audits involve carefully selected areas, outcomes, and samples. Informal review and audits are generally much smaller and performed on an ad hoc basis. (See the discussion of the systems approach in Chapter 1.)

Review design

The review design addresses the basic questions of what is to be reviewed and the depth and type of the review. Typical reviews in the CBR area concern:

- Documentation or charts
- Coding
- Claims and statements
- Reimbursement
- Chargemaster charges
- Charge capture
- Payment system interface
- Various combinations of these items

This list can certainly be extended. The most typical CBR reviews involve examining combinations of documentation, itemized statements, and claims filed. These three elements comprise the key parts of the reimbursement cycle. However, a more focused review may be appropriate, particularly if a specific component such as an itemized statement is questioned or concern is expressed about how supply items appear on itemized statements. This then leads back to categorization of supplies in the chargemaster.

In another instance, a new documentation system may have been implemented for better compliance, and the organization must verify the effective use of the system. A limited combination review may be made of claims relative to HIM coding overriding codes statically placed in the chargemaster.

The review design must also identify the service area and/or support area to be examined. The area can involve a specific department, such as emergency, urgent care, pain clinic, or same-day surgery. A review may also involve a support department and/or system. For instance, a new back-end editing computer system may have been put into place and may utilize a number of edits intended to serve as final checks before claims are submitted. A review may be designed to assure that certain types of claims are indeed identified and changed before they are filed.

The overall objective of a review must be clearly stated. It may be designed to address only compliance errors. On the other hand, it may intend to address all kinds of errors including compliance, payment, and general errors that affect neither payment nor compliance. In some cases, a review may be limited to a specific kind of error. For instance, an organization may have concerns about proper classification of patients as *new* versus *established* in a clinic setting. Thus a review may be designed to check and identify the frequency of incorrect assignments. This type of error may also fall into the category of errors related to proper levels of E/M coding.*

Audit design

After the scope and objectives of the review are determined, it is necessary to design the audit process. The design process depends entirely on the review objectives, and begins after the following are defined:

- Formal versus informal review
- Internal versus external review
- Objective of review
- Area or areas to be reviewed
- Type of review (compliance, payment, other)
- Review personnel and qualifications
- Special considerations

As noted above, the audit design must meet the objectives of the review. The audit may have to be designed to test or examine both a process and its end result. In some cases, only the results will be reviewed or only the systematic process may be under review. Separating the process from the end result may be difficult. For example, certain errors may be found in the course of reviewing claims. The immediate question will then shift to the process that generated the claims. Among audit design considerations are the following:

- Selection of guidelines and/or standards to be used for comparative purposes
- Computer and/or other automated aids
- Determination of size of sample to be taken and/or developed
- Selection and/or development of sample
- Process and techniques to be utilized

The guidelines or standards to be used may be complex. Auditors cannot judge the correctness of a process or end product without a metric or measuring tool. For example, coding documentation reviews and/or medical necessity reviews may depend significantly upon internal organizational standards, external standards, or even benchmarks. If someone is reviewing observation coding and charging related to medical necessity, the hospital's care paths in this area will probably

---

* For provider-based clinics, the definitions of *new* and *established* are different for professional coding relative to technical component coding.

be used as guidelines. If E/M level coding is audited, external E/M coding documentation guidelines would probably be used. If auditing is directed at the capture of charges for injections and infusions, the coding and billing policies and procedures in this area must be used.

Automated tools and special reports, particularly for retrospective reviews, should be used whenever possible. These tools can often identify aberrant cases that will lead to identification of problems to be investigated. These same tools can often be used in an auditing capacity. Likewise, the guidelines and algorithms used to develop automated tools can also be studied and modified for use in compliance audits. Computer reports that show the percentage splits of triples of associated DRG categories, for example, can point to a possible aberration. A computer report that shows the percentage split between one-day inpatient stays and one-day observation stays can also suggest possible aberrations.

Auditing processes and techniques can vary widely. An audit may simply involve a review of certain charts or claims. Obviously, these charts and claims must be pulled and matched. Audit personnel require space to do their work. While this requires coordination and scheduling, more extensive audits may involve interviewing personnel, conducting team reviews, and observing people at work. In these cases much greater attention must be given to scheduling and coordinating. Other audits such as those directed at hospital pricing through an examination of chargemaster entries and associated charge algorithms require a different process.

The selection of sample size and specifications are major issues discussed in the sections below.

Key learning area: The design of a CBR compliance audit requires careful consideration and extensive knowledge of the coding, billing, documentation, and reimbursement processes. Significant variations in design can occur based on the service area to be audited and/or the problem to be addressed. While many audits are fairly standard and involve uniform formats, audit design may advance from an engineering process to an art form in unusual or special situations.

Determining sample size

The discussion of sample size started in Chapter 4. The following discussion takes the issue a step further. For most auditing in the CBR area, the size of the universe is well known. If an audit involves the office visit E/M codes for a clinic over time, the number of encounters involving office visits is known. Similarly, when auditing hospital outpatient surgical claims, the number of surgical cases is known. Of course, any blanket statement has exceptions. If you want to identify all one-day inpatient admissions changed to observation status by the use of Condition Code 44, you may face a challenge in developing the report that will identify the sampling universe.

When picking sample sizes for a universe of known size, an extension of the formula presented in Chapter 4 is used. This formula is not especially sophisticated, but solving it requires statistical software and/or a spreadsheet with appropriate capabilities.

N_p = Size or number of cases in universe
  population
n = Size of required sample
π = Proportion of estimated errors
z = Confidence interval
E = Proportion relative to error rate

The formula for calculating the number of cases is also an extension of the formula used in Chapter 4.

$$N = N_p \left(\frac{z^2 \pi (1-\pi)}{E^2 (N_p - 1) + z^2 \pi (1-\pi)} \right)$$

We can revisit the case used in Chapter 4, but will assume the population of possible cases for review is 2000. Thus,

E = 0.05 (stated proportion relative to errors)
z = 1.960 (95% confidence level
π = 0.5 (worst case)
N_p = 2000

The sample size then becomes 322. The other variables can be adjusted for any particular case. An electronic spreadsheet or advanced calculator is needed for this calculation. This case might occur in the course of a formal audit of office visit E/M coding levels for a group of physicians over a six-month period. See the appendix for information about other sets of sample sizes.

Note: If an outside entity such as an OIG or Medicare auditing team performs an audit, the choice of the sample size may be determined in a way that allows the results of an audit of a sample to be extrapolated to the entire sample universe. This type of sample size determination requires advanced statistical analysis and must be performed with great care. See the discussion of the OIG's RAT-STATS program on the next page.

In many cases, sample size will not be determined through a statistical formula of the type discussed above. You may be performing a probe audit to find a potential problem. A probe audit generally involves a review of 30 cases, although a slightly higher number can be used for an extended audit. Also, your hospital or clinic may conduct some type of annual coding audit that may involve 150 cases or more. In this instance, the defining factor for determining sample size is the amount of time auditors are available and/or the amount budgeted for the review. With fixed sample size studies, the underlying intent is to determine problems, then define required actions.

Key learning area: Determining sample size for a formal audit requires an understanding of the statistical processes underlying the determination. While this may seem intimidating, sample size charts can simplify the process. Additionally, sample sizes for many studies in the CBR area will be defined by the resources and time available for the study.

Note: See also the discussion below of the OIG's RAT-STATS program for determining sample size.

Selecting samples

The sample size may be predetermined or may have to be developed based upon the characteristics of the sample space and the objectives of the audit or review. After sample size is determined, the next step is to select the specific cases or records to be reviewed. This process, at least for formal auditing, must be done on a random or independent basis. While an individual can develop a reasonably workable approaches to this task, it is better to use special software developed for this purpose. One such program is the OIG's RAT-STATS discussed in the next section.

The intent of this and similar programs is to generate a set of random numbers that can then be used to select the cases to be reviewed. This is significant because selecting cases in a truly random fashion is somewhat of a challenge. For instance, if a sampling of 350 cases is to be drawn from a universe of 5000, the random numbers will consist of anywhere from one to four digits (but fewer than 5000). How can we be certain that in choosing the random numbers we included appropriate numbers of each of the one-, two-, three-, and four-digit numbers? This is where the software comes into play. If the parameters are correctly set up, the numbers can be generated in a truly random fashion.

Another technique known as *stratifying* the sampling is useful in situations involving the need to subdivide a large universe into smaller pieces, and then make random selections from each stratum or piece.

For example, in conducting an inpatient audit, we may want to stratify the universe by third-party payer type. Medicare patients will undoubtedly fall into one of the strata; Blue Cross patients into another; and Medicaid patients into a third. A fourth stratum might comprise all other third-party payers. Thus, if we take as the universe all inpatient discharges over a calendar quarter, we can then generate a computer report that subdivides the cases according to the primary payers. Then, within each of the strata, we can perform our random sampling.

In some cases you may want to further subdivide a given stratum. For instance, we may decide to divide the Medicare cases into *problem DRGs* and *all other DRGs* categories and be concerned about examining a representative sampling of problem DRGs along with a random sampling of all the other DRG categories. Almost immediately, we realize that we must now identify the problem DRGs that may comprise single DRGs, pairs, triples, or even quadruples. This will cause further stratification.

For clinics, stratification by third-party payers is only one cut through a sample universe. If a clinic has five physicians and the audit is to review the five main E/M levels for established office visits, we must stratify by the individual physicians and then by the five different E/M levels. Thus, we could have these categorizations:

- By third-party payer
- By physician
- By established office visit E/M level

Stratification could mean four third-party payer categories, five physicians, and five E/M levels for a total of $4 \times 5 \times 5 = 100$ strata. What if we wanted to consider more E/M categories by including new patient visits, consultations (inpatient and outpatient), hospital visits (initial and established), and skilled nursing facility visits? These additional variables could total many hundreds of strata. Because stratification is a flexible tool that can expand random sample size to suit specific needs, it is an important aspect of meeting audit or review objectives. Note, however, that we expanded the overall random selection in a single universe to multiple random selections within all strata of that universe.

Key learning area: Designing formal and informal reviews and audits in the CBR compliance area is a technical undertaking that requires understanding of basic statistical processes and systematic audit processes.

RAT-STATS program of OIG

In the preceding sections we discussed the concepts of determining sample size and random sample selection. The sample selection process may also involve stratifying the sample space. Unless you have studied statistics, these discussions and formulas may seem esoteric and intimidating. While a mathematical discussion of these processes is certainly important, most healthcare compliance personnel including those specializing in the coding, billing, and reimbursement area will never have to use the formulas.

Commercially available programs can perform such calculations. One available at no charge is the OIG's RAT-STATS that can be downloaded in a few minutes. The associated documentation includes extensive discussion of some of the mathematical and statistical bases for the calculations made by the RAT-STATS.

Familiarize yourself with the statistical auditing software that you are going to use. This means taking time to study the documentation, understand the parameters, and experiment with the parameters to see what kind of results you obtain. For actual audits or reviews, keep copies of the reports that generate the sample size and the random sampling of cases selected. These reports will form the basis of justifying the statistical validity of the statistical selection processes included in a review or audit.

Example service area considerations

Now that we have discussed setting up the audit and selecting cases for review or audit, we can turn to specific service area concerns. What follows is a brief discussion of several representative service areas. CBR compliance personnel should take this discussion as *starting point* for developing monitoring and auditing activities in all applicable service areas. The specifics for a particular area can be developed based upon monitoring and auditing activities (focused reviews) conducted by FIs or carriers, investigations conducted by federal and state level law enforcement entities, and also internally identified problem areas. One place to start is the OIG's annual work plan.

Home health services

Home healthcare can involve a wide range of services provided in home settings. Typically, the main sorting criterion for such services is the case* that may involve a number of visits. In other words, the need for home health services may be established at the case level, while

---

* Terminology may vary.

individual services are documented through individual visits. Case study 8-1 illustrates how this works.

Case study 8-1. Home health agency audit. A home health agency has four different locations. It has decided to conduct a formal audit of each of the four agencies with a 95 percent confidence interval and a 3 percent error rate to ensure that errors relative to documentation for homebound status, medical necessity, and billing are discovered. The home health agency (HHA) which is associated with Apex Medical Center conducts a total of 32,000 visits per year, related to 1200 cases. The number of visits per case varies from a low of 5 to a high of 44 over the course of a year. Apex also wants to include a representative sampling from the three main payer sources: Medicare/Medicaid, private/self-pay, and managed care.

The strategy is to identify the number of cases by third-party payer category and then, within these cases, select an appropriate number of visits to achieve an appropriately sized sample. The suspected error rate is unknown so that a value of π will be chosen as 0.5. The overall population size is 10,000. A sample size for this population can then be determined to be 964 which is rounded to 1000. This is 10 percent of the number of visits.

The number of visits is translated into 100 cases (average number of visits per case is 10), and the cases are chosen proportionally from three third-party payers. It is recognized that on occasion the cases selected may not involve enough visits to yield the desired sample size. If necessary, additional cases will be randomly selected within a given third-party payer category. The audit will be conducted according to guidelines relative to establishment of homebound status, 60-day episodes of care based on physician orders, the content of visit documentation, and subsequent billing.

Emergency department

Hospital emergency departments provides a microcosm of both technical and professional services. Thus a number of areas should be routinely audited in connection with these services. Some of the auditing activities will be informal and based on small samplings, while others will be more formal. The emergency department provides outpatient services driven by *encounters*. A typical encounter is generally brief and the documentation and associated billing and claims filing processes must be done quickly. Nonetheless, many perspectives must be addressed:

- Coding—professional, technical, modifiers, E/M levels
- Billing and claims—correct (reflection of services), properly bundled
- Chargemaster—descriptions, revenue codes, CPT and HCPCS charges
- Documentation—complete, legible, time reporting, automation
- Care paths—documented, adherence
- EMTALA—systems, adherence
- Proper use of NPPs
- Proper billing for level of care (emergent versus urgent versus clinic)

CBR compliance personnel must determine what needs to be monitored in connection with emergency department personnel including physicians. The following audit targets are typical.

1. A formal audit of ED claims is to be conducted for the purpose of comparing the coding on 1500 (professional) and UB-04 (technical) claims. The intent of the audit is to determine the correlation (as appropriate) of:
   - CPT surgical codes
   - CPT E/M level of service codes
   - Use of modifiers
   - Diagnosis codes
2. An informal sampling of cases is to be taken to determine whether the EMTALA guidelines are met as documented in the medical records.
3. An informal sampling of ER encounters involving critical care and CPR services is to be conducted to verify proper reporting of time and exact services.
4. A formal audit is to be conducted relative to the medical necessity of services and the associated billing and claims filing process.
5. An informal sampling of the billing for self-administrable drugs is to be made to ensure that the claims filing process works appropriately.
6. A formal audit is to be conducted of fracture care coding, billing, and dispensing of crutches and canes.
7. An informal sampling of the coding and billing for infusions, injections, and associated charges for drugs.

Observation services

Observation services are provided at virtually every hospital and create compliance problems for most hospitals. Part of the problem is whether observation is a status or a location (observation bed). Other concerns involve inpatient admissions that should have been observation admissions and the related concerns about the use of Condition Code 44 on the UB-04 technical component claim form. As Case study 8-2 shows, conducting a comprehensive audit of all aspects of observation services is a major undertaking.

> **Case study 8-2. Annual observation audit.** Apex Medical Center is interested in performing a periodic informal audit of observation services. The annual statistics for observation services are kept as components of the baseline audit process and divide the services by location:
>
> - Emergency department
> - Acute care—direct admit
> - Acute care—post-surgical
> - Acute care—ED admit
> - Intensive care unit
> - Obstetrics
> - Psychiatric unit
> - Other specialty units
>
> Apex has decided to look at 5 percent of the cases but no fewer than ten from each location. The guidelines for the review will involve:
>
> - Signed physician orders
> - Medical necessity documentation through care paths for observation services
> - Correlation of physician coding to hospital coding (CPT and ICD-9-CM)
> - Level of E/M coding relative to history, examination, and decision making documentation

Notes: Patients at some hospitals may go directly to specialty areas such as obstetrics, ophthalmology, and/or psychiatric units. Under EMTALA, these areas may be subject to various rules and regulations requiring maintenance of EMTLA logs. Note also that off-campus provider-based clinics can be subject to EMTALA under certain circumstances. Physician coding and hospital coding may be different because the ED level of service for physicians must be bundled into observation E/M code; hospital coding has no such requirement.* The use of observation in obstetric services must be carefully reviewed based on a history of problems in this area. If unusual problems are

_____
* Check current coding guidelines in this area.

encountered in this informal probe, Apex will develop and pursue a more formal sampling and audit.

Medical clinics

Medical clinics can be small, single specialty practices, large multispecialty practices, free-standing independent, provider-based, and/or parts of larger integrated delivery systems. Thus, to address compliance concerns for medical clinics, significant care and consideration must be given to organizational status; this, in turn, will drive reviews and audits.

For provider-based medical clinics, the compliance concerns are similar to concerns of emergency departments but are likely to be more extensive because medical clinics deal with both technical (UB-04) and professional (1500) components, thus generating concerns about correlation of coding and use of codes and modifiers. Furthermore, a range of different specialty physicians may be involved along with billing for clinic-based laboratory and radiology services. The integration of documentation for the technical and professional components into the hospital (main provider) system is another concern.

For free-standing medical clinics, areas of focus are proper procedure coding, use of modifiers, medically necessary services, and proper generation of 1500 claim forms. While medical necessity through diagnosis coding correlation to procedure codes represents a concern for all forms of medical clinics, it is of special interest for billing because of the direct correlation of diagnosis codes to line item procedures on 1500s.

Note also that the processes for coding and billing for NPP services are different for provider-based and free-standing clinics. It is permissible for a physician or other practitioner to bill incident-to services at a free-standing clinic. A provider-based setting involves no incident-to services because the NPP's payment comes through the technical or facilities payment. NPPs who are practitioners in both settings can obtain their own provider numbers (national provider identifiers) and bill for their services. For NPPs who are not practitioners, questions arise about direct supervision (physician or practitioner on the premises) and indirect supervision (physician available by telephone). Note that a physician in a free-standing clinic may elect to bill for practitioner services on an incident-to basis and then the supervisory rules come into play.

Notes: The issues of coding and billing for non-physician providers and the non-physician practitioner subsets are very complex. If your healthcare organization employs and/or otherwise uses non-physician practitioners and/or non-physician providers who are not practitioners, special auditing and review processes should be considered. Teaching hospitals or hospitals with residency programs face a special set of concerns relative to resident utilization, documentation, and coding. For these hospitals, proper utilization of the -GE and -GC modifiers is especially important.

Issues that can be addressed through formal and informal audits or reviews in medical clinic settings include:

- E/M level coding relative to coding documentation guidelines
- Relative frequency of E/M levels relative to benchmark data by specialty
- Proper documentation relative to coding and billing for consultation services
- Use of preventive medicine codes versus use of regular therapeutic office visit codes
- Coding of all applicable services and diagnoses
- Correlation of diagnosis codes to procedures codes relative to medical necessity
- Proper use of waivers relative to services that may be considered not medically necessary
- Proper coding and use of -54 and -55 modifiers relative to Medicare's GSP
- Proper coding and use of -76 and -77 repeat procedure modifiers
- Proper coding and use of assistant at surgery for physicians and NPPs
- Review of proper coding techniques for NPPs relative to billing for incident-to services
- Proper use of -25 modifier when billing for both E/M level and surgical procedure
- Coding and billing for hospital admissions or observation admissions when services are provided on a different date
- Proper adherence to diagnosis coding guidelines relative to physician and/or outpatient diagnosis coding (e.g., not coding rule-out diagnoses, probable diagnoses, versus diagnoses and/or suspected diagnoses)
- Checking for physician indication of final diagnoses after encounter when diagnostic test results are available, and for associated coding (e.g., determination of malignancy or suspected condition)
- Physician signatures on documentation and requests for diagnostic services
- Accuracy of claim forms relative to full inclusion of diagnosis codes and all procedure codes
- Checking for incidence of potentially bundled codes and the proper use of -59 modifier relative to CMS's CCI,
- Review of supervisory status (direct versus indirect) for billing relative to NPPs
- Documentation of case management services that rely on accurate reporting of time

Note that for provider-based clinics, both professional claims and technical component claims are filed. Some of the issues above relate to both types of claims; others may apply to one component. For instance, physicians use the -54 (intra-operative only) and -55 (post-operative) modifiers because of the global surgical package (GSP) arrangements of Medicare and other third-party payers. On the technical side for a provider-based clinic, these modifiers are not used because follow-up visits are considered new encounters. See Chapter 14 for more discussion of audit and review areas for physicians and clinics. Chapter 12 also discusses the provider-based rules.

Inpatient services

The DRG (diagnosis-related groups) system is the oldest of the prospective payment systems (PPSs). Starting in 2008, CMS implemented the Medicare Severity DRGs (MS-DRGs). The additional severity classifications using major complications or comorbidities (MCCs) will most likely increase up-coding concerns on the part of Medicare. Hospitals must continue to be vigilant in reviewing and auditing inpatient DRG assignments along with the coding processes for developing DRGs. This system depends directly on diagnosis and procedure coding as provided by ICD-9-CM and the forthcoming ICD-10-PCS and ICD-10-CM systems.

Case study 8-3. Annual Medicare DRG audit. Apex Medical Center decides to formally audit DRG assignments for Medicare inpatients from two different perspectives. A smaller general sample will be taken of all cases with the objective of a 90 percent confidence level with a 5 percent error rate relative to proper assignment. A more specific and larger study will cover cases involving the following DRGs and/or diagnoses:

- DRG 177 versus DRG 178 versus DRG 179
- DRG 196 versus DRG 197 versus DRG 198
- Hospital-acquired infection
- Septicemia
- Ventilator management
- Post-operative anemia

The proper present-on-admission (POA) indicator will be checked as will the disposition status of the discharge relative to the Medicare transfer rule under DRGs.

This list of special, problem DRGs is a short one used for illustrative purposes. Such lists are usually much longer in real situations and seem to grow every year. CMS is currently developing and implementing a severity refinement to DRGs, so the overall listing of problem DRGs will change.

At Apex, the number of discharges per year for the Medicare population is 3500. The sample size selected is 200 cases. The audit guidelines to be used are based on and correlated with the current ICD-9 coding guidelines, with special emphasis on physician documentation and clear evidence of diagnoses confirmed by physicians.

It is determined that 825 cases fall into the 6 special categories listed above. A stratified sampling of 120 cases from the special areas will be used; the remaining 80 cases of the 200 will be determined by a random sampling of non-problem cases from the universe.

Case study 8-2 is an overly simplified example, but the decisions Apex made relative to this type of audit are fairly typical. Dozens of issues surround DRGs and other case management systems of private third-party payers. The whole area of skilled nursing services provided after inpatient admissions can create difficulties. Was the inpatient stay three days or more? Will the discharge disposition create an inpatient payment reduction?

Administrative area considerations

Several areas support the overall coding, billing, and reimbursement process including:

- Billing systems
- Documentation systems
- Chargemaster
- Cost report
- Service area organizational structure
- Coding systems

Within these general administrative areas is a specific compliance subset involving the use of computer and/or manual systems to address specific compliance areas. These systems generally fall into (1) prospective and (2) retrospective categories.

Prospective systems check claims prior to submission. For instance, a computer system might be in place to generate advance beneficiary notices (ABNs) or waivers relative to medical necessity of laboratory tests. Another system may be used by coding personnel to edit claims relative to CMS's CCI to determine whether certain modifiers are needed and/or certain codes should be bundled. Yet another system may check for the DRG pre-admission window for bundling relative to diagnostic or non-diagnostic services related to the principal diagnosis for a specific DRG.

These systems or subsystems tend to fall into several categories. The laboratory system that checks for waiver generation may be a stand-alone system or be integrated into the laboratory order entry process. A number of these systems will be separate and not function as front-end or back-end systems. Figure 8.1 illustrates the use of these two types. As shown in the figure, other stand-alone systems may interface to the billing system. Hospitals sometimes have separate pharmacy or surgery systems among other specialty types that can enhance both efficiency for the service area and provide a charge capture interface to the main hospital billing system.

Case study 8-4. Interfacing computer systems. At Apex Medical Center, a review of surgical coding, billing, and claims generation uncovered a disconcerting situation. A number of charges were missing from itemized statements and the resulting claims or incorrect items were

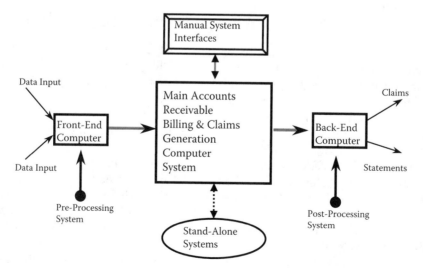

Figure 8.1 Compliance auditing computer systems and subsystems.

charged. The surgery department implemented a new information system about a year earlier. A review of the flow of charge entry revealed that surgery personnel made double entries of charges, once into the surgery system and a second time directly into the hospital billing system. Upon questioning about the double charge entry system that generated errors, the surgery area indicated that the two computers could not "talk" with each other and thus the double charge entries were necessary.

Obviously the situation in Case study 8-4 should never have occurred. Under the HIPAA administrative simplification rules and regulations, HL-7 (health level 7) provides a standard interface that should be required for all healthcare-related systems. This standard ensures that all computer systems can communicate (are properly interfaced) with each other.

Retrospective systems go back to develop data and/or statistics that can then be analyzed and used to assess compliance and/or identify compliance problems. While these systems do not identify problem claims or codes before they are sent out, they do provide a valuable means of monitoring the coding and claims filing processes.

Whether a system is manual or computer-based, it must be understood fully. Personnel must know how it works, the logic behind it, and whether it reliably produces the desired outcome. This is a highly technical form of compliance auditing, especially with computer-based systems. CBR compliance personnel should work with information technology personnel to conduct quality assurance tests to make certain these systems work properly and are fully documented. A simple approach is to send a batch of claims with certain errors through the system to ensure that these types of mistakes are identified and corrected.

The *chargemaster* or charge description master is a key component of the billing system and is heavily involved in coding and the use of modifiers. The chargemaster is in a constant state of change and must be updated to accommodate new codes, new line items, new charges, new service areas, and changing requirements of third-party payers. A chargemaster audit is generally called a review. For compliance purposes, the chargemaster should be reviewed internally every year, generally toward the end of the calendar year to coincide with coding updates. About every three to five years, an outside entity should perform a comprehensive review to ensure that the chargemaster is properly constructed and meets compliance norms. See Chapter 13 for additional information on the chargemaster.

The *cost report* is another important component of Medicare payment systems. Cost report data in the form of cost-to-charge ratios (CCRs) are used to convert charges on UB-04 claim forms into costs to develop weights for DRGs and APCs. Critical access hospitals (CAHs), rural health clinics (RHCs) and federally qualified health centers (FQHCs) are reimbursed directly based on their cost reports.

The complexity and detail involved in development of a cost report vary from organization to organization. The report can target certain compliance issues such as appropriateness of costs or proper capturing of charges that often depend on revenue codes from the chargemaster. From a compliance perspective it is best to have cost reports formally reviewed by an outside consulting firm every three to five years.

Key learning area: The internal auditing processes for both the chargemaster and cost report are called reviews and are performed annually. They should also be reviewed by external consultants every three to five years. Note that annual and other reviews can significantly improve reimbursement if developed appropriately.

Service area structuring involves the way service areas are organized. While a healthcare organization has many ways to organize, the most common structures for compliance purposes are provider-based and free-standing.

The reason service area structuring is of such concern to third-party payers is that structure affects reimbursement. For our purposes, the provider-based entities are hospital-based, that is, areas organized as a part of the hospital (most generally within the outpatient department). Provider-based status allows hospitals to file both UB-04s for technical components and 1500s for professional components. Under Medicare, a site-of-service differential reduces the professional component slightly.*

The term *free-standing* refers to organizational structuring. A clinic or entity may be physically attached to or within a hospital, but may be organized so that it is not part of the hospital outpatient department. In this case, the only claim form filed is the 1500. Third-party payers consider payment for the professional component to include payment for the facilities component.

Because a hospital can generally generate significantly higher reimbursement when a clinic or entity is provider-based, third-party payers, especially Medicare, are concerned about the appropriateness of provider-based structures. Hospitals must meet certain regulations in order for a clinic or other entity to

---

* For details, see the Physician Payment Reform or RBRVS *Federal Register* updated annually late October or early November.

be classified as provider-based.* Because these clinics and service areas and relevant regulations change, it is important for a hospital to periodically review the status of its provider-based entities relative to new regulations. Thus, an annual review of provider-based entities involving information updates that reflect new regulations is appropriate.

The coding, billing, and documentation processes are integral parts of other CBR compliance concerns. However, these processes alone warrant review and audit. Because they involve many perspectives and subprocesses, it is often difficult to audit them comprehensively. As CBR processes involve both organizational and compliance considerations, the use of business process reengineering (BPR) is appropriate. See Chapter 12 for additional discussion of the provider-based rule (PBR).

Assessing personnel competencies

Although monitoring and auditing focus on specific processes or outcomes such as documentation, codes, statements, and claims, the knowledge and skill bases of employees constitute real organizational resources. Regardless of how well a system is designed or implemented, if the people involved lack appropriate training or are not motivated or competent, the system will not work. Thus, CBR compliance personnel must assess and monitor changes in the workforce, especially those connected to technical competencies and ongoing training. Monitoring of this type should addressed carefully with service, administrative, and human resources personnel. Consideration can be given to competency-based testing although this can be very sensitive. Monitoring certifications and continuing education can also be useful.

Additional monitoring interfaces

Specific issue monitoring via reviews and audits addressed in this chapter interfaces directly with baseline audits discussed in Chapter 9. In fact, information gained from baseline compliance audits leads to specially designed monitoring of specific areas. Thus the monitoring activities relative to CBR compliance are driven, at least in part, by the baseline compliance audit process. These monitoring activities can be extended

by scheduling periodic reviews to assess compliance within the baseline audit.

Benchmark data should be used in connection with guidelines and standards for auditing. Benchmark data may come from CMS (data dealing with relative percentages of DRG assignment) or from other healthcare organizations (data dealing with relative frequencies of code utilization or services provided). In the therapy services area. it may be desirable to institute benchmarks relative to frequency of physical therapy modality utilization for certain types of cases and/or the relative frequency of multiple modality utilization. Such data may be national or regional.

Using the services of *external consultants* is recommended in several OIG model compliance guidelines. Although the reasons for using external consultants vary from organization to organization, one primary reason is to obtain an independent and objective assessment of a situation. Another reason for engaging outside consultants is to gain leverage within the organization. Often healthcare organization personnel know what is wrong and those in authority fail to listen to their concerns. If the information these employees have is supported by the findings of an outside consultant, the issue will likely be considered seriously. Another reason is that outside consultants can provide additional expertise and a fresh perspective. Whatever the reasons, external consultants including legal counsel should be carefully integrated into the monitoring process through reviews and audits.

Corrective actions

The results of reviews and audits can vary significantly. In some cases, the results will be generally positive except for a few errors or problems with compliance. Corrective actions in these cases may involve minor adjustments to a system or process or additional training. However, an audit may reveal significant problems. Auditing involves the identification of a problem area. The systems approach to solving compliance problems must be used from the beginning of any corrective action. This means going back to the starting point for problem identification and analysis. Several situations can trigger the need for corrective actions:

- A newly identified problem
- A previously implemented solution does not work
- Internal conditions changed (e.g., personnel turnover may create problems)
- External rules and regulations may have changed, causing new problems

---

* See 42 CFR §413.65 for the CMS provider-based rule (PBR) and the Abbey & Abbey, Consultants, Inc. website, www.APC-Now.com for a comprehensive toolkit of documents relating to the PBR.

Documenting review and audit activities

Although audits and reviews aim to detect problems or confirm that implemented solutions work, they can also establish diligent handling of compliance matters by a healthcare organization. Thus it is important to carefully document all reviews and audits, whether formal or informal, in terms of design, intent, and results. Documentation serves as an important mechanism to show governmental auditors and/or other law enforcement representatives that the organization seriously addresses compliance issues. Obviously, issues identified during an informal study will require a more formal study. If a formal audit identifies problems, a systematic process relative to resolving compliance issues must be initiated and allowed to run its course until such issues are resolved.

Key learning area: Carefully document the design and content of every review and audit. Be certain to document all corrective actions, additional training, development of policies and procedures, and/or other steps taken. Use the approach that documentation is "for the judge." If a compliance situation leads to court action, you will have documentary evidence of decisions made and actions taken over time.

Summary and conclusions

Formal auditing comprises a complex set of activities. The approach recommended in this chapter is to design a review that ties into the overall process and intended outcomes; an auditing process may arise from the review. An audit may be formal or informal, depending on the nature of the organization and/or the issues involved. Most formal audits include the following components:

- Statement of specific objectives and criteria, usually derived from review design
- Specific determination of sample size to be considered (possibly with stratification)
- Specific formal process for randomly choosing sample
- Analysis of selected cases in the sample, based on standard and/or developed guidelines for assessment
- Development of findings and recommendations
- Writing report
- Presentation and discussion of report and action steps

One example of such and audit is a review of physician E/M coding level determinations relative to coding documentation guidelines. Another example might be a review of DRG assignments for inpatient services.

nine

Conducting CBR baseline audits

Introduction

Routine sample auditing of various activities and processes is common in the CBR compliance area. A CBR baseline audit is more comprehensive and has a different objective. The intent is to establish a baseline against which data from future audits can be assessed to (1) verify that remedial actions taken to achieve compliance are effective and (2) discover other potential problem areas. The two approaches to developing a baseline audit are (1) comprehensive organizational top-down and (2) problem-driven specific bottom-up. In practice, a combination of both approaches is used. Because critical resources such as time and personnel are not always abundant, care must be taken in designing a baseline audit to achieve the overall goal while meeting resource constraints.

It is important to recognize that auditing is normally a precise process involving statistical analysis and quantitative measures using established metrics. Organizational auditing requires the use of qualitative data. While qualitative data is not as precise, it can be effective in explaining changes at a hospital, clinic, or IDS. Other disciplines may be used in conjunction with a baseline audit, for example:

- Benchmarking
- Business Process Reengineering (BPR)
- Total Quality Management (TQM)
- Performance Management Improvement
- Six Sigma

This chapter should be viewed as an introduction to a much larger and more encompassing topic.

Baseline audit: Overall objective

The overall objective of a baseline compliance audit is to take a "snapshot" of an organization at a specific point in time. After three, six, or even 12 months, another snapshot is taken. A comparison of both snapshots will reveal differences that can be used as indicators to identify potential problem areas and measure progress toward better compliance.

Obviously, the sizes of the snapshots and the levels of detail can differ significantly. In most cases, a series of snapshots will be taken and a mosaic or panoramic view of the organization from a compliance perspective is compiled. Typically the initial baseline compliance audit takes more time and consideration than subsequent reviews and audits because initial data gathering includes assessments of current organizational structures and infrastructures. In addition, the organization, format, and detail of the information to be gathered must be identified and/or developed. In some cases, the data will be highly quantitative, such as the number and frequency of DRG assignments for various types of inpatients. Another example might be a comprehensive listing of all surgical services by CPT that can be correlated to ICD-9-CM Volume 3 procedure codes. Some of the information gathered will be a little more qualitative. For instance, a complete synopsis of all the physicians on the medical staff of a hospital may include information about specialty, relationship to the hospital, admitting status, number of admissions, and number of surgeries.

Subsequent snapshots will be more routine because the form and format of the data will have been established. However, care should be taken to review the form, format, and process for gathering data. The organization change as will the associated payment systems and even the type and range of compliance concerns. Thus additional data gathering and new areas of investigation may be needed. In the coding area, for example, new codes and modifiers may be required. Because coding is a classification system, new requirements will generate addition information sources. Keep in mind that the development of new codes and/or modifiers is often in response to third-party payer concerns that may be monetary or compliance-centered.

The OIG cited the baseline compliance audit in several of its model compliance guidelines.* The way to accomplish a baseline compliance audit is left to the healthcare provider's personnel, but the process should be conducted at the corporate compliance level. For the purposes of our discussion, we will address only the CBR-related issues.

Figures 9.1 and 9.2 illustrate the time sequencing of a baseline compliance audit. Figure 9.1 shows four of many factors, two quantitative and two qualitative.

---

* See bibliography for OIG model compliance guidance in different areas.

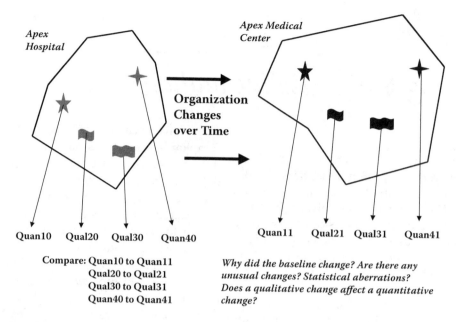

Figure 9.1   Assessing changes over time.

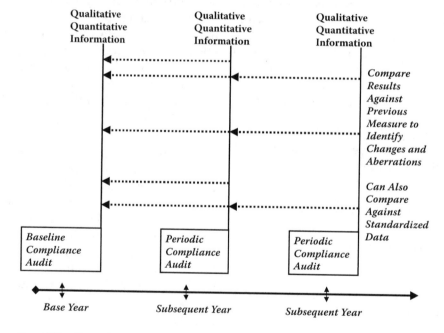

Figure 9.2   Comparative utilization.

Note that between the initial and follow-up snapshots, the hospital underwent a name change (from hospital to medical center). The differences in the polygons represent changes in hospital scope and activities for the four areas indicated. Obviously, the figure is oversimplified. The intent is to track changes over time.

Figure 9.2 illustrates how a baseline compliance audit is used over a two-year period. Note that subsequent periodic audits include new factors for consid-

eration. While a baseline compliance audit may have many objectives, three immediate ones are:

- Identifying aberrations, anomalies, and suspicious changes
- Meeting OIG requirements for auditing, reviewing, and identifying problem areas
- Neutralizing OIG and OIG contractor studies by identifying compliance situations before governmental entities do so

Beginning baseline audit process

The two approaches to designing and conducting a baseline audit are discussed below. Regardless of the approach, a baseline compliance audit may be extensive and require significant resources and several preliminary steps. Consider the following assessments applicable only to the coding, billing, documentation, and reimbursement areas:

- Current standards, polices, and procedures
- Information and documentation systems
- Operational processes
- Computer systems and interfaces
- Legal responsibility and risk
- Agents and relationships
- Knowledge bases and capabilities
- Information sources and flow
- Service areas
- Satellite services and organizational structure
- Coding and billing functions
- Contract issues
- Employee reporting process and organizational environment

This list can be extended and may need to be modified. A free-standing medical clinic, for example, is not as complex as an integrated delivery system that may have multiple locations and a variety of service areas. However, the fundamental concerns remain the same for both entities. The following exercise can serve as a first step in the process of developing a baseline compliance audit.

Exercise: For your healthcare organization (hospital, clinic, IDS), identify all its providers of healthcare services and delineate their exact relationships to your organization. Obtain all written contracts, letters, and/or memoranda of agreement between the healthcare organization and the providers. Limit this data gathering to business or contractual relationships; do not include full credentialing activities.

While it is easy to list the exercise activities, the tasks are demanding. Even a modest-sized hospital has many providers, and multiple relationships may extend to the CBR areas. At Apex Medical Center, the following areas are affected:

- Hospital-based physicians: radiologists, anesthesiologists, pathologists
- Non-physician providers: PAs, NPs, CRNAs, CNSs, CSWs, psychologists, nurse midwives
- Physicians: family practitioners, specialists
- ER physicians
- Therapy services: physical, occupational, speech

Simply identifying all the providers may be a challenge because some are closely associated with the hospital and others are only incidentally associated. Finding the contracts and identifying all billing relationships can also be difficult. For example, the ER physicians may be contracted and the hospital may perform billing (both professional and technical components). Similarly, hospital-based physicians may handle their own billing while they are at the hospital, but questions may arise as to why their billing personnel are located in the hospital and whether rent is charged at fair market value (FMV).

Designing baseline audits: Different approaches

Figure 9.3 illustrates the two main approaches: top-down and bottom-up. In many instances healthcare organizations will use a combination of the approaches. CBR compliance personnel must be flexible by being ready and able to adjust the approaches for given organizational imperatives.

Designing baseline audits: Top-down approach

The top-down approach means viewing an organization as a whole and defining areas for data gathering. For large organizations, this may require division of the organization into parts and then performing individual baseline compliance audits on each part. The results of these audits can be combined if appropriate.

Great care must be taken to define the scope and level of detail to be addressed. It is easy to take too big a bite and end up lost in a sea of details. Also, it is best to focus on quantitative factors because data gathering in these areas can be more easily systematized. For instance, once a computer report relative to CPT utilization has been designed, it is reasonably easy to rerun the report again. Do not omit qualitative or narrative information because it complements quantitative data and often provides revealing insights. See Figure 9.4.

The exercise presented above concerned gathering and organizing information about the medical staff organization.* After this information has been organized and entered in the computer, it should not be overly difficult to update when a new physician starts work at the hospital or when relationships change.

---

* We really should refer to this as the Provider Staff Organization since there are an increasing number of non-physician providers working at various types of healthcare organizations.

Top-Down Approach
Driven by Organizational
Structure - Hierarchical
Provides Overall View/Data
Selective Level of Detail

*The final design of the Baseline
Compliance Audit is typically a hybrid
of the top-down organizational and
bottom-up problem/opportunity
approaches.
Care must be taken to carefully
identify the level of detail for data
gathering and organization.*

Bottom-Up Approach
Problem/Opportunity
Driven
Highly Detailed in
Selective Areas

Figure 9.3   Basic baseline audit design approaches.

Baseline Compliance Audit-Design Approach
Top-Down Approach

- Follow the Hierarchical Organizational Structure

- Determine the Level of Detail - Less Detail - Qualitative
  Integrate Level of Detail with Bottom-Up Problem
  Approach

- Cross Organizational Issues

- Special Service Area Considerations

- Special Quantification Techniques

- Overall Corporate Compliance Program

Figure 9.4   Top-down design approach.

Area overview

The following list outlines areas that should be considered in developing a top-down approach for baseline compliance auditing. It was developed for a medical center but can adjusted to the needs of any healthcare organization. Note that it concentrates on the CBR areas but includes other areas. The outline should be considered a **starting point**. CBR personnel may need to modify, delete, and/or add areas for consideration. Each provider's situation is different and flexibility is important.

Administration and support areas

- Corporate compliance
- Financial services
- Patient accounting
- Health information management
- Information systems or technology
- Marketing and public relations
- Human resources
- Training and education
- Facilities and environmental control

Service areas

- Provider staff organization
- Case management
- Emergency
- Surgery
- Acute care
- Laboratory
- Radiology
- Special care
- Clinic
- Urgent care
- Therapies
- Home health
- Skilled nursing

Corporate compliance program (seven key elements)

- Assess status of implementation—policies, hotlines, personnel
- Quantitative information on number and type of problems reported, hotline utilization, problems resolved, cases involving refunds of money, cases involving self-disclosure
- Establishment of subcompliance programs
- Number and type of personnel directly involved in compliance activities
- Major programs and/or areas of concern
- Availability of information—national, state, local

- Dissemination of information to and from departments
- Availability of legal counsel
- Documentation system for compliance activities
- Settlement agreement requirements and activities

Provider staff organization

- Identify each provider
- Determine exact relationship
- Identify type and level of services provided
- Assess credentials and special capabilities
- Review documentation for relationship
- Document billing and/or financial relationships

Emergency department

- Providers and relationships
- Coding, billing, and claims development—physician and hospital
- Volume, types, and levels of services
- Volume, types, and levels of ancillary services requested
- Documentation system
- Support staff
- Financial assessment

Information systems and technology

- Number and types of personnel
- Vendor relationships
- Overall system identification
- Systems and subsystems relating directly to compliance (prospective versus retrospective) including reporting capabilities
- System and subsystem planning and development
- Involvement level—CBR, compliance (proactive versus reactive)
- Information resource management—database and data warehousing capabilities

Financial services

- Overall sources of reimbursement and income
- General breakdown of reimbursement and income by type of service
- Cost report decisions and information
- Third-party payer contracts
- Analysis of reimbursement and income by patient type and location and payer type
- Budget for compliance activities
- Credit balance reporting
- Co-pay and deductible waiving processes
- Chargemaster design, update, and review processes
- Interface of chargemaster and cost reporting

Health information management

- Number, type, and expertise levels of coding staff
- Documentation system and flow
- Use of computer aids—encoders, groupers, edit checkers.
- Coding policies and procedures development
- Resource and reference material availability
- Credential and training attendance
- Interface to billing and claims development
- Auditing techniques and review of benchmarks in use

Case management

- Observation versus inpatient determination
- Referrals to post-acute care
- Emergency to observation
- Clinic to observation
- Nursing facility oversight
- Care path and clinical path development

Patient accounting

- Billing
- Billing privileges—national provider identifiers and CSM-855 forms
- Use of audit and editing software
- Manual review and audit sampling
- Billing policies and procedure development
- Information and resource availability
- Interface to HIM and service areas

Marketing and public relations

- Advertising program
- Potential incentives—advertising
- Referral patterns
- Post-discharge case management

Human resources

- Number and type of personnel by department or service area
- Labor relations status
- FLSA standards
- EEOC standards
- ADA standards
- Policies and procedures development

Special care units

- Identification of types and levels of service
- Identification of personnel
- Quantification of number and types of procedures performed
- Interface to coding, billing, reimbursement, and documentation

- Identification of covered versus non-covered services
- Assessment of payment patterns
- Financial assessment by unit or area such as chemotherapy, dialysis, subacute units, bone marrow and stem cell transplants, other transplants, and nuclear medicine

Training and education

- Level, type, and expertise of training personnel
- Facilities, equipment, and technology for training
- Compliance training curriculum implementation
- External compliance training coordination status
- Ethics and facilitation training techniques

Facilities and environmental controls

- Environmental protection status
- Safety and risk management procedures
- Disaster planning status
- ADA compliance status

Surgery

- Frequency and types (inpatient by DRG; outpatient by APG, APC, CPT; categorization by patient types, ages, demographics)
- Utilization of observation and/or extended recovery
- Clinical pathways established for post-operative care
- Staffing levels
- Profitability
- Interface to billing, coding, documentation

Acute care

- Levels and types of services
- Categorization of services by DRG
- Staffing levels
- Profitability
- Facility considerations
- Bed utilization statistics

Observation

- Number, level, and location of observation services
- Documentation policies and procedures
- Clinical pathways for admit and discharge decisions

Clinic and urgent care

- Number, type, location, and personnel
- Organizational structuring (provider-based versus free-standing)
- Patient record keeping

- Patient billing and claims filing system
- Accreditation and licensing status
- Level of coding E/M
- Medical necessity through diagnosis codes
- Location, types, and levels of services
- Provider relations
- Organizational structuring
- Utilization of ancillary services (number, location)
- Contractual relationships

Laboratory

- Number and types of tests
- Staffing
- Provider utilization and sources
- Use of ABNs and waivers
- Interface to coding, billing, reimbursement system
- Status of special compliance program
- Internal sampling audit utilization and purpose
- Use of computer systems for compliance and/or editing
- Use of modifiers on claims

Radiology

- Number and types of tests
- Staffing
- Provider utilization and sources
- Use of ABNs and waivers
- Interface to coding, billing, reimbursement system
- Status of special compliance program
- Internal sampling audit utilization and purpose
- Use of computer systems for compliance and/or editing
- Use of modifiers on claims

Therapies

- Location, types, and levels of services
- Staffing utilization
- Provider relations
- Contractual relationships
- Subacute care services
- Documentation
- Interface to billing, coding, and reimbursement system

Home health

- Compliance program implementation status
- Types, levels, and location of services
- Referral patterns and sources
- Staffing utilization
- Provider relationships
- Utilization statistics
- Financial status

Skilled nursing

- Compliance program implementation status
- Types, levels, and location of services
- Referral patterns and sources
- Staffing utilization
- Provider relationships
- Utilization statistics
- Financial status

Chapter 12 discusses gaining and maintaining billing privileges under Medicare. The process requires preparation of five different CMS-855 forms. Based on the organizational structure, multiple copies may be necessary. Completing these forms properly requires an intimate knowledge of the entire organization, all the activities and services provided, and the personnel performing various jobs. A high-level top-down analysis can assist significantly in meeting this compliance requirement. Note that other third-party payers may also require special procedures for gaining billing privileges. Generally, these requirements are not as onerous as those of Medicare.

Designing baseline audits: Bottom-up approach

The bottom-up approach develops mechanisms to monitor specific problems or potential problem areas over time. This approach simply constructs a baseline by addressing a whole series of problem or opportunity areas. As shown in Figure 9.5, the bottom-up approach is problem- or event-driven. The problem can be real, suspected, or potential. Typically, a problem or challenge will be specific to a given compliance issue. Chapter 3 discusses a number of standard problem areas. OIG work plans and advisory opinions, a current compliance audit, and litigation assessment can all be used to identify areas for consideration.

What a baseline audit does is develop a tracking mechanism to see what is happening to a problem over time. For instance, in a clinic setting, a concern may arise about the relative frequency of a physician's use of office visit E/M CPT codes. A preliminary snapshot of the relative frequency can be made by performing a study reviewing claims over a certain period. The intervention may require training sessions, development of written policies and procedures, development of templates, and other steps. After the intervention and allowing sufficient time for changes to take place, a second snapshot is taken for comparative purposes. Note that this example involves only numerical indicators, i.e., relative frequencies.

It is theoretically possible that the numerical indicators may not change, but the level and detail of documentation may have changed and does support the level of E/M coding. An investigation of the medical documentation to support the level would require a different kind of study.

Another area of concern might be medical necessity as provided through diagnosis coding in an outpatient setting. A simple snapshot might present the number of diagnosis codes on various types of outpatient claims, for example, surgery, ER, therapies, medical visits, etc. Making a correct or incorrect assumption that a higher frequency of diagnosis codes will provide

---

**Baseline Compliance Audit-Design Approach
Bottom-Up Approach**

- Problem/Opportunity Driven
- Problem Area Analysis
- OIG Work Plans
- Legislative Initiatives
- Identified Compliance Problems
- Specific Settlement Agreements
- Audit/Analysis Tends to be Detailed/Quantitative
- Integrate with Top-Down Approach

Figure 9.5 Bottom-up design approach.

better medical necessity justification, the average number of diagnosis codes for these various types of claims can be tracked while various interventions are made for provider and coding staffs.

Hybrid approach

Healthcare providers of different types and sizes will approach baseline compliance audits differently. If relatively few resources are devoted to the effort, it is likely that a limited number of issues will be addressed via the bottom-up approach. For organizations seeking a more comprehensive effort, the top-down approach along organizational lines may be best both for identifying and monitoring purposes.

Most healthcare organizations will find it useful to adopt a combination or hybrid approach. Specific problem areas can be tracked, analyzed, and improved through a bottom-up approach. Conversely, an organization may want to tackle specific issues from a top-down approach that facilitates problem identification and also provides evidence for external auditors that the organization proactively addresses compliance situations. A good example of a limited top-down benchmark is in the exercise above in which a hospital must identify all its relationships with providers. These relationships are often sources of legal, financial, and compliance concerns.

Tools, techniques, and processes

The process for a baseline compliance audit is similar to the process discussed in Chapter 8. It can be informal or formal. If a baseline compliance audit is conducted to any degree of detail, it will quickly become large enough to justify careful planning and the use of a team approach. The following steps apply:

- Audit plan preparation and documentation
- Audit team development
- Authority for conducting the audit
- Requirement development for auditing
- Documentation, checklists, guidelines, and log sheets
- Data and information gathering
- Audit analysis, conclusions, and recommendations
- Reports and preparation for future comparisons

The design and documentation for a baseline compliance audit were discussed in the preceding sections. CBR personnel should anticipate that subsequent audit activity will expand over time. In other words, more information will be required and more comparative analyses will be made.

Since a baseline compliance audit can cover a host of areas, it is best to spread the responsibility for the activities among people and also across different areas. Depending on the size of an organization's internal audit capabilities, the personnel on the team may be devoted to internal auditing or may be assigned on a functional basis to the baseline compliance audit team, in which case, the team leader should be directly responsible for the corporate or CBR compliance program.

Even on a small scale, a baseline compliance audit requires full administrative authority. Since the data and information to be gathered may not be readily available and may require access to records and conducting interviews of personnel and people outside the organization, the need for administrative authority is critical.

Requirements, checklists, guidelines, log sheets, and other tools will probably have to be developed. Although some areas audited will be well understood and the information well structured, certain areas may be new and/or sensitive, particularly when the information gathered crosses into patient areas. Another sensitive area is the possible use of information in other ways such as for economic credentialing. The objectives and requirements for baseline compliance audits must be carefully reviewed for potentially sensitive issues and possible abuses.

An initial baseline compliance audit is somewhat different from other auditing activities because the objective is to create an instrument that serves as a standard for comparison. Physicians often establish baselines by ordering laboratory and radiological tests, then determining whether a patient's health stays the same or changes while under their care by comparing changes to the baseline. Such comparisons can easily show when a test parameter does not meet a national norm and is also outside a patient's norm.

Report preparation for baseline audits is molded by the objective. Since the intention is to compare data developed and later compare them to other data in the future, it is vital that the data be as structured as possible. Charts, graphs, data arrays, and other statistical tools are helpful, especially for portraying quantitative data. Data must be structured to make it useful for future comparative analyses.

Utilizing payment system classification

Healthcare payment systems often provide quantitative tools for monitoring. Virtually every prospective payment system (PPS) categorizes services for payment purposes. Fee schedule payment systems also use classifications. RBRVS uses the CPT system; HCPCS codes are used for the DME fee schedule. CPT laboratory codes are used for laboratory fee schedules. All these systems can provide statistics that can be used to monitor activities within service areas. Consider the following systems:

- DRGs and related variants
- APCs and related variants
- RBRVS
- RUGs-III

Every one contains underlying coding and/or documentation systems. DRGs use the ICD-9-CM for procedures (Volume 3) and diagnoses (Volumes 1 and 2). APGs and APCs use a combination of CPT and ICD-9-CM diagnosis codes. RBRVS uses the CPT coding systems. RUGs-III utilizes a documentation process that requires certain information. Other PPSs may use different underlying coding and/or documentation systems to drive their classification processes.

Diagnosis-related groups (DRGs)

DRGs have been in use for more than two decades. CMS recently implemented a severity refinement that increased the complexity of this payment system. The system also has a number of variations such as AP-DRGs (all patient DRGs), APR-DRGs (all patient refined DRGs), and SR-DRGs (severity refined DRGs) in addition to the new base MS-DRG system used by Medicare for hospital inpatient services. The differences in the system result from details and service classification levels. For auditing and monitoring purposes DRGs provide information at (1) frequency analysis and (2) case mix index levels.

Frequency analysis involves arraying every DRG category and its frequency within a certain time period. Monitoring the frequencies over time allows tracking of shifts and variations in services. Unusual variations can then be analyzed. A simple example is a sudden increase in the number of orthopedic surgery cases that could be explained by an increase in the number of orthopedic surgeons on staff.

A case mix index (CMI) number shows the relative severity of cases or services provided on the inpatient side. Hospital CMIs are carefully monitored by third-party payers to identify unusual changes and potentially fraudulent activities. Since overall payment for inpatient services is directly related to the CMI, hospitals are sensitive to keeping their CMIs as high as possible while maintaining compliance.

CBR compliance personnel must be very sensitive when developing rationales for a CMI change. A continuing trend for services to move from inpatient to outpatient status indicates that the DRG CMI for a given hospital should increase over time since lower level inpatient cases have become outpatient cases. Other measures and statistics such as shifts in frequencies of services in different settings can identify anomalies and enable CBR compliance personnel to provide explanations and rationales for changes.

Note: With CMS implementing the MS-DRGs, the development of comparative statistics with previous DRGs is problematic. MS-DRGs use a completely different numbering system and thus we will have to crosswalk statistics between the old and new DRG systems.

Other statistics can also be used with DRGs. A length of stay (LOS) is associated with each DRG. In the Medicare DRG system, this is known as the GMLOS (geometric mean length of stay). The LOS can be monitored for each DRG and then averaged and compared against the GMLOS or other measure. The DRG system typically provides for outlier payments—extra payments for unusually costly services. The number of times that cost outliers are paid and the overall extra payments can also be tracked and analyzed.

Another CMS measure within the DRG system is the AMLOS (arithmetic mean length of stay). The AMLOS was used for day outliers, that is, extra payments if a patient remained in the hospital longer than the AMLOS. While CMS no longer uses this statistic, it is maintained for hospitals and other third-party payers to use.

Ambulatory payment classifications (APCs)

CMS ambulatory payment classifications (APCs) represent a payment system for hospital outpatient services. As with DRGs, services are classified into categories. APGs and APCs tend to be more complex than DRGs. Grouping of outpatient services may involve several categories along with associated services such as laboratory and/or radiology that are paid separately via fee schedules.

Despite various third-party payer implementations, APGs and APCs allow for classification of services. Frequency analysis of surgical, medical, ancillary, and other types of services provides a means of monitoring. Again, unusual changes in frequencies over a period can identify potentially fraudulent activities. A sudden increase in observation services may require determination of the reason for the increase in frequency. Other information from baseline auditing activities may yield an answer.

The APC and APG counterparts of the DRG CMI comprise (1) a service mix index (SMI) and (2) an

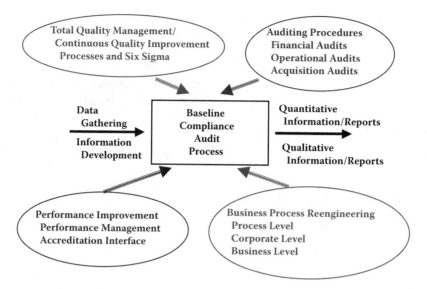

Figure 9.6 Baseline compliance audit-related disciplines.

encounter mix (EMI). Because APG and APC groupings can result in multiple assignments to different categories and associated services may fall outside the categories, the development of indexes becomes more complicated relative to the DRG CMI. The SMI gives an overall measure of severity and can be broken down into areas such as surgical or medical to refine the measurements of activities. The SMI is calculated by considering each APG and APC assignment to be included in the averaging process of adding the APG or APC weights and dividing the total by the number of APGs or APCs.

The EMI is more analogous to the CMI. APGs and APCs are encounter-driven. To obtain a truer measure of severity and thus the level of resource utilization for outpatient services, it makes more sense to develop an index for encounters. The calculation of this average is modified by first adding the APG or APC weight per encounter and dividing the sum of all the weights by the number of encounters (not the total number of APCs and APGs generated).

Related disciplines

As shown in Figure 9.6, closely related disciplines can provide tools, techniques, and a general body of knowledge to aid the baseline compliance audit process. Total Quality Management (TQM), Continuous Quality Improvement (CQI), Six Sigma, and related techniques such as root cause analysis and sentinel events are useful for quality improvement. Business process reengineering is another discipline that can aid CBR compliance. BPR can applied at different levels that often correspond to levels of compliance activities.

Of the related disciplines shown in Figure 9.6, the one closest to the baseline compliance audit is the regular financial and operational audit. The general steps undertaken in an operations audit are relatively close to those of a baseline compliance audit. General audits often take a top-down approach. A significant part of a baseline compliance audit involves the monitoring and assessment of specific problem areas. See the bibliography for additional references concerning these disciplines.

Summary and conclusions

One of the primary justifications for compliance activities is that they improve performance while also improving the ability to manage a healthcare organization. CBR compliance activities almost certainly lead to revenue enhancement when the processes involved are optimized to bring CBR into full compliance with relevant rules and regulations.

The process and techniques involved in conducting a baseline compliance audit, even one limited to the CBR compliance area, are complex. This chapter represents a starting point. A baseline audit can be designed as a bottom-up or problem-driven approach or as a top-down or organizational approach. Most organizations find that a hybrid that combines top-down and bottom-up works best.

Healthcare organizations differ in size and structure and these distinctions influence the development of baseline compliance audits. Regardless of the size or type of organization, conducting even a limited baseline compliance audit requires significant resource utilization. These audits must be carefully planned and crafted.

ten

Integrating CBR compliance into corporate compliance

Introduction

The integration of a CBR compliance program with a corporate compliance program varies significantly, depending on the size and diversity of the healthcare organization in question. For a small hospital or a single medical clinic, both programs may be totally integrated, have common personnel, and share a single compliance manual and associated policies and procedures. The chief compliance officer (CCO) will directly handle CBR compliance issues. For larger organizations including teaching centers, multihospital systems, and integrated delivery systems, the CBR compliance program will most likely be distinct from the corporate program in terms of manuals, activities, and personnel. In these larger settings, CBR compliance personnel may constitute a separate unit that reports to the CCO.

Corporate compliance programs

Figure 10.1 illustrates interfaces to be considered by CBR compliance personnel. The most significant interface at CBR compliance level is to the corporate program. While the corporate level program addresses the full range of compliance issues for the organization, the CBR compliance program concentrates on specialized issues revolving around coding, documentation, billing, and reimbursement. The relationship of corporate program efforts and CBR level specific issues varies from organization to organization.

In a small organization, the CCO will generally also address CBR compliance issues. Even in small organizations, he or she may not be an expert in the full range of CBR issues and may need assistance from technical personnel. The CCO may have an assistant who addresses CBR issues. In somewhat larger organizations, the CBR compliance functions will normally be separated from the CCO's activities. The compliance efforts may well involve a full-time employee who reports to the CCO, but this specialist in CBR compliance areas usually operates fairly independently. In large organizational settings such as multihospital systems or integrated delivery systems, the CBR compliance functions may require a staff to address and coordinate activities. A separate office may even be established for these functions.

CBR compliance personnel will generally not have line authority over administrative and/or service areas. Despite a significant administrative mandate relative to all forms of compliance, the work of CBR compliance personnel is performed at a staff level and not at operational line manager level. As a result, CBR compliance personnel and others involved in various aspects of compliance activities must utilize a variety of team approaches, facilitation techniques, and persuasive skills. Obviously compliance issues can force changes on a healthcare organization. However, it is best to implement these changes in the least disruptive fashion and in a way that can be most readily accepted by the organization as a whole and the specific personnel involved in the services provided by the organization.

Seven fundamental principles

This section briefly reviews the differences between a corporate compliance program and a more specific CBR compliance program. This comparative process can be performed with any specialized program and helps those involved in specialized programs to focus on the relevant areas for prioritization. The seven principles were discussed in some detail in previous chapters relative to coding, documentation, billing, and reimbursement.

Compliance standards and procedures

A corporate compliance plan is usually embodied in a formal system of documents that are crafted with great care usually with assistance from legal counsel. These documents are approved by the organization's board and provide the entire organization with the framework for addressing compliance. They also address the organization's commitment to maintaining compliance in all the relevant healthcare compliance areas. A corporate plan tends to be fairly static and not involve major changes because it details general directions and an overall system for maintaining compliance. While policies and procedures may be

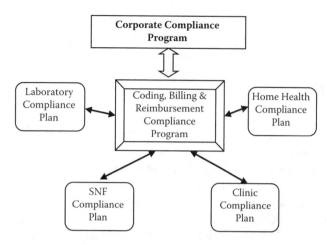

Figure 10.1 Interfaces to CBR compliance program.

specific, they tend to be more prevalent in specialized plans addressing specific areas.

At CBR level, the written policies and procedures take on a different form. The base form of a CBR compliance manual may not change a great deal, but the individual policies and procedures will change as different requirements come into play related to payment systems and legal requirements. Moreover, the CBR policies and procedures will probably be widely distributed and may be used as training tools. Depending on organization size and its program structure, it will most likely have policy and procedure manuals covering billing, coding, chargemaster, utilization review, outcome management, and other issues. Table 10.1

summarizes key differences between corporate and CBR compliance, most of which are shaped by the context in which compliance activities are undertaken. Specific features may vary from organization to organization.

Oversight responsibility

The organizational structure supporting a corporate compliance program will tend to be hierarchical; that is, the oversight responsibility will lie with the COO who will then delegate as appropriate. A large integrated delivery system setting will probably employ a true CCO who will manage compliance officers at the entities (hospitals, clinics, and other service organizations). The great diversity in healthcare organizations means that many types of organizational structures handle compliance activities. Note that the CCO must have independence in reporting relationships.

Whatever the organizational structure, a vital factor is support for CBR compliance activities that dovetail with the overall organizational structure. An integrated delivery system will most likely handle oversight related to CBR issues through an employee or office at corporate level. As appropriate, within each of the subordinate entities, appropriate CBR compliance personnel will be assigned on a part- or full-time basis. The critical criterion in the CBR compliance area is the availability of competent, trained, and technically experienced staff to handle oversight.

Table 10.1 Summary of Seven Principles: Corporate versus CBR Compliance

Principle	Corporate Compliance Level	CBR Compliance Level
Standards and procedures	Established compliance plan is relatively static	Compliance plan and associated policies and procedures are highly dynamic
Oversight	Depends on size of organization; oversight is general, organizational	Oversight is technical; addresses coding, billing, and documentation
Delegation	Delegation is along organizational reporting lines depending on compliance area	Delegation generally functional at technical level with line reporting retained by CBR compliance personnel
Training	Tends to be more general and includes ethics training and organizational sensitivity to compliance	Highly specific relative to technical aspects of coding, billing, documentation, and reimbursement
Monitoring and auditing	Monitoring and auditing activities at organizational level, including baseline compliance audit; specific monitoring within special areas	Targeted at problem areas; include informal reviews and formal audits
Enforcement and discipline	Formal enforcement, disciplinary, and remedial actions broad application across entire organization	Actions generally take form of specific training to remedy systematic problems
Response and prevention	Response and prevention broadly based with specific actions for specialized areas	Specific systematic activities designed to identify and resolve technical problems with coding, billing, and reimbursement

Delegation of authority

The delegation of authority at corporate compliance level is a formal process that is well documented in terms of performance standards, authority, supervisory functions, and the like. Delegation at the CBR compliance level may be formal setting for large organizations. Often, however, CBR compliance is handled at a working or functional level, particularly if personnel work on a part-time or as-needed basis. In this situation, the working arrangements and delegation of authority will be based more on expertise than on formal organizational or hierarchical criteria. Thus the delegation of authority is on a functional basis, not a line basis.

Employee training

The overall thrust of training at the corporate compliance level is on ethics but includes more general training that supports the organization's commitment to maintaining compliance in all required areas and certification that employees have been trained and understand the organization's commitment to compliance. Training at CBR compliance level is far more specific. The level of activity will generally be greater and the range of topics addressed broad and will target employees and non-employees involved in and/or interfacing with CBR processes. This may entail a simple review of the many healthcare payment systems and statutory requirements such as HIPAA and EMTALA; the technical level of training is more intense.

Monitoring and auditing

Monitoring and auditing comprise large segments of CBR compliance activities. Formal audits along with informal reviews and associated activities are the main tools for determining whether compliance criteria are met and whether changes within the CBR process work effectively. Internal activities must be correlated and coordinated with external consulting activities.

Monitoring and auditing activities at corporate compliance level tend to be more general and involve detailed activities within specialized service areas or plans. One comprehensive activity undertaken at corporate level is baseline compliance auditing as discussed in Chapter 9, and most effort is directed at coding, documentation, billing, and reimbursement activities. The techniques used for a baseline compliance audit may be quantitative or qualitative, depending on the area under consideration and the type of data available. CBR compliance activities also involve both types of data although the emphasis is on hard data that can be quantified and thus analyzed.

Enforcement and discipline

At corporate compliance level, enforcement and discipline issues receive careful consideration. Employees and/or areas that conduct conducting activities outside compliance norms must be brought back into conformance. Appropriate discipline (including termination) is applied as required.

The CBR area tends to be more technical and fraudulent activities are generally accidental rather than intentional. Under normal circumstances, employees and/or units of an organization are not deliberately out of compliance. Generally the personnel do not know (and thus the automated systems) simply do not know the correct way to document, bill, and file claims within the compliance norms. As a result, the enforcement and disciplinary actions are usually directed at identifying problems, developing solutions, and instituting appropriate training to implement changes, then ensuring that a problem has been rectified.

Response and prevention

Response and prevention are major issues at both corporate and CBR compliance level. Coding, billing, and reimbursement issues require quick responses after a problem is identified. This may mean not billing or filing claims for certain period until a fix can be effected. After a solution (computer or manual system modification or personnel training) has been developed and implemented, the focus is on preventing recurrence and this requires ongoing monitoring. A manual system may have to be implemented while a longer-term computer solution is developed. Note that with CBR compliance problems, detection and recognition may be difficult. Personnel may have to spend considerable time interpreting data in order to uncover a problem.

At corporate compliance level, response and prevention activities must be broader because the range of types of problems and areas is much greater. For example, medical waste disposal procedures may not conform to environmental standards. The cause may be an OSHA issue related to power wiring or a tax classification that fails to conform to IRS requirements. Often, response and prevention involve a wide range of organizational facilities including computer systems. Many problems at this level will involve organizational structure and relationships. Many teaching hospitals, for example, have close relationships with groups of teaching physicians and the associated financial arrangements can be complex. Such relationships (clinics, for example) may have to be assessed from the perspective of ownership and/or operation of real property. Both corporate and CBR level compliance programs must sometimes rely on interpretive skills to recognize problems.

Key learning area: The seven fundamental principles of compliance apply equally well to corporate and CBR programs. The activities prompted by the principles, however, can be significantly different.

Specialized compliance programs

A number of specialized compliance programs may be necessary for a healthcare organization. At hospital level, in addition to a corporate program, the following specialized compliance programs may be appropriate:

- CBR
- Laboratory
- Pharmacy
- Radiology
- Home health
- Skilled nursing
- Subacute care
- Renal dialysis
- Durable medical equipment
- Other specialized service areas

All these programs must dovetail with the corporate program and will contain CBR components that must also be integrated into the overall CBR compliance program.

The way to accomplish this varies significantly from hospital to hospital. In a smaller setting where not all these services are provided, specialized compliance programs may be included in a master plan. Small hospitals may have limited laboratory services and a few swing beds that compromise skilled nursing services. Only a few items such as crutches and canes may be dispensed as durable medical equipment, and other services may be similarly limited. Rather than separating these special areas, small hospitals find it more logical to deal with them as a separate unit of a corporate plan.

In a larger hospital or multihospital system, these specialized programs may be treated individually. In an integrated delivery system providing a wide range of services, specialty programs at different locations must be integrated into the overall corporate level compliance activities.

Whistle blowers

Most corporate compliance plans address whistle blowing, also called a *qui tam* issue (based on the Latin phrase, *Qui tam pro domino rege quam pro se ipso in hac parte sequitur*, loosely translated as, "He who brings the action for the king as well as for himself.") in relation to the False Claims Act (FCA). This is a complex area where prevention is far preferable to the cure and a proactive approach is critical. Taking steps to prevent spurious whistle blowing will prevent such problems.

Most whistle blowers of the *qui tam* variety are disgruntled current or former employees; a few are employees who genuinely feel that an organization has unresolved compliance problems. One of the best ways to address the situation with current employees is installation of an internal hotline on which employees can report compliance concerns to proper authorities within the organization instead of prematurely contacting authorities outside the organization. Surveys and interviews can be even more proactive. They should be documented as a precautionary measure. The documentation may be useful if a whistle blowing case arises.

An exit interview is an excellent tool for dealing with a whistle blowing on the part of a discharged or resigning employee. The interview provides an opportunity for the healthcare organization to determine whether the employee knows about or suspects fraudulent activities or other compliance concerns. Unfortunately, termination is unpleasant process for both employers and employees and it may be difficult to maintain a good rapport with an employee whose separation from the organization is less than amicable.

Concern about employee whistle blowing is common in the coding, billing, and reimbursement area, and the concern is frequently justified. A concerted effort should be made to provide CBR personnel involved in these complex processes with opportunities to share their thoughts and concerns before they expand into a needless full-blown external investigation. Teamwork, process analysis, information flows, training and education, and similar activities are all designed to address employee concerns before they become crises.

Disgruntled or misinformed employees are not the only whistle blowers. Patient complaints can escalate into whistle blowing via the OIG's hotline. While we have little more than anecdotal evidence, it appears that the two major stress points for patients are the care provided and the ensuing bill. Because itemized statements and explanations of benefits represent challenges even for trained professionals, it is little wonder that patients experience stress when trying to decipher them. This stress and the lack of understanding creating the stress can turn into a complaint that can escalate and become a formal complaint filed with state and/or federal authorities.

Case study 10-1. Autologous blood billing. Sarah, an elderly patient, recently underwent an outpatient surgical procedure. In preparation, Sarah donated two units of autologous blood that fortunately did not have to be used. It is now five weeks later and Sarah received a bill for the collection of her blood. She cannot understand how the hospital could bill for her own blood that was never used. She suspects that something is wrong and contacts Medicare.

Case study 10-1 is a simple example of how Medicare and other patients can easily become confused and suspect that something is amiss in their billings. Patient concerns have escalated in recent years, especially related to what are perceives as excessive hospital and healthcare charges. In response, hospitals are currently taking steps to establish a transparent or rational pricing system that makes hospital charges more accessible and easier to understand. When you consider that patient complaints can serve as the main triggers for visits by federal agents to healthcare facilities, instituting transparent pricing may be a very good idea indeed.

Key learning area: Whistle blowing or *qui tam* cases are delights for prosecutors. Healthcare organizations must take proactive steps to ensure that any potential for spurious or misguided whistle blowing is kept to an absolute minimum.

Managed care: Capitation compliance

This book focuses on a wide variety of coding, documentation, billing, and reimbursement issues that are generally considered in the context of payment systems:

- Cost-based
- Prospective payment
- Non-capitated managed care

Cost-based systems are still used even though Medicare and Medicaid have made significant movement toward fee schedules and prospective payments. Cost reports are also still important although their use is changing. Prospective payment systems (PPSs) such as DRGs, RUGS-III and APCs, along with fee schedule systems such as physician RBRVS, are popular and similar types of payment systems for areas such as home health and rehabilitation and from third-party payers continue to be developed.

Managed care covers an enormous range of meanings and nuances. Most managed care payment systems that do not involve capitation or assumption of significant risk by a provider typically utilize a fee schedule, discounted fee schedule with several types of withholdings, or another form of prospective or case-based payment. Thus, these types of managed care payment systems exhibit the same kinds of compliance concerns: overbilling, overutilization, duplicate billing, medical necessity, etc.

Capitated payment systems create a new environment for compliance concerns. The assumption of risk on the part of healthcare providers created by capitation requires a paradigm shift in the way we think about payment. Compliance concerns related to payment are also significantly different. While a full discussion of these compliance issues is beyond the scope of this book, a few of the concerns are diametric opposites of those that affect cost-based, PPS, and non-capitated managed care payment systems. The concerns include:

- Inadequate care
- Lack of specialist referrals
- Patient dumping
- Non-existent covered lives
- Out-of-plan services

This list can certainly be longer. The basic idea is the shift of economic risk to providers provides a strong economic incentive to reduce costs, including utilization costs. Most compliance concerns in this area involve inappropriate techniques to reduce utilization and consumption of resources that may or may not be covered by fixed payments under capitation.

Since capitated arrangements are relatively new, much is to be learned about the compliance issues they present. The penetration of capitated arrangements, as with all types of managed care, is highly dependent upon geographic location. One growing concern is the relationship between capitated systems and the more traditional cost-based or PPS systems. A patient under a managed care plan may present to a provider that is not a part of the plan, receive services, and express surprise when the services are not covered. Some patients even seek services not covered through their HMOs. Payment to a provider who is not part of a managed care plan can be problematic. Difficulties with payment system interfaces often lead to compliance concerns.

Depending on geographic location and dispersion of a healthcare organization, managed care compliance may constitute great concern or a passing concern if the revenue stream from such payment arrangements is small. CBR compliance personnel must be cognizant of the differences in compliance concerns in this area and make appropriate adjustments to their programs.

Key learning area: Most current CBR compliance problems reside with payment systems based on utilization or fee-for-service arrangements. A developing area of concern is compliance with a special form of managed care involving capitation. Recognizing new compliance concerns requires a mental paradigm shift reflecting changes in payment approaches and a shift of financial risk to providers.

CBR compliance officer

A CBR compliance officer is a key player in developing a program that addresses the many issues surrounding coding, documentation, billing, and reimbursement. A sample job description is provided in the appendix. Human resources must work with the CCO to fill this position, depending on the size and complexity of the healthcare organization. In small hospitals or medical clinics, one part-time person may be assigned to this position. Larger hospitals and multispecialty clinics may require a full-time person. Large integrated delivery systems may include a fully staffed department in which each individual performs one or more specific CBR functions as needed. The basic job functions remain the same; the scope and diversity of CBR situations change.

The relationship of CBR compliance personnel to the corporate compliance program can also vary. The corporate compliance office of a small organization

such as a rural hospital or single-specialty clinic may also handle CBR compliance. Small organizations may have no need for specially designated CBR compliance staffs.

As the size, scope, and diversity of a healthcare organization grow, the need arises to differentiate the responsibilities of the corporate compliance officer from those of the CBR compliance officer. A CCO for a large organizations will normally have some legal expertise; the CBR compliance officer is more likely to have technical skill in coding, billing, and payment systems.

The CBR compliance officer of a large organization reports to the CCO along a distinct chain of command and with appropriate delegation of authority. This ensures that the CBR compliance officer has appropriate access to the administrative ranks, including the board of directors. The office or department dealing with billing compliance often manages personnel at different locations, engages internal auditing staff, and coordinates the work of outside consultants and legal counsel. As shown in Figure 10.2, some overlapping of functions occurs. Such overlapping is natural because it indicates that various activities fall under the scope of CBR.

The top part of the chart shows the interface to the CCO and corporate compliance program. This level also involves interfaces to external consultants and legal counsel. Periodic external reviews by consultants are typical parts of a review and auditing program for a healthcare organization. External consultants provide objectivity. The advice of legal counsel may be needed to handle questions about self-reporting and/or other legal matters. Opinions on such matters

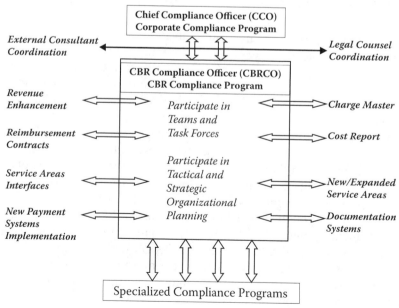

Figure 10.2 Additional interfaces to CBR compliance program.

can come from legal counsel or may be submitted to the OIG with a request for an advisory opinion.

The bottom of the chart shows interface to other (if any) specialized compliance programs. The chart also includes a list of areas in which CBR compliance personnel should be routinely involved.

Chargemaster

The chargemaster is both a direct target of compliance issues and a key component of the CBR process. A hospital at the 200-bed or larger level will typically have a full-time person devoted to maintaining the chargemaster.* Any change made to the chargemaster should involve CBR compliance personnel and the chargemaster should be reviewed by external consultants every three to five years.

Revenue enhancement

Implementation of changes to meet compliance requirements in the CBR area also often increases reimbursement. Any changes made to enhance reimbursement should be carefully reviewed from a compliance perspective, and CBR compliance personnel should be an integral part of any such efforts. Including CBR compliance representatives on teams and committees addressing revenue enhancement is a must.

Reimbursement contracts

Most healthcare organizations have contracts with third-party payers. The wide range of types of contracts impose significant requirements involving coding, billing, reimbursement, and/or special reporting. In addition to basic contracts for specific services or areas, master contracts apply to higher organizational levels. All contracts should also be carefully reviewed from a CBR compliance perspective. At the very least, CBR compliance personnel should verify that all contractual obligations are met. Note that special considerations arise when a third-party payer is also a secondary payer for Medicare. Issues such as discounting may need to be reviewed, with particular attention on how such arrangements might affect (or be affected by) safe harbors for the Medicare Fraud, Abuse, and Anti-Kickback Law.

> **Case study 10-2. Chargemaster review in contract.** Apex Medical Center is renewing a contract with a private third-party payer. This fee-for-service contract basically pays 85 percent

of the charges for both outpatient and inpatient services. A new contract clause allows the payer to audit Apex's chargemaster every three years. The managed care contracting personnel at Apex contracted the Chargemaster Coordinator and CBR compliance personnel to see whether this audit requirement is appropriate.

Whether such a contractual obligation is reasonable is a decision that the hospital must make. If a contract requires audits, the parameters and methodology should be known in advance. This small example shows why it is important to include CBR compliance personnel in contract matters.

Service area interfaces

Compliance concerns proliferate at every service area interface. Status changes from outpatient to inpatient, from inpatient to skilled nursing, from inpatient to subacute care, and various downstream services create the potential for compliance problems. This is particularly true for areas that have distinctly different payment systems. Within Medicare, significant problems can arise from the relationship between Part A and Part B payments. For this reason, CBR compliance personnel must be involved when interfaces among service areas are proposed or changed and/or when problems arise.

Cost reports

Developing cost reports is a highly technical activity. While CBR compliance personnel will probably not be involved in the accounting details of a cost report, they must be involved at a conceptual level. Cost reports are direct targets of compliance investigations. The coordination of cost reports, cost accounting systems, the chargemaster, and the overall philosophy underlying cost report development must be taken into account.

New and expanded service areas

New and expanded service areas continue to develop at a rapid pace, particularly in outpatient areas. CBR compliance and coding and billing management personnel must be involved in strategic planning for new service areas. CBR compliance measures must be addressed before implementation. How such services are organized is of particular concern. The chargemaster structure and billing process are also concerns. All these factors influence a healthcare organization's compliance stance. (See the rules and regulations regarding provider-based status relative to organizing hospital owned clinics.)

---

* See the author's book about the chargemaster; it is listed in the bibliography.

Documentation systems

The cry that "we can't code what isn't documented" can extend easily to "we can't bill for what is not coded." Both statements lead to the conclusion that documentation is the driving force that starts the coding, billing, and reimbursement cycle. Thus, the systematic process whereby documentation is developed is of special concern for CBR compliance personnel. The systems may be manual, partly automated, or fully computer-based. They typically use templates and a variety of forms and flow sheets. All these components can enhance documentation, but if not properly designed, they will introduce systematic deficiencies into the process. To prevent this (or at least indicate potential risk factors), CBR compliance personnel must be involved in discussions about documentation system development and computer automation.

Key learning area: The role of the CBR compliance officer varies from organization to organization. The position can be part-time or may require creation of a new department. CBR compliance personnel must participate in activities such as revenue enhancement, chargemaster updating, reimbursement contracting, and tactical and strategic planning.

Integrating CBR compliance with other compliance programs

The corporate compliance program is the starting point for compliance activities within a healthcare organization—from a one-physician practice to a multihospital integrated delivery system. A CBR compliance program concentrates on complex coding, documentation, billing, and payment system considerations and represents most of an organization's compliance activities. Because of its wide scope, a CBR program must interface to other programs and the interface should include a degree of commonality.

Figure 10.3 shows where and how a CBR compliance program overlaps with other areas. Each program depicted has policies and procedures covering both coding and billing and audit activities for coding, billing, and documentation. As discussed in Chapter 9, all these elements come together when a baseline compliance audit is conducted. Whenever possible, a CBR compliance program should pull together all existing commonalties.

A number of areas bill for services in the form of units, and more specifically, time units. Delineating a consistent standard for coding and billing time units is a compliance issue. Time units are embedded in coding structures in certain areas. Physical therapy

modalities are measured in 15-minute units. Infusion therapy codes use 1-hour units. A hospital may also use time units internally to develop charges for surgery time, recovery time, anesthesia time, etc. The compliance question is, for the last subsequent time unit, how many minutes must a provider render a service before counting a full unit? The most common answer is the one-half time unit approach as developed through Medicare: a service must be provided for one-half of the time unit before a provider can count the last subsequent unit for coding and billing services. The first time unit can also become a coding and billing issue. For example, the first hour of critical care must extend at least half an hour before it can be coded and billed.

Applying the one-half time unit rule for a 15-minute unit translates into 7.5 minutes, generally rounded to 8 minutes. For other time units, the one-half calculation is straightforward. The variations in time units require a policy directing how many units are to be billed for a service. In some cases, Medicare insists that the actual start and stop times must be documented and reported on claim forms. An organization-wide policy and procedure for counting time units will cut across different service areas, some of which may have their own compliance policies and procedures for coding and billing. This is another example of overlap of compliance programs.

All service areas, with or without separate compliance programs, perform compliance activities, many of which are common to all areas. For example, informal reviews and formal audits relative to coding, documentation, and billing will be performed in all areas and their audit guidelines and auditor checklists will be similar. After an audit checklist is designed for one area, it can be fairly easy to adjust the design to make it appropriate for a related area. Similarly, the statistical

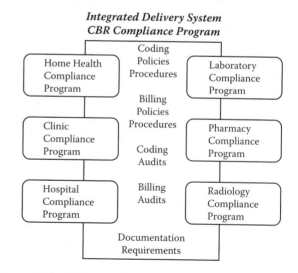

Figure 10.3 CBR compliance plan overlap.

process of selecting cases for review can cut across several areas. While the process will vary somewhat, the statistical basics are already in place.

Another area where uniformity and consistency can come into play is the billing system. While it would be wonderful to have a single system with the capabilities of total billing for all services, the state of the art tends to favor specialized separate systems or subsystems within a single system. While the objective is to generate proper bills and claims, such systems form the bases for powerful databases. However, the abilities to generate similar reports and thus monitor activities from a compliance perspective impose different requirements. A CBR compliance program can help pull these disparate pieces together for organizational consistency and address (1) service area interfaces and (2) payment system interfaces from two perspectives. Both interfaces constitute significant compliance problems within the CBR area and this can lead to concern about the interface to the corporate compliance program. In cases where individual specialized compliance programs are not coordinated or interfaced means that interfaces are addressed only on an ad hoc basis and coordination would occur only when problems or conflicts arise. For instance, a hospital may provide skilled nursing facility services and also hyperbaric oxygen therapy on an outpatient basis. These two types of services may use different payment systems and the service areas must coordinate which one provides which services, when they are provided, and how to bill correctly. Medicare considers hyperbaric oxygen therapy a skilled nursing benefit and thus not payable as an outpatient service.

Key learning area: CBR compliance personnel must fully understand the different payment systems that reimburse for a wide variety of services and must be acutely aware of how these payment systems interface, their special billing requirements, and the need for diverse service areas to work together to achieve coordinated compliance.

Documenting compliance activities and keeping records

Documenting all compliance activities including policies and procedures, training, employee interviews, hotline calls, patient complaints, identified problems, solutions, baseline audit results, annual reports, and other factors is a matter of great concern at corporate

compliance level. This concern is almost immediately passed down to the CBR compliance level.

A great deal of emphasis has been placed on the development of CBR compliance manuals and the associated coding and billing policies and procedures. Beyond these obvious documentation necessities lies a much larger realm of compliance documentation needs. Training should be carefully documented—both the formal (internal and external) and the informal on-the-job and just-a-quick-question instruction. Activities resulting from CBR compliance personnel participation on teams and committees must be documented and minutes and notes of meetings should be kept. CBR compliance personnel participate in telephone conversations, e-mail discussions, fax exchanges, and other communications. To ensure that documentation is complete, they should be encouraged to keep personal logs of telephone calls (who, when, topics discussed, directions given, conclusions reached, etc.). Additionally, e-mail communications should be retained and organized (by person, topic, organization, function, etc.). Other forms of communication should also saved and organized. These efforts will pay dividends if (or more likely when) you are questioned or called into court to testify.

Key learning area: CBR compliance personnel are encouraged to keep extensive detailed records of all compliance activities. They should also maintain logs of telephone calls and meetings.

The use of e-mail requires a special note. E-mail communication over the Internet, organizational intranets and extranets, and even over local area networks has grown tremendously. While most e-mail involves communications that should be kept, filed, and organized, some e-mails should not have been sent, went to the wrong recipient, were only partially completed, unintelligible, or simply wrong. These problem e-mails can cause unanticipated problems for an organization. CBR compliance personnel are advised to communicate electronically with care.

In Chapter 12 we will discuss the HIPAA privacy and administrative simplification rules that engendered elevated concern about removing documents from computer systems so that they cannot be retrieved. These concerns revolve around the concept of protected health information. Among other concerns, can you be certain that a file has been removed from your computer system? Are communications transmitted to and from your computer system secure?

Depending upon your organization's understanding of HIPAA directives, both questions are relatively simple to handle. Deleting a file from your computer system does not necessarily mean that the message has disappeared for good. To ensure that a file cannot be recovered, it is literally necessary to "shred"* the file inside your system by overwriting it with randomly generated characters. Department of Defense Standard DOD 5220-22M covers this process.

The second situation involving the privacy of transmitted messages may require encrypting (by a sender) and unencrypting messages received. This can be complicated but compliance personnel may find it beneficial or necessary to master the technique. Great strides have been made in developing hardware appliances ensuring secure communications.

Key learning area: In times of high compliance anxiety, due consideration should be given to the ability to completely remove documents from computer systems. Additionally, concerns about privacy in communications, particularly e-mail communications, should be addressed.

Record retention

Another area impacting CBR compliance concerns is record retention—a long-standing issue for healthcare organizations, primarily on the clinical side. "How long must we keep medical records?" is a common question. Since implementation of the HIPAA privacy rule, healthcare organizations must carefully define designated record sets. While we are all accustomed to protecting the privacy of clinical records, the HIPAA rules also cover what might be called business records including itemized statements and claims. The entire subject of record retention now affects the coding, billing and reimbursement world as well.

It is imperative to understand that no single answer covers the issue of how long to retain billing, claims, and reimbursement records. General financial and tax guidelines can be applied. An alternative approach is to ask how far back the OIG and Department of Justice will investigate in recoupment and/or criminal prosecutions. They sometimes go back as far as ten years. While this is not the norm, it can be used as a baseline to start thinking about retention times for billing and claims data. You should probably also check state law requirements and the conditions for participation under Medicare.

An associated problem for most healthcare organizations is that most billing and claims filing processes are computer-based. The task of keeping itemized billing statements and associated claim forms can

be overwhelming. Ensuring logical organization of records is an even more difficult task. One alternative is to organize alphabetically, by patient, and then in reverse chronological order.

Other questions involve the amount of billing and claims information kept in clinical or medical records and whether billing information should be correlated to and kept with claims information. While a healthcare organization may not keep itemized statements and claims, it may have a need to regenerated billing information at a later date. This means that the constantly updated chargemaster must be archived so that past claims can be faithfully reproduced. These and similar questions should be carefully considered and policies and procedures covering them must be put into place.

Billing and claims information is computerized and claims are often filed electronically. It is therefore logical that any statement or claim form could be regenerated, but other questions arise. For example, how far back can statements and claims be regenerated? Is it possible that a regenerated claim will differ from the original?

The first question is purely a computer matter. Billing information is typically retained for months and often for several years. However, at some point, the information is archived, typically to a magnetic medium. The issue then becomes whether it is possible to restore the archived data and make it useful. This may not be a straightforward as it appears. The basic charge data may have been saved, but is the chargemaster that generated the statement or claim still the same? In other words was the chargemaster also saved so that it could be used generate archived claims and statements?

A more fundamental question lies with the life cycle of a hospital or clinic billing system. How long does a typical healthcare organization use a computer system without replacing it or making significant upgrades to hardware and software? In today's healthcare environment, system changes are relatively frequent. In some cases, major changes are made almost annually. A more pressing question is whether the computer system currently in use can generate or even read materials archived five or six years earlier.

The question about the chargemaster's ability to generate archived materials is interesting. As an experiment, pull a small sampling of paper statements and associated claims from a year earlier and instruct your system to regenerate the same claims and statements. It is likely that you will find the regenerated claims and statements are different from the paper counterparts. One reason is that one set or the other may have been altered. For example, late charges may have been added only to one set. Errors may have been found

---

* Yes, the analogy is to a paper shredder that can destroy and make paper documents unrecoverable.

and corrected long after the original claims were filed. These are only two examples of thousands of changes that can occur over time. The bottom line is that what a computer system generates today may be different from what was generated years ago.

Key learning area: Record retention is a general compliance issue that takes on new significance in the CBR area. Questions about record retention and/or the ability to regenerate billing and claims information as early as ten years back must be carefully considered.

Investigation and subpoena response planning

One significant concern at corporate compliance level is preparing the organization for formal visits from auditors and law enforcement personnel. A related, if smaller concern, is preparing a response to a subpoena for documents and/or information. This concern is highly applicable to the CBR area. Law enforcement personnel may approach employees working in the CBR area and simply ask for information. In other cases, a formal process will generate legal documents requesting information. In the worst cases, law enforcement officials simply back up their trucks and haul evidence away.

It is extremely important for the corporate compliance program personnel and their counterparts in the CBR compliance program to make certain that the organization and all its employees are prepared to properly respond to investigators and requests for information. In the CBR area, this covers a wide range of employees and job levels. For this reason, it is important that explicit written policies and procedures address all levels of inquiries. Additionally, employees must be fully trained in how to conduct themselves during such investigations and how to respond to requests by auditors and/or law enforcement officials. Emphasis should be placed on contacting supervisors, managers, and administrators, meeting only the legal requirements, and providing only the information requested.

Every inquiry about a healthcare organization's coding, documentation, billing, and/or reimbursement activities should be viewed as a compliance concern. Although requests for records may seem innocent (an FI may simply request copies of ten observation stays or a carrier may ask data on ten new patient visits), be certain to review the situation carefully and assess the potential ramifications of delivering the requested information to the party requesting it.

The HIPAA Privacy Rule defined much of the coding, billing, and reimbursement information to be included under the parameters of protected health information (PHI). Electronic health information under the HIPAA security rule may be referred to as EPHI or electronic PHI. Many inquiries and requests for CBR information must be addressed by policies and procedures covering HIPAA privacy and security concerns.

Key learning area: Every inquiry made of a healthcare organization regarding coding, documentation, billing, and reimbursement must be viewed from a compliance perspective. Generally, CBR information is considered protected health information under HIPAA. Any paper or electronic information should leave the organization only after a careful review by CBR compliance personnel.

CBR personnel, especially at management levels, should also be alerted to the fact that law enforcement agents typically visit healthcare providers during regular business hours. However, in some cases they may visit individual employees at home. Clear standards and procedures to prepare personnel for such visits must be included in compliance preparation.

Key learning area: It is imperative to prepare the organization and personnel about appropriate conduct and communication during visits by investigators, outside auditors, and/or law enforcement officials. Prior planning for such visits should be carefully crafted and all employees trained appropriately.

Summary and conclusions

The corporate and CBR compliance programs are distinctly different but share certain commonalties. The biggest difference lies in context and intent. A corporate compliance program functions at a higher organizational level and is more broadly based in that it addresses all possible compliance areas. A CBR program tends to be more focused and concentrates on highly technical issues. Both programs must address the seven compliance principles and great care must be taken to properly interface the two programs. For very small healthcare organizations, this is typically not a problem because the two programs may be fully integrated and administered by the same person. Larger organizations may maintain the two programs separately and employ a CBR compliance officer or even a department to address the various issues. Additionally, CBR compliance personnel must be involved in related areas such as revenue enhancement, cost reporting, documentation systems, and the chargemaster.

eleven

HIPAA compliance

Introduction

HIPAA, the Health Insurance Portability and Accountability Act, was passed by Congress in 1996 and will affect healthcare delivery and healthcare compliance for many years to come. While many aspects of HIPAA directly impact CBR issues, other features are more incidental to CBR compliance concerns. However, narrowing our focus to the issues involving coding, billing, reimbursement, and associated healthcare payment processes, only slightly reduces the scope and complexity of the rules that this legislation encompasses.

Note: For privacy and administrative simplifcation, the rules and regulations as developed by CMS for implementation of HIPAA are found at 45 CFR §§160, 162, 163. Many of the CBR related Medicare rules are located within the various sections in chapter 42 of the CFR. This is a slight, but important, departure when researching issues at the CFR level.

In this discussion of HIPAA, the general term "provider" will be used to indicate any individual or organization that provides healthcare services or dispenses healthcare related items. CMS, in 42 CFR §424, has a slightly different definition of "provider" (i.e., hospitals and other that have a provider agreement) and differentiates "providers" from "suppliers" (i.e., physicians, clinics, DME companies, and others not classified as providers). Similar distinctions appear in other legislation on related issues, and readers are cautioned to understand the exact context of the information being studied. For example, the Administrative Simplification Compliance Act (ASCA)—Public Law 107-105 provides for an exemption from the HIPAA TSC (Transaction Standard/Standard Code Set) rule for small employers, but the law actually includes two provisions for this exemption—one for providers and one for suppliers.*

HIPAA privacy

The provisions of the HIPAA Privacy Rule went into effect on April 14, 2003, after significant preparation by hospitals, clinics, pharmacies, clearinghouse, insurance companies, and organizations that are gener-

ally are referred to as "covered entities." Interestingly enough, Congress added the privacy portion of this public law at the last minute. Clearly, however, the issue of privacy is certainly an important aspect of healthcare, one that affects not only patients but providers and suppliers and many others associated with the healthcare field.

There are many different facets to the HIPAA Privacy Rule. The basic idea behind all the provisions within the rule is to protect the confidentiality of patient information and to control the disclosure of protected health information (PHI). The regulatory body for privacy is the Civil Rights Commission, a fact that makes the HIPAA Privacy Rule distinctly different from the administrative simplification provisions that are under the control of CMS.†

In creating the HIPAA Privacy Rule, Congress provided for an *extremely* broad definition of protected health information. The definition, in fact, is easier to understand when "health information" and "protected health information" are addressed separately. Let's start by looking at the definition of health information (45 CFR §103).

> **Health information** *means any information, whether oral or recorded in any form or medium, that:*
>
> *(1) Is created or received by a health care provider, health plan, public health authority, employer, life insurer, school or university, or health care clearinghouse; and*
>
> *(2) Relates to the past, present, or future physical or mental health or condition of an individual; the provision of health care to an individual; or the past, present, or future payment for the provision of health care to an individual.*

CFR then defines protected health information as health information that is:

1. Transmitted by electronic media;
2. Maintained in electronic media; or
3. Transmitted or maintained in any other form or medium.

---

* See the August 15, 2003 *Federal Register*, page 48807. (68 FR 48807)

† Note that CMS also administers the Medicare Program. Thus, CMS has a dual role of administering HIPAA Administrative Simplification as well as Medicare. This dual role has the potential of creating conflicts of interest during development of rules and regulations.

A careful reading of the aggregated definition of PHI certainly indicates that almost anything relating to an individual's health falls under this rule. While we tend to think about PHI in terms of medical records or clinical services documentation, CFR's definition goes well beyond the scope of traditional medical records and documents and includes a great deal of information that is normally within the sphere of coding, billing, and reimbursement. We briefly addressed this concept in Chapter 10 relative to record retention under the corporate compliance plan.

This takes us to yet another key term, "designated record set," which is defined below. (See 45 CFR §165.501.)

Designated record set means:

(1) *A group of records maintained by or for a covered entity that is:*
   (i) *The medical records and billing records about individuals maintained by or for a covered health care provider;*
   (ii) *The enrollment, payment, claims adjudication, and case or medical management record systems maintained by or for a health plan; or*
   (iii) *Used, in whole or in part, by or for the covered entity to make decisions about individuals.*
(2) *For purposes of this paragraph, the term record means any item, collection, or grouping of information that includes protected health information and is maintained, collected, used, or disseminated by or for a covered entity.*

This definition clearly states that much of the information with which CBR personnel work is PHI and falls squarely under the HIPAA Privacy Rule. The phrase "business record," in this context, is more or less analogous to "medical record." Thus, a CBR compliance plan must address these privacy issues just as a medical records department would address them at a hospital. A full discussion of the many different aspects of the HIPAA Privacy Rule, even as it applies only to coding, billing, and reimbursement issues, is beyond the scope of this book. However, it is important for any personnel affected by the HIPAA Privacy Rule to be aware of issues such as Business Associate Agreements (BAAs) and various disclosure rules and procedures.

The questions that arise can be quite subtle. One reason for this is that legislation on health information privacy is multileveled. Although the HIPAA Privacy Rule is national, there are also many state laws that address health information privacy. A simple case study shows how questions about privacy issues can arise. The setting for this case study is the fictitious Apex Medical Center featured in previous chapters of this book.

Case study 11-1. Divorce case—Release of information. Steve is the estranged husband of Susan. Steve and Susan are in the middle of a difficult divorce. Steve is responsible for the co-payments on hospital and medical care that Susan has recently received. He is at Apex Medical Center's Patient Financial Accounting office demanding a detailed statement and a copy of the claim form. He has stopped short of requesting the medical record as it pertains to her medical care, but his comments suggest that he will soon be asking for this information as well. Hospital staff are concerned that Steve is trying to obtain information that might be used in the divorce proceedings. Should the information be released to Steve?

A careful analysis of even this little case study requires a great deal of study and no simple solution exists without additional information. For one thing, the question should not be answered without a legal opinion from an attorney qualified to deal with health information privacy as it pertains to the marital issue, especially when a divorce is pending. In addition, it is necessary to review and analyze the provisions of any applicable state laws. This case study clearly illustrates the need for CBR compliance personnel to become familiar with various aspects of the HIPAA Privacy Rule, even though this rule would seem to be only incidental to the coding, billing, and reimbursement functions at a hospital or clinic.

Key learning area: The HIPAA Privacy Rule is a major compliance issue for all hospitals, clinics, and other healthcare providers. While the coding, billing, and reimbursement issues involving health care services may not appear to be affected by the privacy requirements, CBR information is considered to be Protected Health Information (PHI), and all the applicable regulations and procedures must be carefully observed.

See the CD-ROM accompanying this book for additional information.

HIPAA transaction standard/standard code set rule

The HIPAA Transaction Standard/Standard Code Set Rule (HIPAA TSC) directly impacts coding, billing, and reimbursement personnel for all types of healthcare providers. While the overall intent of the code set rule is to standardize and foster EDI (Electronic Data Interchange), there are many distinct facets to this process. Providers and payers alike are to follow the rules, and this includes clearinghouses and other organizations that process and/or otherwise assist in the transmission and processing of claims.

Key learning area: The objectives and purposes of HIPAA TSC are quite appropriate. However, the specific goals associated with this rule can be quite elusive and will probably take years to achieve. From a compliance perspective, whenever circumstances force a provider, such as a hospital or clinic, to deviate from what appears to be an written or legislated standard, care should be taken to document the exception and the reason why any directive was not followed. Written policies and procedures should be used to provide some degree of compliance protection.

The basic concept of the HIPAA TSC Rule is fairly simple. There should be standard code sets used in standard formats for electronic submission and processing. *In theory*, a healthcare provider should be able to provide a service and/or supply items, prepare a claim with the standard code sets in a standard format, and file the standard claim to any third-party payer. By standardizing this whole process, claims can be processed very quickly, there can be secondary claims cross-over that occurs automatically, and payments can be made very quickly.

The HIPAA TSC had a rather unusual start. The official starting date was October 16, 2002. However, an extension was granted to every covered entity that filed an extension plan. This extension plan provision ensured that the HIPAA TSC would be operationally intact and in place by October 16, 2003.

The sections below explore some of the key components of the HIPAA TSC Rule. This discussion will be relatively brief and will concentrate on the impact of the HIPAA TSC relative to coding, billing, and reimbursement compliance.

Standard code sets

There are numerous code sets that are used on claim forms. The 1500 claim form (CMS-1500 for Medicare) and the UB-04 claim form (CMS-1450 for Medicare) have many different fields, and thus a number of different code sets are used. Because everything is now supposed to be electronic, it seems logical to address the electronic formats for these claims, that is, the Form 837-P for professional claims (P for Professional)

and the Form 837-I for technical component claims (I for Institutional). However, for the purposes of this book, this discussion focuses on the paper format and associated fields.

For any standard code set, the key issues are:

1. The code set itself,
2. The standard code set maintainer.

Thus, for compliance purposes, let alone claim filing, healthcare providers must be intimately familiar with the various code sets that are used on claim forms and also with the organization that maintains the given code set. Guidance for the use of any given code set is to be issued by the standard code set maintainer. Since there is uniform guidance, everyone can use the code set the same way. Thus, providers can file uniform claims and third-party payers know the format of claims and the codes that will be used.

One of the code sets routinely used by physicians and hospitals is CPT or Current Procedural Terminology. This is a classification code set that has been designed, developed, and used by physicians to codify the services that physicians perform in various settings. There is an extensive set of modifiers, and this code set is updated each calendar year. Guidelines for the use of CPT come from the American Medical Association (AMA), which is the standard code set maintainer.

Note that the time period for any given code set to be in place is strictly limited. For CPT, this means one calendar year. Thus, on January 1 of each year, the new or amended codes go into effect immediately. There is no grace period, and healthcare providers and third-party payers using CPT must adjust their systems just as the New Year starts. In practice, this process may not always work. Healthcare providers should be prepared for possible claims adjudication problems with the implementation of an updated code set.

The CPT code set also underscores one of the challenges faced by CBR compliance personnel. As noted above, CPT is used by physicians, but it is also used by hospitals for filing outpatient claims on the UB-04 or Form 837-I. However, the basic coding process involved is different for hospitals and physicians. While this situation, in and of itself, is not necessarily a problem, one compliance issue that arises is who is to provide guidance on the use of CPT for hospital outpatient coding. A great number of guidelines related to CPT can be found in the CPT Manual, but most of these are for physicians. How are hospitals supposed to interpret this guidance on the hospital or technical component side?

Because hospitals are required to use CPT coding, the HIPAA TSC Rule mandates that the standard code set maintainer provide guidance for the use of CPT codes for hospital claims. However, because the CPT code set has been developed for physician utilization, this means timely guidance for hospital utilization of CPT may not be available. This becomes a major CBR compliance issue because the absence of formal guidelines makes it necessary for hospitals to make decisions about how to code, bill, and file claims. In such cases, hospitals must make considered decisions and ensure that carefully crafted policies and procedures are developed and carefully maintained until official guidelines become available.

Note: This issue of formal guidance from the standard code set maintainer is a major issue. While the code sets may be properly developed and maintained, these code sets are used by third-party payers within the context of a multitude of payment systems. Often third-party payers will issue guidance relative to their specific payment system that mandates the use or non-use of certain codes in a particular manner. This guidance may not be universal for all third-party payers and also may go beyond guidance provided by the standard code set maintainer.

A second major classification system is ICD-9. ICD-9 has been scheduled to be replaced by ICD-10 or maybe even ICD-11 for several years. Whichever new version is finally adopted, this is a major system consisting of both diagnosis codes and procedure codes. This code set is updated on a Federal Fiscal Year basis, that is, on October 1 of each year. The diagnosis portion of this code set is maintained by the American Hospital Association in the United States, although the World Health Organization is the international sponsor of this code set. The procedure coding system is maintained by CMS. Virtually all healthcare providers use this code set, at least the diagnosis portion. The procedure coding system is generally used for hospital inpatient claims filing.

The coding guidelines are embedded within the ICD-9-CM Manual and in a separate document that provides official coding guidelines separated into hospital and physician or outpatient guidelines. A quarterly publication, the *Coding Clinic*, which is issued by the AHA, provides additional information about ICD-9-CM.*

CMS has also developed another classification system, namely the HCPCS (Healthcare Common Procedure Coding System) codes. This code set is maintained by CMS, except for the dental codes, which are maintained by the American Dental Association. Major updates to this code set are made at the beginning of each calendar year, and there are also quarterly updates. Although this coding system is developed by and used mainly by CMS, other third-party payers also use it. As with ICD-9-CM there is a publication, *Coding Clinic for HCPCS*, published through the AHA that provides guidance on interpreting HCPCS codes.

Moving beyond the CPT, HCPCS, and ICD-9-CM code sets, there is a vast range of other code sets that are used on various claim forms. We will look briefly at three of these code sets, just as examples. CBR compliance personnel should be very careful to understand each and every one of these codes sets and learn to "read between the lines" to interpret any nuances.

Revenue codes

The revenue codes are used on the UB-04 claim form, that is, by hospitals. These codes are usually embedded in the hospital's chargemaster or charge description master (CDM). Technically, this is a four digit numeric code; in practice, however, hospitals often refer to the three digit version. For instance, revenue code 450 refers to services in the Emergency Department of a hospital; revenue code 510 refers to clinic services; and revenue code 360 refers to the operating room.

This code set is maintained by the National Uniform Billing Committee (NUBC).† A manual is available on an annual basis and is distributed by the American Hospital Association through State Uniform Billing Committees that are generally sponsored by state hospital associations. There is also a national level manual, *Official UB-04 Data Specification Manual*, directly available from NUBC that provides a great deal of information.

The definition and descriptions of the revenue codes tend to be somewhat cryptic. Although actual use of many codes is fairly straightforward, there is rarely any explicit guidance on how codes are to be used in any unusual circumstances. In practice, the third-party payers will sometimes provide claims adjudication requirements relative to revenue code utilization that can conflict with official guidelines. This runs counter to the whole philosophical thrust of standardization of the HIPAA TSC Rule, and is a situation that must be addressed by hospitals.

Because hospitals may be required to use different revenue codes to meet the specific demands of various third-party payers, there are immediate CBR compliance concerns. Whenever decisions are made to use revenue codes in different ways, this process should be documented and embedded in written policies and procedures.

---

* A quick reading of the official ICD-9-CM coding guidelines will reveal that this document has actually been prepared to provide guidance in coding for the DRG payment system. Additional guidance for physicians, outpatient services, and present-on-admission (POA) has been added over time.

† See http://www.nubc.org.

Condition codes

This is another code set used on the UB-04. The official code set is developed and maintained by the NUBC. Thus, the NUBC is supposed to provide the "official" guidelines and definitions for these codes. However, as with revenue codes, third-party payers may make requirements that go beyond the official definitions. (One such situation is illustrated below.) CBR compliance personnel are urged, once again, to address these situations through written policies and procedures.

Condition Code 44 is used on the UB-04 to indicate that an encounter initially classified as an inpatient admission is being changed to an outpatient encounter, generally for observation services. The NUBC definition is:

> *Condition Code 44: Inpatient admission changed to outpatient—For use on outpatient claims only, when the physician ordered inpatient services, but upon internal review performed before the claim was initially submitted, the hospital determined the services did not meet its inpatient criteria.*

As you can see, there are two critical criteria included in this definition:

1. The change from inpatient to outpatient must be made before the claim is filed, and
2. The hospital is to determine if the services did not meet inpatient criteria.

The development of this Condition Code by the NUBC was very much welcomed by hospitals because it made it easier for hospitals to address situations that were sometimes difficult to classify for coding purposes and subsequent claims filing—i.e., situations in which a patient was admitted, care was provided, but at a later time (generally within a few days) the hospital determined that the services were actually observation services and that inpatient criteria were not met.

However, when this Condition Code was published, CMS decided to establish a much more stringent definition for the use of Condition Code 44. In Transmittal 299 to the Medicare Claims Processing Manual, dated October 10, 2004, CMS mandated the following requirements:

> The change in patient status from inpatient to outpatient is made prior to discharge or release, while the beneficiary is still a patient of the hospital;
>
> The hospital has not submitted a claim to Medicare for the inpatient admission;

> A physician concurs with the utilization review committee's decision; and
>
> The physician's concurrence with the utilization review committee's decision is documented in the patient's medical record.

A careful reading of this expanded policy definition indicates that the change must occur while the patient is still in the hospital and the physician must agree with the change in status. In practice, hospitals generally find these more restrictive requirements to be onerous and even unworkable. The result can be that services are provided to Medicare patients and there is no reimbursement at all!

The question that is raised is: Who really sets the definitions and policies for the use of Condition Code 44 within the condition code set? It would appear that, according to the HIPAA TSC Rule, the NUBC is the official source of guidance. However, in this case CMS appears to be overriding the NUBC definition and thus hospitals are thrown into situations that create significant compliance concerns.

Note: This is only one example of a very large and complex issue. CBR compliance personnel must be watchful to recognize when there are special requirements being made by third-party payers that go beyond the official guidance provided by the designated code set maintainer.

Place of service codes

The POS code set is used on the 1500 claim form to indicate where services were provided. This code set is under the purview of the National Uniform Claims Committee (NUCC).* However, the code set is maintained by CMS. This code set can be found at the CMS website and is also published as part of the CPT Manual. For the most part, there is relatively little guidance on exactly how the POS codes are to be interpreted. For instance, POS 11 is described as "office." Does this include clinics? What about services that a physician might provide away from the office, even though they are office related?

Much of the terminology in this area relates to various Medicare rules and regulations. Some third-party payers use this code set as part of the claims adjudication process while other do not use it at all. From a compliance perspective, these types of ambiguities create potential concerns for physicians filing professional claim forms or for hospitals filing professional claim forms on behalf of physicians.

The important point with the POS codes is to understand how third-party payers use this code set in the

---

* See www.nucc.org for additional information.

adjudication of claims. For some third-party payers, there may be differences in the amount of payment made for the same service in different locations, that is, sites of service. Probably the best known and most extensive of these site-of-service differentials is with the Medicare program. Physicians can provide a service in their own freestanding clinics or may go to the hospital on an outpatient basis to perform a service. If a physician is performing the service at the hospital, then his or her overhead has been reduced. Thus, arguably, the physician's payment should be reduced since the hospital will also file a technical component claim on the UB-04. (See Chapter 12 for an additional discussion of the provider-based rule and provider-based clinics.)

The Medicare Physician Fee Schedule (MPFS) has been developed through RBRVS (Resource Based Relative Value System) to accommodate this reduction in payment or the so-called "site-of-service differential." For the reduction to be properly applied, the POS indicator used must show that the services were provided in a facility setting. Most typically this is indicated by using POS 22 or "hospital, outpatient." If a physician provides the services at the hospital but indicates POS 11 for "office," then improper payment will result, that is, the site-of-service differential will not be applied.

While the use of the POS code set might appear to be straightforward, there can be circumstances in which great care must be taken to understand the code set itself and then, most importantly, how the code set will be used. A simple example involving Apex Medical Center illustrates this point.

Case study 11-2. Urgent care clinic place of service. Apex Medical Center has decided to establish an urgent care clinic about five miles from the hospital. This clinic will be open from 5:00 a.m. to 11:00 p.m. seven days a week. The hospital has hired several physicians and practitioners to provide services. Thus, the hospital will be filing both a 1500 claim form for the professional component and a UB-04 for the technical component. (This means that this clinic has been organized to be provider-based for Medicare purposes at least.)

In establishing the 1500 claim generation system, it has been decided to use POS 20 for Urgent Care Facility. The full definition is: Location, distinct from a hospital emergency room, an office, or a clinic, whose purpose is to diagnose and treat illness or injury for unscheduled, ambulatory patients seeking immediate medical attention.

The choice of POS 20 appears to be quite correct since this description fits Apex Medical Center's urgent care clinic. However, a further check is needed, at least for the Medicare program. The question is whether or not this particular POS is classified as "facility" or "non-facility" for the site-of-service differential under RBRVS. A careful check will show that this POS is classified as a non-facility for RBRVS payment purposes even though the word "facility" appears in the description. If Apex Medical Center were to use this POS 20, there would be improper payment for the professional component claims.

Key learning area: There are many standard code sets used by healthcare providers to file claims and receive reimbursement. Each of these code sets has an organization that serves as the standard code set maintainer. The guidelines for using a particular code set reside with the standard code set maintainer. Thus, healthcare providers using a given code set should be able to use the code sets in the same way. In practice, this process is hampered by special requirements or different interpretations on the part of third-party payers.

See CD-ROM accompanying this book for further information.

Standard transaction formats

The HIPAA TSC Rule establishes a number of standard transaction formats. These generally fall under the ASC X12N standards. Below is brief listing:

- Health Claims
  - Institutional—ASC X12N Health Care Claim (837-I)
  - Professional—ASC X12N Health Care Claim (837-P)
- Enrollment & Disenrollment in a Health Plan
  - ASC X12N Benefit Enrollment & Maintenance (834)
- Eligibility for a Health Plan
  - See ASC X12N—270 and 271
- Health Care Payment & Remittance Advice
  - ASC X12N Health Care Claim Payment/Advice (835)
- Health Care Premium Payments
  - See ASC X12N—811 and 820
- Health Claim Status
  - See ASC X12N—276 and 277
- Referral Certification and Authorization
  - ASC X12N Health Care Service Review Information (278)
- Coordination of Benefits—See Form 837

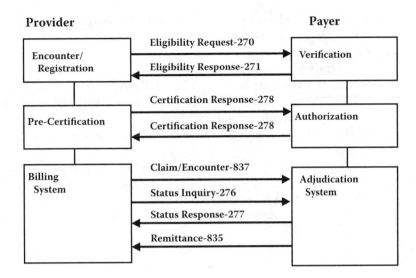

Figure 11.1   Transactions flows with EDI.

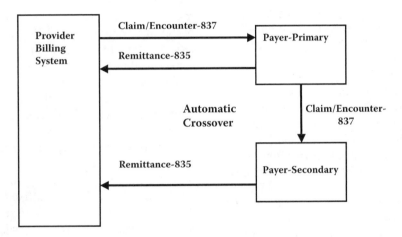

Figure 11.2   Secondary claim automatic cross-over.

Each of these standard formats has an extensive set of computer specifications that involve hundreds of pages of technical information. From a CBR compliance perspective, the main objective is to make certain that claims and other transmissions faithfully follow the technical specifications. The ability of a hospital or clinic or other healthcare provider to meet these various formats is embedded in the billing systems. In many cases healthcare providers may also use clearinghouses to further process their claims to make certain that all the standards are being met.

The basic concept behind this standardization is to allow for EDI or electronic data interchange. Figures 11.1 and 11.2 show the types of information flow that can and/or should occur. Presuming that this can be accomplished electronically and that the standard formats are used and all the necessary information from the standard code sets is provided, the claims adjudication processing should be very quick at both

the primary claim level and the secondary claim level.

Figure 11.1 shows an idealized flow using electronic data interchange or EDI. Since standard transaction formats and standard code sets are utilized, the sequence of events for filing a claim, having the claim adjudicated, and then receiving payment should be accomplished very quickly and with great efficiency.

Figure 11.2 shows the same flow when there is a secondary third-party payer involved. The cross-over claim should occur automatically, again with EDI.

Key learning area: The HIPAA TSC Rule is extensive and complex. This rule directly impacts CBR compliance. CBR compliance personnel must become fully conversant with the many different provisions of this rule, including the various standard code sets and standard transaction formats and associated claims

processing. Care should be taken to understand the organization that is the designated standard code set maintainer and also make certain that the official guidelines for the use of a given standard code set are available and up-to-date.

See the CD accompanying this book for various *Federal Register* entries and associated HIPAA TSC information.

HIPAA security

The implementation of the HIPAA Security Rule lagged behind both privacy and the transaction standards. Implementation finally occurred on April 21, 2005. The final rule was narrowed to address only Electronic Protected Health Information or EPHI. Since this rule was narrowed to just EPHI, the question of security for non-electronic PHI reverted back to the HIPAA Privacy Rule.

A very succinct comparison of the privacy and security rules appears in the February 20, 2003 *Federal Register* on page 8335 (68 FR 8335).

The security standards below define administrative, physical, and technical safeguards to protect the confidentiality, integrity, and availability of electronic protected health information. The standards require covered entities to implement basic safeguards to protect electronic protected health information from unauthorized access, alteration, deletion, and transmission.

The Privacy Rule, by contrast, sets standards for how protected health information should be controlled by setting forth what uses and disclosures are authorized or required and what rights patients have with respect to their health information.

For CBR compliance programs, the HIPAA Security Rule has the least direct impact. Hospitals, clinics, and other healthcare providers are required to meet certain standards for computers, networks, and telecommunications in general. Some of these standards are mandatory while others are simply "addressable" at the provider's discretion. The HIPAA Security Rule is in the domain of information technology. CBR personnel must follow the various directives in using their computer systems. Particular attention must be focused on secure telecommunications processes.

The HIPAA Security Rule applies only to EPHI or Electronic Protected Health Information. The trigger for HIPAA Security to apply is either or both of the following:

- Store PHI electronically
- Transmit PHI electronically

In the current world of electronic computer systems and telecommunication, this means that the HIPAA Security Rule applies to virtually all healthcare providers of almost any type.

The HIPAA Security Rule provides for the overall objectives of security, although the specific way in which the security is to be achieved is often left to the individual providers. Some examples of objectives are:

- EPHI must be secure from unauthorized access
- Backup procedures must be in place
- Electronically transmitted EPHI must be secure
- Disaster recovery procedures must be established

This listing goes on at some length, and, as previously noted, the HIPAA Security Rule delineates requirements as being "mandatory" or "addressable." Obviously, the mandatory issues must be addressed although the way in which a given issue is addressed may vary somewhat. The addressable issues are optional to some degree. Providers are to perform a risk assessment to determine if a given addressable issue should and/or can be addressed.

For CBR compliance personnel the HIPAA Security Rule is not, in and of itself, a major compliance issue. However, this rule does affect everyone that uses the provider's computer system. For instance, the whole area of passwords is an interesting example. Everyone should expect passwords to become longer and be more frequently changed. And, no, you cannot put your password on a sticky note affixed to your workstation! As noted above, the HIPAA Security rule applies only to EPHI while the security for paper-based PHI resides with the HIPAA Privacy Rule. However, security personnel will generally address both the electronic and non-electric circumstances. One example of security policy is putting all PHI into locked storage when an office closes for the day. But for a busy patient financial accounting area, securing all the documents (i.e., claims and other financial documents) that are being processed can be a time-consuming logistical challenge.

Case study 11-3. Contract coding staff. Apex Medical Center has decided to use off-site coding personnel since there is a shortage of qualified coding personnel in Anywhere, USA. The necessary records are scanned and then transmitted to the personal computer of the individual performing the coding. After the coding is completed, the coder sends the result back and then deletes the files from their personal computer.

From a HIPAA Security Rule perspective, there are many questions surrounding this type of arrangement.

For instance, how will the transmissions of these records be kept secure? How will security be maintained at the remote site? Who will have access to the computers at the remote site? When the contract coder is finished with a given file, is the question becomes "how can we be assured that the records are *really* deleted from the coder's personal computer?" Simply hitting the delete key does not erase the files. We briefly addressed this question in Chapter 10 when discussing records and record retention policies and procedures. As indicated there, the solution is to obtain an eraser program that overwrites the file a specified number of times. The Department of Defense (DOD) has a standard for different levels of erasing files. (See DOD 5220 Standard.)

Key learning area: The HIPAA Security Rule has an indirect impact on the coding, billing, and reimbursement functions for a healthcare provider. Only Electronic Protected Health Information (EPHI) is covered by this rule. The requirements are categorized as mandatory or addressable. Non-electronic PHI, generally paper-format PHI, certainly creates security concerns, but any HIPAA security requirements are found within the HIPAA Privacy Rule. The HIPAA Security Rule is very much the domain of information technology personnel, however, CBR compliance personnel will be drawn into situations involving the HIPAA Security Rule.

See the CD accompanying this book for copies of *Federal Register* entries and other information concerning the HIPAA Security Rule.

HIPAA National Provider Identifiers (NPIs)

HIPAA legislation includes provisions for the development of various types of identifiers. Only the provider identifier system has been developed in the form of NPIs or National Provider Identifiers. Under this straightforward system, every provider obtains an identifier number that is recognized and used by all third-party payers. There is a single number assigned for the life of the individual or organization that is used and updated as appropriate.

This new system is designed to simplify the legacy system in which a provider, such as a physician, may have dozens of provider identifying numbers. For instance, on the physician and practitioner side, the UPIN or Unique Physician/Practitioner Identifying Number is replaced by the new NPIs.

While this is a reasonably simple concept, complications can arise. If you are dealing with a single physician who is in practice and organized as a sole proprietor, then only a single NPI needs to be (or for that matter can be) obtained. This is an individual NPI.

However, as the organizational structure become more complex, as in the case of hospitals and systems of hospitals and clinics, the analysis of who and what organizational subunits are to have NPIs can become quite daunting. In this case, organizational NPIs can be obtained.

Note: Providers in complex organizational structures may identify and obtain NPIs for various subunits. Obtaining an NPI does not necessarily mean that a given health plan has to recognize all the NPIs obtained in this manner. As noted on page 3441(69 FR 3441) of the January 23, 2004, *Federal Register*:

> *If an organization health care provider consists of subparts that are identified with their own unique NPIs, a health plan may decide to enroll none, one, or a limited number of them (and to use only the NPI(s) of the one(s) it enrolls).*

Moreover, a health plan cannot require a provider to obtain additional NPIs. This is also addressed in the January 23, 2004, *Federal Register* (page 3441):

> *A health plan may not require a health care provider or a subpart of an organization health care provider that has an NPI to obtain another NPI for any purpose.*

For identifying subunits, there are a number of elements that come into play. First, there are the **providers**, such as physicians, hospitals, clinics, etc. Then there is the **business organization**, which can include sole proprietors, partnerships, limited liability companies, and corporations of various types. Third, are the **tax identification numbers** (TINs) or financial identifier numbers (FINs). The overall organizational structure must be aligned appropriately for the TINs and NPIs. For a large integrated delivery system, this alignment can become a challenge.

While decisions must be made as to who and how many NPIs are appropriate, from a compliance perspective there is the secondary concern related to keeping all of this information up-to-date. Hospitals and other healthcare providers tend to make frequent changes in their organizational structure, and new facilities may be developed and/or acquired. At the same time, databases of various physicians and practitioners must be maintained and updated so that claims can be properly filed. Updating a provider NPI data base will, again, require time, effort, and some sort of organizational infrastructure.

Chapter 12 focuses on the Medicare Provider-Based Rule (PBR) and the Medicare Conditions for Payment (CfPs), both of which also involve reporting requirements.

Case study 11-4. Acme medical clinic. Acme Medical Clinic is a freestanding, physician-owned clinic with six physicians, one nurse practitioner, and two physician assistants. For business organization purposes, the clinic is a Professional Corporation. How many NPIs are needed by Acme Medical Clinic?

As with so many questions in healthcare organizations, the answer will depend upon specific additional information. Certainly the clinic itself (that is, the Professional Corporation) will need an organizational NPI. Each of the physicians will also need an NPI. Now, what about the mid-level practitioners? The real question is whether or not any of the mid-levels will be billing independently to various third-party payers. Keep in mind that this is a freestanding clinic so that all the work of the mid-levels can, if desired, be billed as incident-to a physician (i.e., as if the physician performed the service). Actually, the questions here almost seem to multiply because even if the mid-levels do not file claims under their own NPIs, do the mid-levels still need to obtain NPIs in order to have their services identified as a rendering practitioners?

> **Key learning area: The National Provider Identifiers (NPIs) are designed to replace multiple identification legacy systems with a single, unified provider identification process. Obtaining an NPI is relatively easy. However, determining exactly how many NPIs and associated business subunits that a provider should identify may become quite complex. The information on file with the NPI enumerator must be kept up to date. For healthcare providers that have large, complex organizational structures, keeping track of all the NPIs and keeping them up-to-date can be a significant job.**

Summary and conclusions

This chapter has briefly discussed the very large topic of HIPAA Privacy and Administrative Simplification law and the rules that have been developed by Health and Human Services to implement this law. There are thousands of pages of *Federal Register* entries and associated explanatory documents relating to HIPAA issues. The four key areas addressed in this chapter are:

- HIPAA Privacy
- HIPAA TSC or Transaction Standards/Standard Code Sets
- HIPAA Security
- HIPAA NPIs or National Provider Identifiers

The Office of Civil Rights is in charge of the HIPAA Privacy implementation. As noted, there are also security aspects in the HIPAA Privacy Rule since the HIPAA Security Rule addresses only Electronic Protected Health Information (EPHI) and leaves security for non-electronic PHI to the privacy area.

CMS is in charge of the HIPAA TSC, Security and NPI implementation, which is lumped into the administrative simplification category. The goal of the HIPAA TSC is quite laudable in that healthcare providers should now be able to file uniform, consistent claims using the different standard code sets in a standard transaction format. In fact, this should all be electronic which is the goal of EDI or Electronic Data Interchange. How quickly we will all be able to achieve this goal is yet to be determined. CBR compliance personnel must be watchful for aberrations and exceptions that occur in the coding, billing, and reimbursement areas. When there are exceptional cases, written policies and procedures should be developed to provide an explanation of why exceptions were made.

twelve

Special regulatory areas

Introduction

Special regulatory areas in healthcare can address a wide array of issues, most of which are at the statutory level. This chapter covers several regulatory areas and provides guidance on the kinds of issues you may want to include in your organization's CBR compliance plan. Fully exploring each of these issues is difficult because of the level of detail involved and because the issues change over time. The choice of topics is somewhat generic and not intended to cover all subjects in every situation. You may work in a specialized area that presents unusual concerns and may need to add or amend topics accordingly.

For instance, you may be involved with compliance for an ambulatory surgery center (ASC) that converted into a specialty hospital located inside another hospital so that the special CMS rules and regulations for a hospital within a hospital (HwH) may apply. Another example might be a free-standing, physician-based clinic in which the physicians decided to opt out of the Medicare program, thus establishing contracts with Medicare patients for services may become important. Another issue is the provision of urgent or emergent care for Medicare patients even after the physicians opt out of Medicare.

We will consider only a representative sampling of special healthcare compliance issues at the federal level. You may also have special state level concerns because licensing of healthcare operations is under the purview of individual states and special licensing concerns must be correlated with federal requirements. This discussion will be continued in the sections that delineate various types of special audits that focus on specific regulatory and/or contractual issues.

Provider-based rule (PBR)

The PBR is a regulation promulgated by CMS; it appears in the Code of Federal Regulations at 42 CFR §413.65. (See the accompanying CD-ROM containing this CFR section.) You are encouraged to read the rule, but it is not easy to read or understand. In simple terms, a provider-based facility or organization is truly a part of a provider, which is most often a hospital. One question arising from the explanation is: What does it mean to be a part of a hospital?

A provider-based (or hospital-based) entity is a Medicare concept. However, other private third-party payers may also recognize this status for reimbursement purposes. The most typical example of this concept is the hospital-based clinic. For claims filing purposes, both a professional claim form (for Medicare the CMS-1500) and a technical component claim form (for Medicare the CMS-1450) are filed. For private third-party payers, filing would involve the 1500 claim form for professional service and the UB-04 for the technical component. How these two claim forms are adjudicated by a private third-party payer depends on recognition of the provider-based status by the third-party payer. Note also that the Medicare rules allow hospitals to split-bill (i.e., file both 1500 and UB-04) only for Medicare beneficiaries. A single 1500 claim form can be filed with other third-party payers.

Note: Depending upon specific organizational circumstances, a hospital may file 1500 claim forms. For instance, a hospital may have a specialty clinic in which specialty physicians work several times a month. A specialty clinic may be organized as provider-based, that is, the hospital files a UB-04 claim. However, the specialty physicians may file their own 1500 claim forms.* Conversely, the hospital may file a UB-04 that has no corresponding 1500 professional claim form, e.g., a hospital (provider) may establish an off-campus, satellite radiology operation for which only the technical component is provided.†

Note that even for Medicare, a *provider* may be something different from a hospital. A skilled nursing facility (SNF) or nursing facility (NF) might establish a clinic that would be provider-based; in this case, the main provider is the SNF or NF. The claims filing process and associated reimbursement adjustments when applied to payment processes would generally be the same as those used by hospitals.

The primary impetus for formally establishing the PBR came from the proliferation of hospital-based clinics in the 1980s and 1990s. Both a professional claim

---

* In this situation, the physician must use the POS (place of service) code indicating that the services were provided in a facility or hospital setting. They generally use POS 22 (hospital, outpatient).

† A general operational definition of a provider-based service is one for which a UB-04 claim is being filed.

and a hospital claim could be filed, and thus payment for a hospital-based clinic was higher than for a more traditional physician-based free-standing clinic that filed a claim only on the professional side. During the late 1990s, CMS (then HCFA) developed a payment process that reduced the professional reimbursement when the services were provided in a facility setting, that is, in a hospital-based setting. This reduction is referred to as the site-of-service (SOS) differential. The basic idea is that since the physicians involved in providing the services have no overhead (the facility or hospital takes care of it), their reimbursement should be appropriately reduced. However, the technical component billing, now under APCs, more than makes up for the SOS reduction. A simple example shows how this works:

Physician service—free-standing reimbursement → $60.00

Physician service—provider-based reimbursement → $40.00

Facility service—technical component reimbursement → $50.00

The SOS in this example is $60 – $40 = $20. However, the facility or technical component payment more than makes up for the SOS reduction. The total reimbursement for a provider-based clinic is $40 + $50 = $90. The total reimbursement for a free-standing clinic is $60. This constitutes a net gain of $30 for the provider-based clinic for a single encounter and/or service within an encounter. For a modest-sized clinic with a reasonable percentage of Medicare patients, this can add up to a significant additional reimbursement.

Needless to say, hospitals (and other providers) have an economic incentive to establish provider-based clinics and/or other provider-based services. Whenever an economic advantage may be gained, almost certainly a form of regulatory guidance will appear. Thus, the PBR concept and the regulations must be included in CBR compliance planning, particularly for hospitals.

While the impetus for the PBR was the increased reimbursement available from clinics, the final evolution of the requirements in this rule applies to the entire hospital, both inpatient and outpatient areas. Basically, if a CMS-1450 or UB-04 is filed, a provider-based situation applies and the rules must be followed. Meeting the specific requirements is mandatory. Moreover, *all* the requirements must be met; providers cannot fall back on a "preponderance of evidence" showing that most of the rules were followed. True compliance means total compliance in this case.

Note: A hospital must meet all the conditions set forth in the PBR in order to file technical component claims, but this point raises additional questions. What if

a facility or organization meets all the conditions in the PBR? Does this mean that the hospital must file a technical component claim? Probably not. A hospital clinic may simply be the hospital doing business as a clinic. The clinic may be fully integrated financially and operationally with all the PBR requirements met. However, the hospital may still choose to file claims only on the professional side, that is, treat the clinic as free-standing. Does this mean that the compliance and regulatory issues to be followed are those that apply to a free-standing clinic?* For instance, is incident-to billing allowed? If the clinic is off-campus, does the physician supervision obligation still exist?

Summarizing and interpreting the requirements under this rule is difficult. The following information should be considered as a starting point for your study. First, separate your thinking into three relatively distinct geographic divisions:

1. Inside hospital
2. Outside hospital, but on hospital campus
3. Off hospital campus

Off-campus situations present the greatest concern.

Next, think about hospital departments or service areas in which the same services could be provided in an equivalent free-standing structure. For example, most hospitals provide physical therapy (PT) and occupational therapy (OT) services in a hospital (provider-based) setting or in a free-standing, independent clinic. Is there the potential for a payment differential between the provider-based and free-standing analog? Certainly, as the discussion above showed, a payment differential exists between provider-based and free-standing clinics.

What about our PT/OT example? Depending upon whether the PT/OT payment cap† is in place, the potential of a payment differential is present and thus the potential payment differential criterion again comes into play. Of greatest concern are situations that involve off-campus services *and* potential payment differentials. For compliance purposes, these situations often require the most attention.

Remember that the PBR applies to all inpatient and outpatient departments, service areas, facilities, and organizations. It prohibits providing services totally under arrangements.‡ This prohibition applies to any hospital (provider) department or service area. Another

---

* When this book was written, this issue had not yet been tested in court and/or explicit guidance provided by CMS.

† Over the past several years, the PT/OT cap for payments to freestanding PT/OT operations has been in limbo, depending on directives from Congress.

‡ At the time this book was written, the exact interpretation of how this prohibition is to be interpreted is still pending.

requirement mandates that hospitals must report all changes that may affect provider-based status. Exactly to whom, when, and how this reporting is to be accomplished is not completely clear. (See the related reporting requirements for NPIs and CMS-855 forms.)

It should be clear that the PBR applies to the entire hospital, and this is a good place to return to the critical situations—the off-campus, provider-based situations with potential payment differentials. What about these situations is so critical? The main answer lies in the special rules and requirements in addition to the general requirements for provider-based situations. Let us first look at the general requirements, all of which must be met in order for a facility to be provider-based:

- Common licensure with main provider
- Operation under ownership and control of main provider
- Administration and supervision
- Clinical services
- Financial integration
- Public awareness
- Location in immediate vicinity of main provider

The nuances of these requirements can be explored, depending on the specific circumstances. Let's consider two of these general issues in term of provider-based clinics: 1) public awareness and 2) location.

Public awareness means that every patient entering a provider-based clinic must know he or she is entering premises of the main provider, which, as stated above, is generally a hospital. If the facility is located off the campus of the hospital, the name of the facility must clearly reflect that the facility is part of the hospital. Thus, names and signs are important. Also, think about what this means in terms of the EMTALA concept of a patient going to a hospital. If the clinic is indeed a part of a hospital, what is supposed to happen if the patient with an emergency, presents to its provider-based clinic? Patients with emergency medical conditions certainly may be rushed to clinics. The PBR provides guidance for establishing policies and procedures in this area.

The second issue that we will discuss is the geographic location of a clinic—how close must it be in order to be considered a part of a main provider or hospital? This question has some history. CMS has maintained that a clinic should be close to its hospital. Congress ruled a default distance of 35 miles.* Thus, if the clinic is within a 35-mile radius of the hospital, the geographic closeness criterion is met by default. Obviously, the 35-mile default limit is artificial for a heavily

populated area where the limitation is unlikely to be exceeded. However, in sparsely populated areas, 35 miles may be almost meaningless; facilities may be separated by hundreds of miles. Other statistical tests may be applied. One is a ZIP code overlap test that can establish the degree to which a clinic and hospital share a patient population. Three special considerations or obligations apply to off-campus facilities:

- Physician supervision
- Notice of two co-payments
- EMTALA policies and procedures

In off-campus facilities, a physician or practitioner must provide supervision (be present in the office or clinic). For on-campus or in-hospital situations, a physician is presumed to be available. EMTALA comes into play if the off-campus facility is truly a part of the hospital and a patient with a potential emergency condition may present to the hospital by presenting to the off-campus, provider-based facility. Thus, appropriate policies and procedures must be in place to handle such situations. The notice of two co-payments may or may not apply. A medical clinic will involve two co-payments, and the notice must be given. However, if a hospital has a satellite radiology center, only one co-payment applies as it would inside the hospital.

Based on this brief summary of the PBR, what are hospitals required to do to maintain compliance? The rules governing this issue evolved over a period of about ten years and the compliance requirements have changed. Today, this rule is ostensibly voluntary. In theory, a hospital need only make certain that all the provisions of the PBR are met. The penalties for non-compliance involve reimbursement of all overpayments based on incorrect provider-based designations.

If you are planning to establish an off-campus provider-based facility or operation, it is generally recommended that you request and receive a formal designation from your fiscal intermediary (FI) and CMS regional office (RO). The formal designation allows the burden of proof to be moved from the hospital to the CMS. For all other provider-based facility, operations, organizations, departments, etc., filing an attestation with the CMS and retaining all necessary documentation confirming that your organization meets all provisions of the PBR are generally recommended. For off-campus situations, a further recommendation is to provide supporting documentation along with the attestation.

Case study 12-1. Purchase of medical clinic. Apex Medical Center decides to purchase the Acme Medical Clinic located about two blocks from the hospital. The plan is to organize Acme

---

* The 35-mile limitation appears to be arbitrary. The same limitation appears to the sole community hospital designation.

as a provider-based clinic and hire the physicians and practitioners who currently provide services there. What steps must Apex take relative to establishing provider-based status?

Apex will need to meet all the provider-based rule requirements and observe the obligations for an off-campus situation. Also, it is strongly recommended that Apex seek a formal determination of the provider-based status after the reorganization. Obviously, other tasks must be handled, including physician contracts, filing CMS-855 forms, and the like. Split-billing, that is, filing both 1500 and UB-04 forms, will also require changes to the billing system and establishment of a proper set of charges for both the hospital and the professional component.* See the accompanying CD-ROM for additional information and various forms relative to the provider-based rule.

Key learning area: The PBR is complex; it was developed by CMS in response to establishment of provider-based clinics by hospitals to gain increased reimbursement. The final form of this rule, as developed over about ten years, is comprehensive and extends beyond clinic situations. Adherence appears to be voluntary, but recommendations for compliance purposes include requesting formal determinations, filing attestations, and keeping all necessary documentation on file.†

Billing privileges

Virtually all healthcare providers will formally obtain billing privileges with third-party payers. Most of these arrangements will be parts of contracts negotiated with third-party payers. As noted in Chapter 1, a provider may file claims with third-party payers with which it has no formal arrangements. Typically the number of such claims filed will be minimal. However, a provider must still meet normal industry practices‡ such as proper use of NPIs and complying with general HIPAA transaction standards and the TSC rule. At governmental level, the Medicare program developed an extensive set of forms required to gain and maintain billing privileges or meeting conditions for payment (CfPs).§ The CMS-855 series includes five different forms:

- CMS-855A—Institutional Providers
- CMS-855B—Clinics/Group Practices and Certain Other Suppliers
- CMS-855I—Physicians and Non-Physician Practitioners
- CMS 855R—Reassignment of Medicare Benefits
- CMS 855S—Durable Medical Equipment, Prosthetics, Orthotics, and Supplies (DMEPOS) Suppliers

Additionally, rules and regulations can be found at 42 CFR §424. See the accompanying CD-ROM in which this CFR section is provided along with current CMS-855 forms.

Practitioners use CMS-855R to reassign Medicare benefits, and this form is relatively brief. The other forms are more extensive and sometimes require sensitive information. Much of the information required concerns issues that you would anticipate being queried about. CMS must know certain details about your organization before granting billing privileges. For instance:

- What is your official name?
- Who are you?
- What kinds of services to you provide?
- Where are you located?
- Who owns you?
- Who has financial control over you?
- Who has management control over you?
- Have adverse legal actions been instituted against you?
- Who is the official contract person?
- Who is the official signatory?

It is important to note that some of the information requirements raise sensitive issues. CMS-855A is generally used by hospitals, and assuming that the hospital has a board, the board members and their social security numbers must be identified. The CMS-855S is used by DME suppliers. Dispensing location information must be provided and a location requires a separate CMS-855 form.

One major concern is that these forms must be updated, and changes must be reported within specified periods. Certain changes must be reported within 30 days; others must be reported within 60 days. CMS is particularly interested in ownership, management control, and financial control. From a compliance

---

* For those interested in an actual case, see the *Virginia Mason* case at: http://www.healthbusinessandpolicy.com/PricingLawsuits.htm.

† Most of the required information and supporting documentation overlaps with the documentation requirements for the various CMS-855 forms.

‡ The *normal industry practices* phrase can be variously interpreted. Great care must be exercised when using this language, particularly in formal legal proceedings.

§ See 42 CFR §424.

perspective, the key issue is who knows what changes have taken place? Hospital organizations can become very complex, and changes often surprise hospital employees. It is not unusual for employees to learn that a new service area or practice location has been established by reading an article in a local newspaper rather than from a formal announcement issued by their employer. Every healthcare provider must establish a mechanism to centralize required information and all of the associated documentation. Compliance personnel must certainly be involved.

The regulatory burden imposed by maintaining the CMS-855 forms will depend very much on the type of organization and also the rate at which changes occur. If your organization is a free-standing, physician-based clinic with only a few physicians and minimal changes, you may not need to update the CMS-855 forms for years although Medicare imposes a normal five-year revalidation cycle. Multiple forms will still apply, most likely, one for the clinic (CMS-855B), one for each physician (CMS-855I), and reassignment forms (CMS-855R) required for all physicians to reassign benefits to the clinic. Since such changes may occur relatively slowly, the task of keeping the CMS-855 forms updated is minimal.

For a more comprehensive example, consider a hospital that has a skilled nursing facility (SNF), a home health agency (HHA), and several provider-based clinics with several dozen employed physicians. The number of CMS-855 forms increases dramatically in this situation, In some cases, the number of CMS-855 forms may easily exceed a hundred. The potential rate of change also increases significantly.

A third level might be a teaching hospital with several hundred physicians or a system of hospitals with multiple operations and clinics. It is not inconceivable that a thousand such forms might have to be maintained, and the potential rate of change is almost daily. A system that could address this level of complexity will require careful planning and considerable resources.

Note that the CMS-855 forms also dovetail with other regulatory concerns, particularly the NPIs and the PBR. NPIs require modest data, but the information must be updated to correlate with the CMS-855 forms. Also, the PBR requires reporting all changes that might affect provider-based status. Although this requirement is fairly general, due consideration must be given to ensuring that any changes are appropriately reported.

Case study 12-2. Update of CMS-855 forms. Continuing Case study 12-1, assume that the clinic has six physicians, one nurse practitioner, and two physician assistants. Acme Medical Clinic will be renamed Apex Medical Center's Family Practice Clinic. Officially, the business name is Apex Medical Center doing business as (DBA) the Family Practice Clinic. Based on this information, how many CMS-855 forms must be newly filed and/or updated?

To answer the question definitively will require more information. As a general answer, all the practitioners must update their CMS-855I and CMS855R forms. A CMS-855B must be filed for the clinic and the hospital's CMS-855A must be updated. Thus, approximately twenty forms will have to be filed or updated—and this only meets requirements of the Medicare program. What about establishing billing privileges and/or contracts with other third-party payers?

Key learning area: CMS-855 forms must be constantly updated and refiled as appropriate. Since any given healthcare provider may utilize multiple CMS-855 forms, a carefully organized process to gather the necessary information, organize and retain the necessary it (including attachments), and submit changes within the specified times is mandatory. This is not a trivial task and the process must be coordinated with additional issues such as NPIs and the PBR reporting requirements.

Emergency Medical Treatment and Labor Act (EMTALA)

EMTALA involves multiple requirements. Only hospitals that participate in Medicare program and have emergency departments are subject to the provisions of EMTALA. Of course, this covers most hospitals. As with many regulatory provisions, the definitions of EMTALA must be fully understood. A brief sampling is provided in this section to help you understand the compliance implications of EMTALA. The section also explains basic EMTALA concepts and how they relate to CBR compliance.

Basically, EMTALA requires hospitals under its jurisdiction to provide services to anyone who presents to them. This, of course, is a gross over-simplification. In fact, almost every word of the requirement must be examined! For example:

- Does the requirement really cover everyone?
- What services must be provided?
- What does it mean to "present" to a hospital?
- What constitutes a hospital?
- What is an emergency department?
- When does an individual become a patient?

Let us look at just two definitions taken from 42 CFR §489.24(b):

- Dedicated Emergency Department. Means any department or facility of the hospital, regardless of whether it is located on or off the main hospital campus, that meets **at least one** of the following requirements:
  - (1) It is licensed by the state in which it is located under applicable state law as an emergency room or emergency department;
  - (2) It is held out to the public (by name, posted signs, advertising, or other means) as a place that provides care for emergency medical conditions on an urgent basis without requiring a previously scheduled appointment; or
  - (3) During the calendar year immediately preceding the calendar year in which a determination under this section is being made, based on a representative sample of patient visits that occurred during that calendar year, it provides at least one-third of all of its outpatient visits for the treatment of emergency medical conditions on an urgent basis without requiring a previously scheduled appointment.
- Hospital Property. Means the entire main hospital campus as defined in §413.65(b) of this chapter (42 CFR), including the parking lot, sidewalk, and driveway, but excluding other areas or structures of the hospital's main building that are not part of the hospital, such as physician offices, rural health centers, skilled nursing facilities, or other entities that participate separately under Medicare, or restaurants, shops, or other non-medical facilities.

Certainly these definitions are convoluted and require careful reading and study. Note that that the definition of a dedicated emergency department (DED) includes any hospital-based clinic that provides urgent care along with emergency care. The definition also alludes to unscheduled visits, which, if certain frequency tests are achieved, provide a means for meeting the definition and thus a need to meet EMTALA rules. This definition ties directly back to the discussion of provider-based clinics that may be designated as urgent care centers and would thus meet the criteria described here. See Case study 11-2 concerning properly establishing the place of service (POS) indicator.

The concept of hospital property is convoluted because CMS attempts to separate areas into those that are truly part of the hospital from those that are not. For instance, a coffee shop located off the lobby of a hospital is not considered hospital property. If an individual in the coffee shop suddenly develops a medical problem, the protocol for addressing this type of situation may be different from the protocol for a patient collapsing in a hallway outside the coffee shop because the hallway is considered hospital property. This chapter addresses only a few of numerous CBR-related compliance issues to provide a representative sampling of concerns.

Emergency department levels

For 2007,* CMS developed the concept of two different levels of DEDs:

- Type A—Available 24 hours a day, seven days a week
- Type B—Available fewer than 24 hours a day, seven days a week

Both types of emergency departments are fully licensed and subject to EMTALA requirements. CMS determined that Type B EDs should be paid less than Type A EDs because they experience lower costs (i.e., are not open 24 hours a day). Thus, Type B EDs are paid at clinic levels rather than at the higher ED levels under ambulatory payment classifications (APCs).

Advance beneficiary notices (ABNs)

ABNs are used in cases where a service may be considered not medically necessary. ABNs are generally associated with Medicare. The basic idea is to inform the patient that the service may not be paid by Medicare and if not paid, the patient, will be liable for payment. The problem in emergency departments is that patients may feel that they have been coerced. Thus, the use of ABNs in the emergency department requires careful consideration and appropriate training of personnel.

Leaves against medical advice

Virtually every hospital has situations in which patients present, are subsequently triaged and/or receive full medical screening examinations (MSEs), and leave before definitive services can be provided. While careful clinical documentation of services received is required and the EMTALA log must be maintained, billing and coding concerns also arise. Should patients who leave against medical advice (LAMA) be billed for services? While this is a hospital policy decision, the approach taken should be carefully documented in a written policy and procedure.

---

* See November 24, 2006 *Federal Register* for discussion.

Non-emergency care

Hospital emergency departments are often used for non-emergency encounters. In theory, even under EMTALA, after a hospital has determines (via an appropriate MSE) that no medical emergency exists, the hospital is permitted to direct the patient to another healthcare provider. Many hospitals provide any needed services, but the services are provided at clinic level, not emergency level.

From a third-party payer perspective, a reasonable question is whether the clinic level services should be reimbursed at ED levels or at lower clinic levels. In fact, revenue codes delineate such services, for example:

- 0450—Emergency room—general
- 0451—Emergency room—EMTALA emergency medical screening services
- 0452—Emergency room—ER beyond EMTALA screening
- 0456—Emergency room—urgent care

Hospital chargemaster personnel may also want to establish clinic level charges for certain situations. For instance, a patient may return to an emergency department for a subsequent injection in a series. The ED may also encounter patients who would normally go to an outpatient area for a service, particularly when the outpatient department is closed. In these cases, ED personnel may require a mechanism to charge at clinic level for the encounter rather than at the higher ED level. The whole issue of non-emergency care in the ED can and will generate significant discussion for CBR personnel. While different approaches can be developed, keep in mind the EMTALA requirements related to developing CBR policies and procedures.

> **Case study 12-3. Urgent care clinic.** Apex established a provider-based urgent care clinic across town. It is open from 6:00 a.m. until 11 p.m. seven days a week. A mid-level practitioner is always present and a physician also present from 11 a.m. to 7 p.m. A limited number of patients may make appointments, but most patients simply present without appointments. The question is whether this urgent care clinic is a dedicated emergency department (DED) under EMTALA.

Based on the definition presented earlier, this provider-based clinic would be considered a DED and all EMTALA rules and regulations apply, including the need to maintain an EMTALA log, perform MSEs, etc. The mid-level practitioners must be qualified by the medical staff organization (MSO) to be able to perform the MSEs. In addition to EMTALA concerns, a number of coding and billing questions apply. If ED E/M codes are to be used, the example clinical is a Type B ED under Medicare and special coding requirements come into play. The regular clinic visit codes will likely be used although this is a coding and billing policy decision. See the CD-ROM for additional information about EMTALA.

> **Key learning area: EMTALA is a major and complex compliance issue for hospitals. CBR issues dovetail with EMTALA in a variety of forms. In many cases, policy decisions must be made and then established as written policies and procedures. This chapter addresses only a small sampling of situations that are of concern.**

Non-physician providers (NPPs)

Among the many types of NPPs, a special subset includes non-physician practitioners. Because the NPP acronym may refer to practitioners and non-physician providers who are not practitioners (e.g., nurses), be certain that you understand the context of any discussions about non-physician practitioners and/or the more general non-physician providers. The most common non-physician practitioners are:

- Nurse practitioners (NPs)
- Physician assistants (PAs)
- Clinical nurse specialists (CNSs)
- Nurse midwives (NMs)
- Clinical social workers (CSWs)
- Clinical psychologists (CPs)
- Certified registered nurse anesthetists (CRNAs)
- Physical therapists (PTs)
- Occupational therapists (OTs)

Depending on the context, lists may differ slightly. Medicare allows certain practitioners to opt out and treat Medicare beneficiaries under private contracts. As of the writing of this book, the most current listing appeared in the December 1, 2006 *Federal Register* updating 42 CFR §405.400 by adding registered dieticians and nutrition professionals.

> Practitioner means a physician assistant, nurse practitioner, clinical nurse specialist, certified registered nurse anesthetist, certified nurse midwife, clinical psychologist, clinical social worker, registered dietitian or nutrition professional, who is currently legally authorized to practice in that capacity by each State in which he or she furnishes services to patient or clients.

Similarly, for EMTALA-mandated MSEs, NPs, PAs, and CNSs are deemed qualified medical persons whereas other practitioners are not. Generally, non-physician practitioners have the ability to obtain Medicare billing privileges and thus file professional component or CMS-1500 claim forms. Reimbursement is reduced from the full physician fee payment. While Medicare recognizes these NPPs, other third-party payers may or may not recognize them as qualified providers, and this will clearly impact payments for services. A number of significant variations affect payment and billing privileges. Looking beyond the practitioners, a multitude of non-physician providers cannot bill professionally, at least under Medicare. The following is a small subset of such non-physician providers:

- Registered nurses
- Respiratory therapists
- First surgical assistants
- Certified enterostomal nurse technicians
- Certified medical assistants
- Radiology technicians
- Certified nurse technicians

Payment for the services of these NPPs is provided as part of the facility or technical component as billed on the UB-04 or the CMS-1450 for Medicare claims. The utilization of non-physician practitioners and non-physician providers who are not classified as practitioners is increasing in the healthcare industry. Sometimes these NPPs are used as physician extenders; at other times they provide services independently. In some cases, they may file professional claims forms even when restricted to technical component coding and billing.

From the perspective of CBR compliance, non-physician providers and the special subset of practitioners create significant challenges. The overall issue relates to coding and filing claims for services they provide. One aspect of this issue is *incident-to services*. This phrase is used at the Social Security Act (SSA) level in two very different ways. The bifurcated use of this phrase is then translated and interpreted through the *United State Code* (USC), then through the *Code of Federal Regulations* (CFR), and finally through Medicare manuals and instructions.

The overarching issue is how billing for services of NPPs is to be done: indirectly or directly. The organizational context is vital. First, consider a free-standing physician-owned clinic. The physician is allowed to code and bill for services of subordinate personnel (nurses, practitioners, technicians) as if the physician actually performed the services. This is commonly referred to as *incident-to billing*. However, if we change

the organizational context by making this clinic provider-based (hospital-based), the coding and billing requirements change.

The SSA clearly indicates that hospitals are paid for all services and items that are *incident-to* the services of a physician. Thus, a physician may direct the services of nurses, practitioners, and technicians, but the physician is not allowed to code and bill for the services. The hospital must bill for them through the technical component claims process on a UB-04.

In other words, a physician in a hospital or facility setting can only code and bill for services personally performed. Of course, this is an over-simplification. Keep in mind that practitioners can gain professional billing privileges on their own. Thus, a practitioner in a hospital setting working under the direction of a physician can professionally code and bill for services performed. Of course, a number of circumstances further complicate this issue. Every situation or circumstance must be carefully considered from the perspective of maintaining compliance within the coding and billing process. Two case studies showing how complicated this perspective can be represent only the tip of the iceberg.

Case study 12-4. Nurse practitioner performing pre-surgery H&Ps. Apex Medical Center has problems with patients presenting for surgery without meeting pre-surgery history and physician (H&P) requirements. As a result, the center hired a nurse practitioner (NP) to perform pre-surgery H&Ps in the mornings. These services are typically provided in a pre-surgery room or examination room close to surgery. How should the center establish this process organizationally, that is, how can it code and bill for the services of the NP?

As with many situations in hospital settings, what appear to be reasonably straightforward situations can become convoluted. The first decision is whether the NP is to bill professionally. If the decision is to bill professionally, the NP will have to obtain billing privileges from Medicare and other third-party payers that recognize NPs as qualifying for professional billing. The NP will also require an NPI. The POS will most likely be 22 (hospital, outpatient). Medicare will impose a site-of-service reduction. Most likely the NP will reassign Medicare payments to the hospital, that is, the employer; that will require a CMS-855R filing.

Note that the hospital may decide not to bill professionally for the NP's services. This, however, will result in lost reimbursement since such services are generally reimbursable. Also, cost reporting implications arise. If the NP bills professionally, then the salary and fringe benefits of the NP should not be included on the cost report. However, if the hospital elects not to bill professionally, the costs of the NP can be included on the cost report.

Since the NP provides services in a hospital setting, a technical component E/M level can be coded and billed. Appropriate mapping of the resources utilized into an E/M level will be required. For Medicare, the -25 (significant, separately identifiable service) code will have to be used because the UB-04 claim will contain a services-by-surgeon code and then the E/M level as performed by the NP.

Case study 12-5. Joint E/M service in ED. Apex Medical Center hired several nurse practitioners to work in the ED along with ER physicians. Often, a patient will present, be worked up by an NP, and then be seen by an ER physician. How should the center code and bill for these joint E/M services?

Surprisingly, CMS, in Transmittal 1776 dated October 25, 2002, issued guidance relative to the *Medicare Carriers Manual* that allowed a physician and non-physician practitioner to jointly perform E/M services in the ED or hospital setting, allowing *either* the physician or the NPP code and bill for the E/M services under certain circumstances. The NP in the example can perform most services as long as some, albeit minimal, face-to-face contact is maintained between physician and patient. This is an isolated exception to the rule that physicians can code and bill only for services personally performed.

Case study 12-6. Nursing staff providing injections. Apex Medical Center owns and operates a free-standing medical clinic and is discussing making it a provider-based clinic. Frequent clinic services involve nursing staff encounters to provide series of injections ordered by physicians. Currently, an E/M level plus the injection code plus the drug are charged under the physician's name. If the clinic becomes provider-based, the center wonders how the coding and billing will change, and, in particular, whether the change will have financial implications.

This case study also illustrates how seemingly simple situations become complicated. To simplify it, assume that a physician or qualified non-physician practitioner works at the clinic, whether it is organized as free-standing or provider-based. Assume also that the patient presents only for an injection and the encounter will involve only a nurse.

For the free-standing clinic situation, the nurse will perform an assessment to assure that the patient is

ready for the injection. This will probably be coded as 99211. Assuming the patient is ready, the injection will be provided and coded. Another charge will cover the drug or drugs provided. A claim will be developed just as if a physician performed these services, and a 1500 claim form will be developed and submitted. Note that the -25 (significant, separately identifiable) modifier will be used to separate the E/M level from the injection.*

What about the provider-based situation? The nurse is not a practitioner so no professional claim form is needed. However, the UB-04 generated will contain the same codes and modifier as would the professional claim form in a free-standing situation.

Note: Technical component E/M coding in situations of this type is still being fully defined under the Medicare APC (Ambulatory Payment Classification) payment system. Situations of this type are fairly common. Check the latest guidance from CMS if one arises.

Additional compliance concerns surround non-physician practitioners. One is scope of practice. State laws dictate the services that a practitioner can provide, and the services may vary somewhat. The question of prescribing drugs has been an ongoing issue for practitioners over the years. Certain practitioners, mainly NPs, may establish independent practices if state laws permit it and all special conditions are met. An NP establishing a practice must go through the same processes such as gaining billing privileges as would a physician. From a compliance perspective, NPPs represent major issues that require careful thought at several different levels including organizational structure, state laws, and federal regulations.

Key learning area: Non-physician providers in general and the special subset of non-physician practitioners represent significant compliance concerns for proper coding, billing, and reimbursement. Accurate interpretations of rules and regulations require careful analysis and complete understanding of the organizational context. Particularly with clinics, care should be taken to assess whether they are free-standing or provider-based.

Stark law issues

For more than a decade, the physician self referral laws have been in development. The regulations resulting from these laws are often referred to as the Stark regulations because the initial impetus to develop them was

---

* See the new parenthetical guidance in 2007 CPT under code 90772 relative to injections without physician supervision.

made by Representative Pete Stark of California in the 1980s and 1990s. As with many healthcare compliance issues, the Stark regulations continue to be developed and discussed. While certain themes are consistent, the exceptions are numerous. Thus, these regulations tend to be complex and require careful study.

The Stark law prohibits physicians from making referrals to an entity for certain designated health services (DHSs) for which payment may be made under the Medicare or Medicaid programs if the physician or his or her immediate family has a financial relationship with the entity. From this basic description, the primary concerns under the Stark regulations tend to be organizational structuring and the referral of patients to other entities.

This is an area of indirect concern for CBR compliance personnel working with physicians. However, CBR personnel are often called upon to establish billing procedures. All situations and special arrangements should be analyzed with consideration for the Stark regulations. While the Stark regulations are physician-centered, hospitals can become enmeshed in the regulations via their sometimes convoluted relationships with physicians. A simple case study illustrates this point.

Case study 12-7. Joint ambulatory surgery center. A group of surgeons on the medical staff at Apex Medical Center approaches the hospital's CEO and CFO concerning a joint venture to establish an ambulatory surgery center (ASC) on the hospital campus. The hospital would be a 50 percent owner and the group of surgeons would own the other 50 percent. The hospital would perform all billing and claims filing and provide support personnel for the venture. Services would be provided by the group of surgeons and any other community surgeons who might want to provide services in the new facility. Primary care physicians on the medical staff are also showing interest in participating in the venture. They would refer patients to the ASC although they would not generally provide services there.

This case study has many variations. A careful legal analysis of such arrangements is required. One concern is the Stark legislation. Also, the provider-based rule must be carefully considered. Assuming that such an arrangement is legal, the CBR issues can then be considered.

The Stark regulations are generally found at 42 CFR §§411.350 through 411.361. These regulations continue to be developed and constant updating is required. The development of the regulations has spanned more than 15 years. The general chronology is:

- 1991—Stark I Statute—Clinical Laboratory Services
- 1992—Proposed Stark I Regulations
- 1995—Stark II Statute—Additional Designated Health Services
- 1998—Proposed Stark II Regulations
- 2001—Start II, Phase I Regulations
- 2004—Stark II, Phase II Regulations
- 2007—Stark II, Phase III Regulations

The difficulties in developing the regulations are apparent from this chronology. The basic idea is that physicians should not be able to self-refer for services from which they will receive benefits that normally accrue from ownership. The regulations contain many exceptions or safe harbors. The anti-kickback safe harbors can be found at 42 CFR §1001.952. The regulations prohibit receipt of inducements for the provision of healthcare services. Of course, this is an over-simplification. A simple case addresses this issue.

Case study 12-8. Professional courtesy. Apex Medical Center employs a number of physicians for whom health insurance coverage is provided. When services are provided, claims are filed. However, the overall medical staff, including community physicians not employed by the hospital, want the hospital to provide professional courtesy for community physicians. Is this arrangement feasible under the Stark and anti-kickback regulations?

To answer this question fully, more details and a legal opinion are necessary. A quick analysis indicates significant concerns. The professional courtesy exception involves a number of requirements to be met. The above scenario would appear to present difficulties. From a coding and billing compliance perspective, all the physicians or none of the physicians must be billed. Associated claims will be filed or not filed accordingly.

Key learning area: The Stark regulations involving physician ownership and self-referral have been developed over the past 15 years and must be considered in connection with the anti-kickback regulations. While these CMS regulations indirectly involve CBR issues, the regulations must receive due consideration in dealing with physician ownership and self-referrals.

Summary and conclusion

This chapter briefly discusses five topics in the context of CBR compliance:

- Provider-based rule (PBR)
- Billing privileges and conditions for payment (CfPs)
- Emergency Medical And Labor Act (EMTALA)
- Non-physician providers and practitioners (NPPs)
- Stark law issues

Each of these topics could be expanded easily into an entire book. CBR compliance personnel must thoroughly understand all these issues along with associated issues. Adding to the challenge are the constant changes in the rules and regulations and their interpretations by various entities.

thirteen

Compliance considerations for hospitals

Introduction

Previous chapters discussed many different CBR compliance concerns along with the process of structuring a compliance plan. Many of these issues cut across various types of healthcare organizations and providers. Virtually all healthcare providers must be able to code, bill, and file claims. This means that billing privileges must be obtained from Medicare program and other third-party payers. Other compliance topics discussed include major compliance areas such as EMTALA and the provider-based rule that are mainly applicable to hospitals.

This chapter continues to focus on hospital CBR compliance issues. Hospitals are multifaceted organizations that tend to become more complex as they grow in size and scope of services. In today's multihospital systems, compliance becomes even more difficult based on size and number of services provided. Simply keeping up with organizational and service area changes in a hospital setting can be challenging from a CBR compliance view.

> **Key learning area: Hospitals are multifaceted healthcare providers to which many compliance concerns apply. A number of concerns involve coding, billing, and reimbursement. Hospitals also tend to develop and/or otherwise become involved with other types of healthcare services. Thus, interfaces among different types of payment systems further complicate CBR compliance issues.**

Chargemaster

The chargemaster is an integral part of the billing system and fits squarely in the middle of the reimbursement cycle. Figure 13.1 is a generic reimbursement cycle flowchart. *Reimbursement cycle* as used here indicates generation of an itemized statement along with a claim to be filed to a third-party payer. The reimbursement cycle is a subset of the revenue cycle that also involves payments from self-insured or uninsured patients for which claims do not need to be filed.

Figure 13.1 illustrates that the chargemaster is involved with the coding and billing processes by which itemized statements and claim forms are generated. The chargemaster should be viewed from two perspectives when considering compliance issues: (1) as a static file and (2) as part of a dynamic process.

The objective of a hospital billing system is to generate clean, complete, and accurate claims. When a charge is entered into the billing system, a line item from the chargemaster is triggered and it will appear on an itemized statement. The itemized statement information is further amalgamated, generally based on revenue codes, and produces a claim. In some cases, entering a single charge may trigger multiple charges and cause what is called a *charge explosion*. For example, a single entered charge in a coronary catheterization laboratory may result in three separate charges and associated codes appearing on the itemized statement: catheter placement, injection procedure, and radiological supervision and interpretation.

Thus, both the information (static) provided by the line item in the chargemaster and the way in which this process (dynamic) takes place can create compliance concerns. The chargemaster may also be structured with embedded logic to be used by the billing system. For example, the chargemaster may contain several revenue codes based on patient classification or even on the third-party payer involved for any line item.

Obviously, the chargemaster contains all hospital charges. In recent years, the pricing of hospital services has come under increasing scrutiny both at the patient/public and regulatory levels. This scrutiny has also been directed at the way charges are developed. As indicated in Chapter 1, the main compliance concerns are (1) statutory and (2) contractual. Both concerns are very important for the chargemaster.

Additional requirements for the chargemaster and associated pricing are imposed at federal regulatory level and through contracts with third-party payers.

This chapter includes a brief discussion about the somewhat nebulous Medicare charging rule—a major federal regulatory guideline on establishing charges. For contractual relationships, the compliance playing field can vary. If your hospital has a fee-for-service contract whereby it is paid at 85 percent of its charges, the third-party payer will be very interested in your charge structure and the way it is updated. This may result in a contractual obligation that allows audit of the chargemaster to ensure that charges faithfully reflect costs.

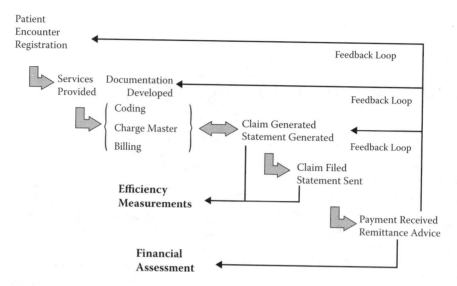

Figure 13.1   Reimbursement cycle flowchart.

This section begins by examining the chargemaster as a static file and then explores compliance considerations related to the dynamic process. It concludes with a brief discussion of the Medicare charging rule and associated charging issues under private third-party payer contracts.

Static file

The chargemaster is basically a huge file that contains a listing of all the charge items for a hospital. This file is actually a database of line items. Each line item has a number of fields. The type of database and precise file layout will vary among billing systems. The billing system can be adjusted to use or not use certain fields that are available for all line items. Certain fields are critical; others provide additional or optional information. While a number of potential compliance concerns surround the chargemaster as a static file, we will look at some of the more common challenges. The four main data elements are (1) description, (2) revenue code, (3) CPT/HCPCS plus optional modifiers, and (4) charge. Additional important information may include general ledger classification and/or other data relative to classifying charges for cost reporting.

The description for a line item should be intelligible. This simply means that a person reading a description will know whether a line item is a supply, procedure, diagnostic test, or service. Stock numbers for supply items can be used if the description is sufficient to show that the item is a surgical supply, implantable device, expensive catheter, etc. The descriptions are somewhat abbreviated and care should be taken to use descriptions that accurately describe the services provided or items supplied because such descriptions will appear on itemized statements. Thus, including

information such as a CPT or HCPCS code should be considered carefully because codes change and a line item description may contain a code that does not correspond to a regular code field.

The selection and use of revenue codes (RCs) may be difficult but is usually straightforward. If a surgical procedure is indicated as a line item, RC 360 would be common. For emergency department services, RC 450 is typically used. However, in some cases the choice of RC is open to interpretation. While RCs represent a standard code set under the HIPAA TSC rule, third-party payers may have specific requirements for the use or non-use of RCs.

The inclusion of a CPT or HCPCS code with a line item is optional. Up to two modifiers can be included with a code. Great care must be taken in designing the chargemaster relative to coding interfaces. In some cases, the CPT/HCPCS codes are placed in the chargemaster. Entry of a charge drives a line item which, in turn, drives the selection of the code. In other instances, professional coding staff may develop the CPT/HCPCS code so that it need not be placed in the chargemaster. In this case, presuming that a CPT/HCPCS code is required, the selection of a line item from the chargemaster drives only the charge, description, and revenue code. The code developed by coding staff must then be associated with the charge (or charges) generated through the chargemaster.

Also possible are hybrid approaches that combine static and dynamic coding. For instance, a default CPT or HCPCS code is placed in the chargemaster. If professional coding staff review the case and determine that a different code should be associated with the charge, the default code can be overridden. If such hybrid approaches are used, care should be taken to verify that the intended codes appear on final claims.

Case study 13-1. Double coding. Apex Medical Center just completed a claim review. Included in the review were several interventional breast procedures, mainly biopsies. To the surprise of auditors, all five claims reviewed showed repeats of the surgical portion—the same surgical code appeared twice even though only a single biopsy was involved in each case. Each claim form showed only one associated radiology code. A further investigation revealed that the surgical and radiological coding was performed through the chargemaster by service area personnel via charge entry. Professional coding staff also performed surgical coding and then transferred the codes into the billing system that finally reported both codes.

Of course, the charge associated with the line item must also be present. The charge development process will be examined separately. Now that we have the key elements of a line item in the chargemaster, the main compliance concern is the appropriate correlation of the four elements cited above. The description should be correctly associated with the CPT or HCPCS code; the CPT or HCPCS code must be associated with the proper RC, and the charge should be reasonably appropriate for the service or item described by the line item.

Case study 13-2. Intravenous solution charges. The chargemaster at Apex Medical Center was recently reviewed by an outside consulting company. While the results were generally favorable, the reviewers raised several questions. One involved charges for intravenous (IV) solutions. Despite concern as to whether these solutions should be separately charged because they are stock items, the larger question involved the actual charge. A typical IV solution was charged at $60 while service area personnel indicated that the cost was much closer to $3. The consultants indicated that this type of mark-up was inappropriate and certainly not consistent with charge formulas used in other areas of the chargemaster.

When the chargemaster is reviewed as a static file, this is the type of correlation that should be checked along with judgments concerning appropriateness of the data (correct code, reasonable charge, correct RC, etc.). However, chargemaster audits involve more than simple examinations of individual line items.

Dynamic process

The chargemaster is an integral part of the reimbursement cycle, as illustrated in Figure 13.1, and is used to develop itemized statements and subsequent claim forms. Thus, the chargemaster operates on many dynamic levels. First, it should reflect the services and items provided in a service area. Thus, making certain that all the necessary entries are in the chargemaster is a major ongoing effort. Even if all the proper line items are programmed, care must be taken to ensure that all appropriate charges are captured. This charge capture interface is a dynamic process.

Secondly, if CPT/HCPCS codes are developed outside the chargemaster, care should be taken to ensure that the correct codes and properly associated charges appear on final claim forms. This involves the coding interface to the chargemaster, which, again, is a dynamic process. Finally, we should not forget the cost report. Charge information is accumulated by some means for use in developing cost reports. This information is also key to developing cost-to-charge ratios (CCRs). The question for the chargemaster as part of a dynamic process then becomes, do these interfaces work properly?

Clearly, many dynamic or process flow interfaces to the chargemaster should be considered from a compliance perspective. Also, while we tend to think in terms of Medicare and Medicaid (statutory compliance), serious concerns surround chargemaster requirements at the private third-party payer contractual level.

Charging and charge development

In recent years pricing has become a major and highly visible issue. Various concepts and buzzwords have come into use, for example, strategic pricing, transparent pricing, market pricing, and geographic pricing. These are really different objectives for establishing charges entered into the chargemaster and represent hospital pricing. Note that virtually every hospital's chargemaster is set up somewhat differently because different design strategies were used. Thus, comparison of charges across chargemasters often makes little sense. The level at which comparisons can be made is the overall encounter level that involves the amalgamation of different types of charges. For instance, cataract surgeries are fairly common, and a patient might want to know the difference in pricing for a cataract extraction and insertion of an intraocular lens (IOL). Even at this specific surgical level, the chargemaster may generate different charges.

Case study 13-3. Time-based surgical charges. Sylvia, the chargemaster coordinator at Apex Medical Center decided to develop surgical charges based on 15-minute time units along with a standard base charge. This charge development approach was chosen due to the simplicity of maintaining the chargemaster and the ease of charge entry by service area personnel. The cataract surgery charge entry simply requires counting the number of time units along with charging for supplies, pharmacy items, and, of course, the IOL.

Using a time-based charging approach, the same cataract surgery performed by different physicians could produce significantly different charges. One physician may take only 30 minutes to complete the procedure while another might take more than an hour. Similarly, anesthesia and recovery charges may differ. Thus, different charges will accrue for most cases. Additionally, IOLs of many types are available including the new technology IOLs (NTIOLs). Thus pricing for these items will also vary significantly. Making pricing visible at the chargemaster level, even in this highly delimited area, may not be instructive to patients.

Note the variability in the terminology in establishing pricing formulas. *Strategic pricing* is a process of modeling charge structures to optimize reimbursement under private contracts. *Transparent pricing* relates to making pricing visible and understandable to the public, that is, potential patients. Considering the variability of chargemasters, transparent pricing is a very real challenge. Highly trained healthcare consultants are often challenged when reviewing chargemaster details; making chargemaster data available to the public may not produce much benefit. *Market pricing* relates to setting pricing at an appropriate market level; *geographic pricing* is simply an objective of making the pricing consistent with other hospital pricing in the same geographic area.

On the compliance side, at the regulatory level, is the so-called *Medicare charging rule*. This somewhat ill-defined rule involves two different hospital pricing requirements, one under the auspices of the OIG and the other a cost reporting requirement: (1) Medicare beneficiaries cannot be charged more than other patients and (2) charges must be consistently based on costs. From the OIG comes the following excerpt from 42 CFR § 1001.701:

> *Excessive claims or furnishing of unnecessary or substandard items and services.*
> *(a) Circumstance for exclusion. The OIG may exclude an individual or entity that has—*
> *(1) Submitted, or caused to be submitted, bills or requests for payments under Medicare or any of the State healthcare programs containing charges or costs for items or services furnished that are **substantially in excess** of such individual's or entity's **usual charges** or costs for such items or services . . . [emphasis added].*

This CFR entry provides exceptions in case there is a need to charge Medicare beneficiaries more than other patients:

> *(c) Exceptions. An individual or entity will not be excluded for—*
> *(1) Submitting, or causing to be submitted, bills or requests for payment that contain charges or costs substantially in excess of usual charges or costs when such charges or costs are due to **unusual circumstances** or medical complications requiring additional time, effort, expense or **other good cause** . . . [emphasis added].*

The challenge for this entry from the CFR is for the OIG to state exactly what the key phrases mean. What, for example, is "substantially in excess?" What are a hospital's "usual charges?" And, when are "unusual circumstances" or "good cause" present? Over the years, the OIG has issued proposed rules. One of the latest was included in the September 15, 2003 *Federal Register* in which the OIG discusses proposed definitions. However, no comprehensive final rule has been published* And the interpretation of the language remains an open question. Consider a simple real-life pricing situation: brachytherapy sources that are paid on a pass-through† basis under Medicare's APC outpatient payment system.

Case study 13-4. Brachytherapy source pricing.
The Chargemaster Coordinator at Apex Medical Center is pricing a new brachytherapy source. The acquisition cost for the source is $3000 and Apex's CCR (cost-to-charge ratio) is 0.40 as noted in its cost report. Three different prices have been developed:

1. For Medicare the price is calculated by dividing $3000 by the CCR of 0.40 or $7500.
2. For a self-pay patient, the price is set at 1.5 times $3000 or $4500.
3. Under a private contract, the price must be set at 10 percent above the acquisition cost or $3300.

---

* The September 15, 2003 *Federal Register* entry was the third in a series of discussions making proposals as to proper interpretation. See also April 2, 1990 (55 FR12205, 12215) and January 29, 1992 (57 FR 3298, 3307).

† Note that "pass-through" can be interpreted in slightly different ways. A direct pass-through payment is made on the specific cost reported through the charge. For brachytherapy sources, CMS developed an averaged pass-through payment mechanism.

On the surface, it appears that Apex is violating Medicare charging rule since it charges Medicare beneficiaries more than it charges other patients. The $7500 charge to Medicare is necessary because Medicare will convert the $7500 into what CMS thinks is the hospital's cost, that is, $7500 times 0.40 or $3000. If the hospital charges less, CMS will calculate an incorrect cost.

The $4500 charge is derived from a pricing formula used by the hospital for expensive supply items. Even at this level, the self-pay patient will probably consider the charge to be high. The $3300 charge is a contract obligation and allows no choice. The real question is whether this type of situation meets the requirements of differentially lower pricing for "good cause" or "good reason."

The second part of the Medicare charging rule requires that charges in the chargemaster be consistently based on costs. This cost reporting requirement appears in the *Provider Reimbursement Manual* at §2203:

> To assure that Medicare's share of the provider's costs equitably reflects the costs of services received by Medicare beneficiaries, the intermediary, in determining **reasonable cost reimbursement**, evaluates the charging practice of the provider to ascertain whether it results in an equitable basis for apportioning costs. So that its charges may be allowable for use in apportioning costs under the program, **each facility should have an established charge structure which is applied uniformly to each patient as services are furnished to the patient and which is reasonably and consistently related to the cost of providing the services.** While the Medicare program cannot dictate to a provider what its charges or charge structure may be, the program may determine whether or not the charges are allowable for use in apportioning costs under the program. [Emphasis added.]

Again, the key issue is the proper interpretation of the language, with the admonition that charges should be uniformly based on costs. Thus, CBR compliance personnel must be reasonably certain that the charge formulas in use do indeed meet this requirement. Note the exception process in that cost reporting personnel can "gross up" charges below the usual Medicare charges to equalize the cost report.

Case study 13-5. Cost-to-charge ratios. Apex Medical Center's CBR compliance personnel have been studying chargemaster charge structures and formulas. Charges were developed in a number of ways. Apex does not have the luxury of a cost accounting system. The following CCRs are noted for different departments:

Service Department	CCR
Operating room	0.65374
Recovery room	1.10045
Delivery and labor room	0.92834
Ultrasound	0.55641
Laboratory	0.66730
IV therapy	0.88452
Respiratory therapy	0.45885
Physical therapy	0.87043
Observation	0.34650
Emergency room	1.05478

Do these CCRs suggest that the center's charges are consistently based on costs throughout the chargemaster? Obviously, these CCRs vary widely and suggest that charges at Apex were not uniformly developed from costs. These figures came from the Medicare cost report which is not truly reflective of all the costs incurred by the hospital, but the variation is so significant that compliance concerns are raised.

Key learning area: The hospital chargemaster is a large, complex file that is integral to billing and claims generation. The chargemaster involves many interfaces including the coding and the charge capture interfaces. The chargemaster is a direct and indirect target of compliance concerns. In recent years, concerns have escalated significantly relative to hospital charges and pricing through the concept of *transparent pricing*. Additional interfaces of increasing concern are cost reporting and cost-to-charge ratios (CCRs).

Special Medicare hospital designations

Probably the most common perception of a hospital is what is now known as the short-term, acute care hospital. Most of the compliance concerns discussed in this book relate to this type of hospital. Medicare developed several new prospective payment systems for long-term care hospitals and rehabilitation hospitals. Additionally, specialty hospitals are increasing although, at least for Medicare purposes, they are generally short-term, acute care hospitals. Medicare also made several other hospital designations that can affect CBR compliance. The following designations are briefly addressed in this section.

- Critical access hospitals (CAHs)
- Sole community hospitals (SCHs)
- Medicare-dependent hospitals (MDHs)
- Rural referral centers (RRCs)

Each of these designation accrues special benefits and demands that certain requirements be met. CBR considerations apply to all designations, and thus all these types of hospitals face CBR compliance concerns.

Critical access hospitals are generally small facilities in rural areas. The number of beds is strictly limited to 25 (acute plus skilled). Patient stays are limited (average 96 hours or less). Medicare imposes special conditions of participation (CoPs). A CAH must be part of a hospital network so that patients can easily be transferred if needed. Several requirements apply to CAH status and compliance must be constantly monitored. CAHs are reimbursed by Medicare based upon reasonable costs, that is, Medicare cost reports. A number of hospital coding and billing rules are not applicable to CAHs, for example, the DRG pre-admission window. A CAH bills for outpatient services, then starts billing for inpatient services when a patient is admitted. Special prospective payment system rules generally do not apply. On the outpatient side, while short-term acute care hospitals use the APC (ambulatory payment classification) system in which the National Correct Coding Initiative (NCCI) edits are in place, CAHs do not have to worry about the edits or use of the -59 (separate procedure) modifier.*

Note: RHCs and federally qualified health centers (FQHCs) are also cost-based reimbursed. Both of these special types of clinics are also frequently located in rural areas, sometimes associated with a CAH.

As the name implies, a *sole community hospital* is generally the only one within a certain geographical area. Specific rules and regulations cover distances and associated population distributions. Compliance with these requirements generally falls outside CBR areas. This status brings a number of payment incentives. The DRG transfer rule does not apply, that is, no payment reduction applies to movement of a patient from inpatient status to skilled nursing status or to home health for selected DRG categories.† CBR compliance personnel at a SCH may need to modify audit concerns relative to provisions for increased reimbursement. From a financial view, SCH status can produce significant reimbursement gains for a hospital.

Medicare-dependent hospitals are similar to SCHs in that they accrue increased payment opportunities. These hospitals treat high percentages of Medicare patients. Typically, they are located in rural areas although the geographic constraints for SCHs and MDHs are different. CBR compliance staff will face auditing concerns relative to the differences in Medicare payment processes.

Rural referral centers are larger hospitals that serve as networks for smaller hospitals in a certain geographic region. They must have more than 275 beds and 50 percent of their Medicare patients must be referred, generally by smaller hospitals in the network. Congress established certain preferential payment processes for RRCs. Despite some payment differences, most CBR compliance issues for short-term, acute-care hospitals are applicable to RRCs.

Key learning area: Medicare has several special designations for hospitals. These designations potentially provide increased reimbursement under Medicare and the facilities must meet special requirements. The critical access hospital designation provides for cost-based reimbursement. This is different from typical prospective payment systems and fee schedules Medicare uses for other hospitals. The sole community hospital and Medicare-dependent hospital designations provide increased reimbursement by changing certain claims filing and/or associated payment processes. CBR compliance personnel should note such special designations when designing audits and reviews.

Medical staff organization and credentialing

While medical necessity is an overarching compliance issue for coding, billing, and achieving reimbursement by third-party payers, healthcare providers must also meet the mandate that a service or item provided must always be based on a physician's order. Also, qualified non-physician practitioners may also meet the physician's order criterion. Whenever a claim is filed, a physician must have ordered the service and/or, in Medicare language, the services rendered or item supplied must be incident-to those of a physician's services.

CBR compliance personnel and plans for achieving compliance are not usually concerned with the medical staff organization (MSO). Physicians and other qualified practitioners are generally credentialed through a rigorous process. Other issues may arise. For instance, certain nursing staff members may be qualified by the

---

* Some claim that the CCI edits generate correct coding so that for CAHs and other hospitals, the edits should be observed even to the point of using the -59 modifier.

† For certain DRGs, movement to a skilled nursing facility or to home healthcare is considered a transfer instead of a discharge followed by admission to the SNF or to an HHA. While the listing of transfer DRGs changes over time, DRG updates usually appear in the *Federal Register* issued on or about August 1 of each year.

MSO to perform EMTALA-mandated medical screening examinations (MSEs). Radiologists may have standing orders to perform certain additional tests based upon the results of an earlier test.* This is fairly common with diagnostic mammography and certain laboratory tests.

MSO bylaws may address situations such as those mentioned above, and CBR processes may well by affected by such protocols or standing orders. CBR compliance staff should carefully review current and proposed bylaws that affect coding, billing, and claims filing. Although credentialing is not normally a major concern for CBR compliance, exceptions can arise, as noted in this case study.

Case study 13-6. Physician assistant credentialing. Apex Medical Center's chief compliance officer has just been informed that a physician assistant has a deficiency in credentials. The PA never completed the last course in the required curriculum and has worked at Apex for three years. Professional claims have been routinely filed under the PA's NPI.

Key learning area: The MSO and credentialing processes are not normally major issues for CBR compliance. However, in order to code, bill, and file claims for services, all services provided and items supplied must have been ordered by a qualified practitioner or physician. Thus, physicians and practitioners must meet credentialing requirements. Also, the MSO may establish standing order protocols that can affect coding and billing.

Managed care contracts

This book uses *managed care* in a broad sense to indicate any entity that contracts with healthcare providers to provide payment. Payment usually depends upon filing a claim although capitated payment arrangements pay providers on a fixed basis, typically per member per month.

The range of managed care arrangements is enormous. In some cases, the managed care organization (MCO) has little to do with managing care and may simply function as a third-party administrator (TPA) that adjudicates claims and makes payments. In other cases, an MCO may be heavily involved with managing participants' healthcare services by limiting unnecessary services, promoting preventive programs, and other measures.

Even the Medicare has *advantage* plans involving several different types of managed care arrangements.

The concern with MCOs from a CBR perspective centers on contractual compliance. In many cases, healthcare providers enter into contracts with MCOs, generally referred to as private third-party payers. These contracts can be lengthy and complex or relatively brief, containing references to other documents and companion manuals that define the claims development rules, claims adjudication, and payments to be made.

Note: In some cases, healthcare providers must file claims to private third-party payers with which they have no relationships. No contractual obligations apply to the provider or the payer. General laws such as the state's Uniform Commercial Code may apply and some guidance may be obtained from the code sets and claim forms through the HIPAA TSC rule. As a practical matter, many healthcare providers file claim to non-contractual payers and then accept whatever payments are made.†

This book cannot discuss all the possible types of contractual arrangements and associated payment systems. From a CBR compliance perspective, the biggest single concern is *to have knowledge of and full access to all negotiated contracts*. To ensure compliance with contractual obligations and for coding and billing issues that may be referenced in the contracts, CBR compliance personnel must have access to the contracts and know the requirements for claims filing and adjudication. CBR compliance personnel should be involved in contract negotiations. In many instances favorable coding, billing, and claims filing conditions can be negotiated with little extra effort.

Hospitals and other healthcare providers generally concentrate on meeting statutory obligations and then secondarily work to ensure that contractual requirements are also met. Operationally, this means that contractual requirements will be prioritized based on the volume of claims with a third-party payer. If a hospital or other provider deals with two or three major private third-party payers, resources should be allocated to ensure that audits and reviews of key contractual requirements are performed. Fortunately, many contractual concerns are similar to statutory obligations with respect to proper coding, claims filing, charge-master set-up, and pricing.

---

* Also referred to as "reflex testing."

† In many instances a non-contractual third-party payer will adjudicate a claim based upon the patient's healthcare plan: treat the claim as if filed under a contractual arrangement. In theory, a claim to a non-contractual payer should be paid in full.

Key learning area: CBR compliance personnel should be knowledgeable about all managed care contracts with private third-party payers. While the contract requirements may be secondary to statutory obligations, appropriate resources should be made available to address all special requirements of contracts. If possible, CBR compliance personnel should be involved in negotiations of managed care contracts.

Associated entities

Many different types of healthcare providers may be formally or informally associated with a hospital. For example, physician offices and clinics are often clustered in the general vicinity of a hospital. The clinics may be free-standing or provider- (hospital-) based. Chapter 12 covers the provider-based rule. Other associated facilities may be ambulatory surgery centers (ASCs), home health agencies (HHAs), skilled nursing facilities (SNFs), and independent diagnostic testing facilities (IDTFs). Most of the entities are formally defined based on Medicare rules and regulations.

All of these entities utilize different payment mechanisms under the Medicare program. Extending the payment considerations to all other third-party payers increases the numbers and types of arrangements to a bewildering degree. CBR compliance is an issue for every type of healthcare provider. Because such entities are often closely associated with hospitals, hospital CBR personnel may become involved with compliance issues of associated entities. This section briefly discusses several types of associated providers. Each discussion is an overview rather than an exhaustive explanation.

Medical clinics: Free-standing versus provider-based

Hospitals often establish provider-based clinics to gain additional reimbursements available from Medicare. The payment increase issue was discussed in Chapter 12. Because of the payment increase, Medicare auditors and the OIG want to be certain that all criteria that allow provider-based status are met. Thus, CBR compliance personnel must conduct audits and reviews to verify compliance with all facets of the provider-based rule (PBR). Chapter 15 discusses this auditing process in detail.

Note that the concept of a provider-based clinic goes beyond a hospital setting. Other providers can also establish provider-based clinics. The following case study illustrates how this works.

Case study 13-7. Nursing facility provider-based clinic. The Summit Nursing Facility is a large, free-standing operation that provides skilled nursing services and nursing services. It has attained a size that can support on-site physicians and practitioners. A decision has been made to establish a provider-based clinic inside the nursing facility; one physician and two non-physician practitioners will provide services. Most patients will go to the clinic area for services. In other instances, the physician and practitioners will go to the bedsides of patients.

As with hospital-based clinics, both CMS-1450 and CMS-1500 forms are filed. Billing privileges must be established via appropriate CMS-855 forms. Billing will require extra care because the facility provides skilled nursing and nursing services. Both types of services are paid differently, depending on the third-party payer, generally Medicare or Medicaid. As an example, both SNF and NF patients may receive parenteral and enteral nutrition (PEN) therapy. For patients under the care of skilled nurses, PEN is part of the SNF PPS payment. However, for NF patients, PEN is separately billable to Medicare through a special process and filing claims on CMS-1500s.

Rural health clinics (RHCs) and federally qualified health centers (FQHCs)

RHCs and FQHCs are often grouped with CAHs because they are cost-based reimbursed and generally located in rural areas. These special clinics can be free-standing or provider-based. One difference between RHCs and FQHCs is that Medicare patients in FQHC settings are not subject to co-insurance. Medicare imposes very specific requirements for RHCs and FQHCs including requirements for the use of NPPs such as physician assistants and nurse practitioners.

CBR compliance personnel face number of potential issues, particularly for a provider-based RHC. The main provider may be a short-term, acute-care hospital or a CAH that established the RHC. Most likely the hospital will employ NPPs to work at the RHC. The NPPs may also be on call to the emergency department of the CAH. The CAH may be reimbursed for on-call expenses, but limitations apply to NPPs working at provider-based RHCs. CBR compliance personnel must become experts in understanding the specific organizational structures with which they work and any considerations for cost report development.

Ambulatory surgical centers (ASCs)

Ambulatory surgical center designates a specific type of Medicare entity and, in a general sense, identifies a facility that simply provides ambulatory surgery. Under Medicare, an ASC must meet certain criteria and be certified. Only certain types of surgical procedures may be performed at an ASC, at least under Medicare. Private third-party payers may be more liberal in classifying the services for which they will pay ASCs.

As this book was written, Medicare was in the process of switching ASC payment to a slightly modified form of ambulatory payment classifications (APCs). Basically, the ASC codes services as a hospital would, but the payment amount will be a percentage of what hospital outpatient departments receive for the same services. Other third-party payers utilize various payment mechanisms for ASCs including fee schedules and modified APCs. Claims are generally filed on 1500 claim forms (CMS-1500 for Medicare) and utilize CPT for reporting services provided.

Hospitals often become involved with ASCs either by directly establishing them or through joint-ventures with physicians. ASCs are often specialized to certain types of services such as orthopedic or cataract surgery. An ASC may be converted to a specialty hospital to provide higher quality care and also improve reimbursement.

Case study 13-8. Hospital outpatient services provided at ASC. Apex Medical Center is in a joint venture relative to an ASC on its campus. Suggestions have been made that Apex should contract to have hospital outpatient services provided at the ASC because of reduced overhead costs. Apex could then bill the services to receive hospital reimbursement through an arrangement with the ASC.

Needless to say, this type of arrangement will run contrary to the provider-based rule because the ASC is a special organization with very specific rules and regulations under the Medicare program.

Home health agencies (HHAs)

As the baby boom generation matures, needs for home healthcare are increasing. Although a market for private home health services exists, most home health services are used by elderly patients under Medicare and Medicaid. Medicare utilizes a special prospective payment system designed only for HHAs. Hospitals often own and operate HHAs although HHAs are independent in some areas. One of the major compliance concerns is that Medicare beneficiaries must have freedom of choice in selecting HHA services.

For CBR compliance personnel, the major concerns center on the development of proper documentation to support the data-driven Medicare HHA-PPS. Copious numbers of data sheets must be generated to drive the proper categorization of and subsequent payment for services. HHA patients are generally home-bound and the overarching issue of medical necessity is very much in play.

Home health patients have frequent encounters with providers. Nursing visits and home health aide visits may occur several times weekly. A physician-ordered plan of care must be established via form CMS-485. CBR audits should concentrate on documentation more than on coding. Classification for the HHA-PPS is driven by data developed through documentation.

Case study 13-9. OIG Probe audit of HHA services. The Chief Compliance Officer at Apex Medical Center has been informed that an OIG agent arrived at the hospital's home health agency and requested thirty cases at the individual visit level. The agent was sent to conduct a probe audit after a complaint by a patient. The agent will review the thirty visit notes and check the associated physician plans of care, after which patients will be called to verify that a nurse or home health aide actually provided services on the dates and times indicated in visit notes.

If you were involved in home health services, how would you fare under such a probe audit? While your documentation might be in perfect order, would patients remember specific visits? How would you verify that a nurse or home health aide actually provided the services?

Independent diagnostic testing facilities (IDTFs)

As with the other entities discussed in this section, the IDTF is a Medicare concept. They provide radiological and other diagnostic services and must meet certain licensing and quality standards. Payment is based on the Medicare Physician Fee Schedule (MPFS) and implemented through the RBRVS (Resource-Based Relative Value System). Claims are filed on CMS-1500 forms for Medicare and generally on 1500s for other third-party payers. Payment is generally through a fee schedule based on CPT and Level II HCPCS codes.

Special supervisory considerations come into play relative to coding and billing compliance. Medicare defines three levels of supervision. Program

Memorandum B-01-28 relates to physician supervision of diagnostic tests:

General supervision means the procedure is furnished under the physician's overall direction and control, but the physician's presence is not required during the performance of the procedure. Under general supervision, the training of the non-physician personnel who actually performs the diagnostic procedure and the maintenance of the necessary equipment and supplies are the continuing responsibility of the physician.

Direct supervision in the office setting means the physician must be present in the office suite and immediately available to furnish assistance and direction throughout the performance of the procedure. It does not mean that the physician must be present in the room when the procedure is performed.

Personal supervision means a physician must be in attendance in the room during the performance of the procedure.

For CBR compliance personnel, the issues are ensuring the supervisory rules are followed and appropriately coding and billing for services.

Note: Direct physician supervision has been a long-standing compliance issue, particularly under Medicare. Generally, *direct supervision* is interpreted as "in the office suite and immediately available." *Indirect supervision* generally means that a physician (or other qualified practitioner) is available by telephone or other communication device.

Comprehensive outpatient rehabilitation facilities (CORFs)

The CORF or ORF (outpatient rehabilitation facility) is another special type of Medicare-certified operation. Medicare has imposed special requirements for establishing such facilities and extensive coding and billing guidelines. Medical necessity issues along with requirements for establishing plans of care (POCs) are similar to those for physical, occupational, and speech–language therapies in hospital settings. The most common issues for such facilities relate to NPPs. Claims are filed with fiscal intermediaries (FIs) via CMS-1450s or UB-04s, generally using Bill Type 75X.

Hospitals become involved with CORFs in different ways. As with other Medicare entities, a hospital may establish a CORF or enter into a joint venture to establish one. Informal networking arrangements may also exist. If a hospital is involved in developing and filing claims, CBR issues will arise as they do for other special types of providers. While the CORF/ORF concept is rooted in Medicare, other third-party payers recognize such facilities in different ways, and this can affect billing and claims filing.

Key learning area: A hospital may be associated with a number of healthcare facilities at different levels of formality including ownership, joint venture, and network affiliation. Most of these special types of facilities are defined through Medicare rules and regulations. They are also subject to special compliance concerns, many of which involve coding, billing, and reimbursement.

Special hospital programs and provider-based clinics

Hospitals typically sponsor special programs that provide certain clinically coherent sets of services. These programs may be small and self-contained or grow to the point of requiring separate facilities. Typical examples are:

- Cardiac rehabilitation programs
- Pulmonary rehabilitation programs
- Partial hospitalization programs

All these programs provide specific clinical services, must meet specific medical necessity criteria, and must follow special coding and billing requirements. Pulmonary rehabilitation programs can serve as generic examples. Such a program typically has a medical director who may see patients. Respiratory therapists, physical therapists, and/or nursing staff can make different types of assessments and monitor therapeutic exercises. Most services will be provided by non-physician providers who are not considered practitioners, so all coding and billing will come from the hospital side, that is, through technical component claims. Medicare issues specific instructions through local coverage decisions (LCDs) that cover proper use of CPT and HCPCS codes, diagnosis codes, revenue codes, the types of services that may be performed by different personnel, and frequency delimitations.

While we have touched only upon one special program, the need for CBR compliance should be evident. Acquiring expertise only in Medicare-associated requirements for a single program can be a major challenge.

The PBR was briefly discussed in Chapter 12, which also addressed the financial advantages for provider-based clinics under Medicare. Hospitals across the country have been developing and operating provider-based clinics for the past 20 years. A bewildering array of different types of provider-based clinics have appeared—the typical ones such as family practice, orthopedics, ophthalmology, and dermatology and the special ones such as medication management or cholesterol control. Even small hospitals in rural areas may have specialty provider-based clinics.*

Operationally, a facility or organization is provider-based if a UB-04 claim form (or equivalent electronic claim) is filed. Hospitals may also have clinics it simply owns and operates but are organized to be free-standing, that is, they file only professional claims without corresponding UB-04 claims. Thus, a hospital or system of hospitals can consist of different combinations of free-standing and provider-based clinics.

Regardless of the organizational specifics, owned and operated free-standing clinics and full-fledged provider-based clinics generate significant CBR compliance concerns. For instance, a free-standing clinic owned or operated by a hospital is subject to the Medicare DRG pre-admission window. Provider-based clinics generally file two claims. For off-campus provider-based clinics Medicare requires issuance of a notice of two co-payments for Medicare beneficiaries. Also, because two claims forms are filed, a split-fee schedule is involved. Care should be taken to charge Medicare and non-Medicare patients the same amounts. While a hospital may decide to split-bill† all types of patients and third-party payers, many third-party payers do not distinguish provider-based from free-standing clinics for payment purposes. Thus hospitals may elect to split-bill only the Medicare program.‡

As with many hospital coding, billing, and organizational issues, clinics and programs generate multiple compliance issues. Hospitals with provider-based clinics face increased CBR compliance concerns.

Key learning area: Hospitals typically have special programs such as cardiac rehabilitation and pulmonary rehabilitation. Many have associated clinics that can be organized as free-standing or provider-based. These special programs and particularly provider-based clinics generate CBR compliance concerns.

Summary and conclusion

This chapter discussed a number of special hospital compliance areas. The chargemaster serves as a direct and indirect target of compliance concerns at both statutory and contractual levels. In recent years, concerns about setting charges and hospital pricing have increased and led to movements advocating transparent pricing and consumer-driven healthcare. We briefly covered medical staff organizations that may involve certain coding and billing issues. Many hospitals are associated with home health agencies, ambulatory surgical centers, and other facilities. All these special types of healthcare facilities can raise the bar for coding, billing, and associated reimbursement compliance concerns.

Special Medicare hospital designations may entail certain obligations. Critical access hospitals are popular in rural areas. They are cost-based reimbursed and thus present another set of specialized CBR concerns. Sole community hospitals enjoy certain reimbursement enhancements under Medicare, but also must meet certain requirements.

Hospitals participate in contractual arrangements with private third-party payers, also known as managed care organization (MCOs). Hospitals should ascertain that CBR compliance personnel have full access to and knowledge of any contractual obligations assumed through such contracts.

Key learning area: Hospitals vary in size and complexity. A small rural hospital may provide limited services. A specialty hospital may concentrate on a few surgical procedures. A regional hospital may provide a wide range of services and be involved with other types of providers such as home health, skilled nursing, and clinics. Hospital systems and teaching hospitals provide the greatest challenges in organizational complexity and range of services. The complexity and diversity of CBR compliance challenges correlate directly to facility size and scope of services provided.

---

* Small hospitals may elect to rent space to specialty physicians at fair market value. Because the physician rents the space, the same specialty clinics may be free-standing; thus only the physician files a professional claim.
† Split-bill in this context means that both UB-04 (CMS-1500) and 1500 (CMS-1500) forms are filed.
‡ See the April 7, 2000, *Federal Register*, page 18519 (65 FR 18519).

fourteen

Compliance considerations for physicians and clinics

Introduction

Some specialized compliance programs are applicable to physician groups and medical clinics. While the diversity of compliance concerns for clinics is not generally as great as it is for hospitals, clinic compliance concerns are just as important. At the integrated delivery system (IDS) level, physicians and clinics play an important role relative to structuring and interrelationships with other providers such as hospitals, skilled nursing facilities, and home health agencies.

Most concerns for medical clinics carry over into other types of free-standing service providers such as therapy services, dialysis centers, nuclear medicine operations, and other types of independent diagnostic testing facilities (IDTFs). Keep in mind the distinction between free-standing and provider-based clinics. (See discussion of the provider-based rule in Chapter 12.) The main Medicare payment system for physicians and clinics is through the Medicare Physician Fee Schedule (MPFS) developed through the Resource-Based Relative Value System (RBRVS). For provider-based situations, ambulatory payment classifications (APCs) also affect the reimbursement picture.

CBR compliance personnel must always be watchful for issues involving physicians, particularly if physician ownership is involved. Chapter 12 briefly discussed the Stark rules that address such situations. Physicians often become involved in owning IDTFs, ambulatory surgery centers (ASCs), and, more recently, specialty hospitals. Physicians as owners are subject to extra scrutiny based on conditions for payment (CfPs) and the CMS-855 forms also discussed in Chapter 12.

Clinic organizational structuring

The simplest medical clinic is physically and organizationally free-standing—physically separate from other healthcare providers and organizationally free from outside ownership and management arrangements. Typically such clinics are owned by the physicians who provide services there. Billing and claims filing at free-standing clinics are generally handled via 1500 claim forms; the place of service (POS) is the clinic or office.

At the other end of the continuum is a clinic that is both physically and organizationally integrated with another provider such as a hospital. The physical facility may be in and/or attached to the hospital. Organizationally, the clinic is part of the hospital outpatient department and billing within this structure is very different: The 1500 is used for the professional component and UB-04 for the technical component. The place of service (POS) on the 1500 is listed as hospital, outpatient.

Falling between these extremes are other arrangements. Some clinics may be physically free-standing and organized as provider-based. The reverse also occurs: A group of physicians may rent space for an urgent care clinic from a hospital. Thus, the clinic is physically inside the hospital. Because the physicians rent the space, the clinic is considered to be organizationally free-standing, and claims are filed only on form 1500. These arrangements can generate additional concerns. If a clinic is provider-based and off the campus of the main provider, it faces concerns about the Emergency Medical Treatment and Labor Act (EMTALA). The following case study illustrates an EMTALA issue. See Chapter 12 for further information on EMTALA.

> **Case study 14-1. Urgent care center across the hall from ED.** A group of physicians have rented space at Apex Medical Center. This space is across the hall from the hospital's emergency department. The arrangement works well for the hospital and the physician group. When a patient presents to the ED, registration personnel quickly assess the situation. If it is not a medical emergency (a minor injury or condition), the patient is sent across the hall to the urgent care clinic rented by the physicians.

Case study 14-1 illustrates the need to assess organizational structuring and patient flow. Although the arrangement described in the case study is probably efficient and results in lower charges to patients, it poses significant problems, particularly from EMTALA, which clearly specifies actions to take when a patient presents to a hospital ED. A medical screening examination (MSE) must be performed by a qualified medical person. The patient information has to be entered into the EMTALA log, and services must be provided if an emergency medical condition is present. If the hospital performs all these services, charges must be imposed and a claim must be filed. If no emergency is present, the patient may be referred to another provider such as the free-standing clinic across the hall.

Another example of organizational structuring is a specialty clinic. The typical arrangement is to have a specialist visit a "host" hospital on a regular basis, perhaps twice a month, to provide services. The specialist may pay rent at fair market value (FMV); in other cases, the hospital bills a facility fee and does not charge the physician. In the former case, the clinic is considered to belong to the physician who bills on a 1500. In the latter case, the clinic is considered provider-based, and both UB-04 and 1500 forms are filed. Note that the POS on the 1500 is critical because it drives the site of service (SOS) differential for Medicare under RBRVS. The site of a specialty clinic may be another clinic. In this situation, the specialty physician typically rents space and handles billing. However, even in this scenario, billing is not always straightforward. What happens, for example, if the clinic in which the specialist provides services is provider-based? In this situation the clinic is part of a hospital and we must consider a rental approach or treat the specialist as provider-based.

Other levels of organizational structuring may be even more complex. What occurs with billing and claims filing if both the hospital and the clinic in question are owned by a parent organization? Although the hospital and clinic may have no direct relationship, common ownership may raise significant compliance concerns such as the DRG pre-admission window triggered by ownership or control. What if the clinic (or other provider) was a joint venture established by two or more organizations? Each of these scenarios will test the knowledge and skill of CBR compliance personnel. Clearly, the answers to such questions must be based on a thorough understanding of entity interfaces and several other factors.

The organizational structure and physical location of a medical clinic or other type of clinic provider can be complex. These issues serve as starting points for building and implementing a workable and appropriate CBR compliance program that accommodates the specific organizational structure of a medical clinic.

Key learning area: From a compliance perspective it is critical to have full information about clinic ownership, management, and physical and organizational relationships. Additionally, any relationships of a clinic with other healthcare providers must be fully known before compliance concerns, including related CBR issues, can be effectively addressed.

Physician relationships

Physicians at clinics typically have multiple relationships. While some physicians have completely clinic-based practices, most work at one or more hospitals, participate in special clinics, work with residents, run drug trials and tests, and handle many additional responsibilities. All these functions and associated relationships must be well defined, both for the physician and the entity with which the physician works.

Consider the fact that most physicians have relationships with several hospitals. This means that the physician is on the medical staff of each hospital, has been credentialed at each hospital, and may serve as a medical director of some area. Every one of these relationships should be examined for possible compliance and/or legal liability on the part of the physician and the associated clinic.

Regardless of the kind of relationship, one issue exerts a direct impact on CBR processes: the activities of physicians at hospitals. Since services are provided at the hospital but the billing for these hospital-based services is performed at the clinic, definite concerns arise about the information flow back from the hospital, particularly about the documentation supporting the services.

Physicians must be vigilant in establishing information flow mechanisms between the site of service and the clinic handling billing. Definitive written records must indicate services performed, for whom they were performed, and the dates of performance. Third-party payers are instituting documentation guidelines that specifically request information about times of services (i.e., start and stop times or duration times). While the physician may provide the clinic with information necessary for coding and billing, it is likely that the written record will remain at the hospital. Thus coding personnel will have no opportunities to review the documentation relative to the level of coding.

Case study 14-2. Physician service information for hospital visits. The physicians at Acme Medical Clinic use an index card (3 × 5") system to track hospital visits and services provided at the hospital. At the end of each week, the physicians bring their cards to coding and billing personnel who then code and enter charges. The coding staff is concerned because the physicians simply indicate the level of hospital visit (level 2 or 3) and several physicians are providing minor surgical care and not reporting the services on their cards.

Case study 14-2 illustrates the compliance issues surrounding physicians who code at levels different from services documented. Coding personnel should always express concern when coding is not based directly on documentation.

Case study 14-3. Nurse assisting physician on hospital rounds. Several physicians at Acme Medical Clinic have started taking nurses along on hospital rounds. The nurse typically sees patients, performs assessments, and develops documentation of the encounters. The physician sees patients and confers with the nurse. The physician is basing the level of service on the combined efforts of physician and nurse.

The basic facts in Case study 14-3 appear to be fully appropriate for complete, quality care of patients, but raise significant compliance issues related to incident-to billing. Physicians can perform incident-to billing if they work in their own free-standing clinics. If the services are performed at another facility or institutional setting, incident-to billing is generally not allowed. The hospital or facility is paid for the nurse's services because they are incident-to the physician's services. Incident-to services constitute a complex and subtle compliance issue. One exception to the general rule is when a physician and a mid-level practitioner jointly perform services. See Case study 14-10.

Key learning area: A significant issue for clinic compliance in the CBR area is documentation related to hospital-based services provided by a clinic physician. Care should be taken to ensure accurate and timely information flow from the site of service to the clinic for coding purposes. Additionally, periodic audits should be conducted to assess the documentation relative to the code selection level.

Another area involving multiple interfaces is the ordering of diagnostic tests. In many cases, clinics operate their own laboratories and radiological services. However, clinic physicians may order tests that will be performed elsewhere. Note that diagnostic information is required when a physician orders diagnostic tests.* The entity performing the tests may want additional information about the medical necessity of the tests in order to consider issuing an advance beneficiary notice (ABN). The entity performing the tests may want the physician to obtain the ABN. The number of potential interfaces of physicians and clinic or non-clinic laboratories, and the associated information required by such laboratories, can create many compliance concerns.

Physicians also become involved in hospital compliance issues when they admit patients for inpatient care. Timing and bundling issues may create compliance concerns. Timing issues can arise if a patient is admitted to the hospital late in the evening and the attending physician does not see the patient until the next day. This may comply with medical staff bylaws but it creates a situation requiring the physician to properly code for encounters relative to the actual dates and times when services are rendered. Physicians should understand that dates of service must be accurate for CBR purposes.

Case study 14-4. Admission by ER physician under attending physician's name. ER physicians at Apex Medical Center do not have admitting privileges to inpatient or observation status. If a patient presents in the evening, the ER physician prepares the paperwork and admits to inpatient status or observation status under the attending physician's name. The attending physician (in theory) sees the patient the next morning.

The basic facts in Case study 14-4 may not pose a compliance issue. The attending physician, upon seeing the patient the next morning, must ensure that the coding and billing cover services on the date he or she provided them, not the date reflecting services rendered by the ER physician the previous evening. In other words, the physician cannot charge an initial service for the evening and then a regular hospital visit the following morning because the physician did not see the patient during the evening.

Case study 14-5. Inpatient status to observation status. The coding and billing staff at Acme Medical Clinic note a problem. The clinic physicians admit patients to inpatient status and coding staff handle coding and billing to reflect this process. However, on several occasions, hospital utilization review personnel have talked the physician into changing the admission to an observation stay instead of an inpatient stay. This information is not filtering back to the clinic coding staff until claims have been filed.

This case study illustrates the use of Condition Code 44. Hospitals are becoming more fastidious about classifying certain inpatient admissions to observation status. While this is appropriate on the part of the hospitals, such changes may impact coding and billing by physicians.

Another interface of possible concern, at least for physicians not employed by a hospital, is the receipt of anything from the hospital that might be construed as

---

* See Balanced Budget Act of 1997 (BBA 1997).

an inducement. Any inducements can be considered to violate the Medicare Fraud, Abuse and Anti-Kickback Laws. While education, training, and food are often covered by medical staff organization dues, physicians and hospitals must be certain that the dues represent the fair market value (FMV) of the goods and services received.

Case study 14-6. Discounted hospital services for staff physicians. Physicians on the medical staff at Apex Medical Center are unhappy. A competing hospital about 50 miles down the road allows discounts on hospital care to its physicians. Basically, the program involves waiving all co-payments, deductibles, and other patient cost-sharing items up to $3000 per year. Of course, this applies to non-Medicare claims.

This type of situation raises significant concerns. Any such arrangement should be carefully reviewed by legal counsel. The facts as stated in Case study 14-6 appear to violate the $300 *de minimis* amount treated as an exception under the anti-kickback laws.

Physician ownership

Physician ownership of a facility or entity creates special kinds of relationships and raises a variety of compliance concerns. Much legislation, mostly associated with the Stark laws, has been enacted in this area. Great care should be exercised whenever a physician becomes involved with a healthcare organization and/or healthcare provider as an owner. In many cases, ownership issues go beyond the physician and may affect his or her immediate family. In light of this, before proceeding with ownership arrangements, physicians should consult legal counsel and financial advisors.

Physician ownership, besides its potential personal risks, also creates compliance concerns. Medicare, for example, is greatly concerned with any arrangement in which physicians may refer patients for tests and services for which the physician receives payment. The underlying reason for concern is the potential for abuse and the fear that physicians will be influenced to order unnecessary tests or services.

Case study 14-7. Physicians establishing IDTF. A group of ten physicians from different practices decides to jointly establish an independent diagnostic testing facility that will provide a wide range of services including laboratory tests and radiology. Services for Medicare and Medicaid patients will be somewhat limited. A significantly wider range of services will be available for non-Medicare patients.

While IDTFs are certainly viable forms of healthcare providers, they face definite coding, billing, and reimbursement concerns that should be fully explored before they start providing services. One of those concerns is the Medicare requirement about supervision of tests and three levels of supervision. See the IDTF section in Chapter 13.

Case study 14-8. Joint venture ASC to specialty hospital. Over the past several years, physicians at Acme Medical Clinic and Apex Medical Center jointly developed an ambulatory surgery center (ASC) on the campus of Apex. The volume of services has grown significantly and the physicians now want to change the arrangement to make the ASC a specialty hospital. A new wing is to be built onto Apex Medical Center, and the operation will become a hospital within a hospital (HwH).

This case study presents a very complex situation. CMS has established rules and regulations over the years covering joint ventures and HwHs. In situations of this type, legal counsel should be consulted about organizational structuring and associated concerns. After the structuring and relationships are determined, proper coding and billing procedures can be established.

Note: CBR issues should be addressed **before** the organizational structuring is completed. The opposite is often true: the business is set up and coding and billing issues are handled after the fact.

Case study 14-9. Partnership of professional corporations. A group of physicians have decided to work together. All the physicians have their own practices and are incorporated as professional corporations. The group of physicians has established a partnership composed of their professional corporations. The partnership provides all the common administrative functions, including patient registration, maintenance of medical records, financial accounting, and coding and billing.

The organizational structure in Case study 14-9 may appear reasonably straightforward, but it presents a number of potential coding and billing compliance issues. The partnership acts as a management service organization for the individual physician professional corporations. Thus, CMS and possibly other third-party payers will be interested in how coding and billing services are handled. If payments are made to the partnership, CMS will want to know about contracts between the professional corporations and the partnership.

Key learning area: Any ownership interest of a physician in a healthcare organization and/or provider requires great care in navigating the Stark laws. Keeping the fundamental concepts of self-referral arrangements in mind can facilitate reasonable interpretations as to the propriety of such arrangements. Be certain to consider CBR issues *prior* to finalizing organizational arrangements.

Non-physician providers (NPPs)

The use of NPPs is growing rapidly. While a number of clinical and other care issues arise, the focus of this discussion will be on the coding and billing of services. NPPs generally fall into two broad categories: (1) those who can file claims for services on CMS-1500 forms and (2) those whose services must be billed as non-professional, i.e., billing via UB-04 (hospital setting) or as incident-to the services of a professional (physician or practitioner).

Note: Professional is used purely relative to the ability of an NPP to file professional claims on form 1500. This discussion in no way addresses the fact that the services are provided on a professional basis.

Currently, the NPPs or mid-level practitioners who are typically recognized for 1500 claim filing include:

- Physician assistants (PAs)
- Nurse practitioners (NPs)
- Clinical nurse specialists (CNSs)
- Clinical social workers (CSWs)
- Nurse midwives
- Psychologists
- Physical therapists
- Occupational therapists
- Certified registered nurse anesthetists (CRNAs)

In addition to these NPPs who are recognized for billing purposes, many other certified NPPs perform special services, for example, certified enterostomal nurses (CENs), first RN assistants (FRNAs), suture technicians (STs), and others. NPPs not yet recognized for separate payment via CMS-1500 are billed in two different ways depending on the organization in which they work. See Chapter 12 for a discussion of provider-based clinics.

For hospitals and provider-based clinics, payments for these NPP services come through the technical or facility component billing on form UB-04. In free-standing (not provider-based) clinic settings, the physicians bill for these NPP services on an incident-to basis as if they, the physicians, performed the services. Two approaches apply to NPPs recognized for

professional billing and their use depends upon the organizational structuring and setting. The two main approaches are:

1. The practitioners bill for their services on 1500 claim forms. All supervision or collaborative agreements must be in place and the POS must be carefully delineated between clinic (generally POS 11) and hospital, outpatient (generally POS 22). Payment for practitioner services is generally 85 percent of what the physician would be paid.* The Medicare site-of-service differential will be applied if the setting is a provider-based clinic.

2. The organization bills for the practitioners' services. In a hospital or provider-based setting, payments accrue from UB-04 claim forms. In a free-standing (not provider-based) setting, the services would be billed on form 1500 on an incident-to basis. Supervision must be direct (the physician or qualified practitioner is to be present in the suite and immediately available).

This is only a brief synopsis and does not address associated employment rules or specialized billing rules. PAs may bill for their services only through their employers. NPs may set up separate practices and bill under their own auspices if state law allows. (See Chapter 12 for a further discussion of non-physician providers and practitioners.) Also, scope-of-practice considerations are promulgated at state level so differences exist among states.

In Case study 14-3 we briefly addressed the situation in which a physician takes a nurse to a hospital to perform what may be inpatient visits or inpatient consultations. In the following case study, a physician and a mid-level practitioner perform joint E/M services in a hospital setting.

Case study 14-10. Joint physician and practitioner E/M services. Acme Medical Clinic now has several mid-level practitioners. One of the physicians will often take a nurse practitioner (NP) along for joint hospital rounds and/or performance of minor procedures. Sometimes, only the NP or the physician will see a patient. On some occasions, both the physician and NP see a patient. The obvious question is how these services should be properly coded and billed.

Case study 14-10 illustrates that coding and billing may not be straightforward when a patient is seen by physicians and non-physician practitioners working jointly.

---

* The percentage of payment under Medicare varies somewhat among different types of mid-level practitioners.

If a physician provides a service alone, the physician will code and bill. If the NP in the case study sees a patient alone, the NP will code and bill under his or her NPI. If the service is joint, only one of them can code and bill, and a decision must be made as to who will do so. The general consideration in such cases is that the physician will receive full payment (at least under Medicare) while the NP will receive a reduced payment (generally 85 percent). Thus, for a joint service (fully documented, of course), the physician will bill and the NP will not bill.*

Special situations affect residency programs, RHCs, and FQHCs. These situations are governed by different rules that require special compliance considerations.

Key learning area: Because the use of NPPs in various settings is growing, the CBR compliance issues for NPPs are becoming increasingly complex and interlaced with organizational structuring. Always fully analyze the distinctions in coding and billing for mid-level practitioners who can file claims on form 1500 versus other non-physician providers who cannot file 1500 claim forms.

Coding documentation guidelines

For physicians and clinics, a major area of a CBR compliance program involves coding and concomitant documentation. The two major coding systems are CPT and ICD-9-CM.† Both systems are complex. The purpose of CPT coding is to report what procedures or services a physician has performed. A number of modifiers must be used to accurately report additional information about the services. The -25 modifier indicates that a significant, separately identifiable E/M service was performed in conjunction with a surgery or medical procedure. The obvious question for this modifier is when it should and should not be used. While following the CPT definition, a third-party payer may impose additional rules and regulations.

Diagnosis coding is different from CPT coding and imposes a number of guidelines. In a clinic or hospital outpatient setting, it is not permissible to code rule-outs, probable, suspected, or versus diagnoses. It is, however, permissible to code these diagnoses in hospital inpatient settings. Other related rules cover addressing chronic and acute conditions.

The two systems also interact. For instance, if a -25 modifier is used, some third-party payers want what

are called *differential diagnoses*. This means that payment will be made for the E/M service only in the event of a diagnostic condition that was different from the diagnosis for performing the surgery.‡ Since payment for physicians and clinics is driven by CPT coding that may be linked to diagnosis codes, it is logical to understand the emphasis on the coding relative to compliance. As coding staff are quick to point out, the codes cannot be better than the documentation. The generation of documentation and its subsequent interpretation by coding staff are critical elements for both payment and compliance.

While surgical coding is certainly important, the vast volume of non-surgical coding and a significant proportion of payments arise from E/M coding. The proper choice of E/M level is governed by various guidelines. The first level of guidelines comes from the CPT manual. The first set of documentation guidelines appeared in 1995 after the introduction of E/M codes in 1992. A significantly revised and more detailed set was issued in 1997 and withdrawn after numerous complaints from the medical community. A proposed draft revision to the 1997 guidelines was released in 2000 but no further action has been taken to formally update the E/M guidelines. Physicians may currently use the 1995 or the 1997 guidelines.

Whatever the specifics of E/M coding, a major part of a clinic CBR compliance program is assurance that documentation meets the standards for any level of coding. Many E/M codes contain a series of levels. To attain a certain upper level, the history, examination, and medical decision making levels must first be achieved. Adding to the complexity is the process of coding by time. Some E/M codes have associated average times. If "counseling and coordination" of care are involved, the coding can be done by time if more than 50 percent of the encounter constitutes counseling and coordination of care. Some items such as critical care and prolonged services must be coded by time, typically based on the first hour and each subsequent half hour.

While meeting documentation standards for E/M codes, it is also necessary to ensure that the correct series are used. For instance, consultation codes generally pay better than the more common office visit codes. Since providers have an economic incentive to use the consultation codes, meeting consultation requirements becomes a compliance concern.

Clearly, coding guidelines and documentation processes are major thrusts for compliance, but steps for monitoring compliance and taking corrective actions if non-compliance occurs must be in place. Formal and

---

* This is the so-called joint E/M service exception relative to incident-to billing in a hospital or facility setting. See Transmittal 1776 dated October 25, 2002.

† Soon to become ICD-10 or possibly ICD-11.

‡ In theory, the requirements for differential diagnoses have been eliminated due to changes of wording in the CPT manual.

informal auditing processes are the norms. Additionally, specialized and routine training of coding personnel and physicians must be ongoing and mandatory.

Case study 14-11. New versus established patient E/M levels. Determining whether a patient is new (not seen within three years) has been an ongoing problem at Acme Medical Clinic. As a result, a number of claim forms showing established patient visit levels (99211 through 99215) must be changed to reflect new patient levels (99201 through 99205). Billing staff simply map levels from established patient E/M codes to new patient E/M codes. For instance, a 99213 code is changed to a 99203, a 99214 to a 99204, etc.

A careful reading of CPT will clearly indicate that the established visit and new patient levels do not correlate directly. The process used in Case study 14-11 will lead to incorrect coding and billing for the E/M levels.

Case study 14-12. Use of 99211 code for injections. The coding and billing staff at Acme Medical Clinic are confused about new CPT language introduced in 2006 relative to intramuscular and subcutaneous injections. Parenthetical language indicates that the 99211 (nursing service) code is to be used in the absence of direct physician supervision. Thus, it appears that if a nurse provides an injection without a physician present, the 99211 can still be used. Is this correct?

This is an example of a new coding guideline that needs further explanation or interpretation. This language appears in the CPT manual, but CPT does not define direct physician supervision. Physician supervision is generally a Medicare concept that has its own related complexity. The coding and billing personnel at Acme should seek further advice, possibly including a legal opinion, about how to correctly code under these circumstances.

Key learning area: CPT and ICD-9-CM govern the ways physicians and clinics are reimbursed. As a result, most compliance issues in this area stem from various coding guidelines.

Establishing medical necessity

For most healthcare organizations, the single biggest compliance issue may be medical necessity: bills and claims must reflect charges only for services that are medically necessary. Additionally, the levels and types of services provided must be appropriate for the care and appropriately documented.

A major difference between hospital outpatient claims (UB-04) and physician professional service claims (1500) is that the 1500 provides a formal mechanism for correlating up to four diagnosis codes back to line item charges. This allows the direct ability to check for medical necessity even at the line item claim level. The choice, sequencing, and correlation of diagnosis codes are this extremely important.

One of the main concerns in establishing medical necessity is the full development of all relevant diagnosis codes. Since clinic work and most hospital outpatient services are encounter-driven, it is important that physicians document all signs, symptoms, and other defined (or sometimes ill-defined) conditions along with more definitive diagnoses. While clinic coding personnel must conform to existing diagnosis coding guidelines, it is also important to develop as many diagnosis codes as possible. Obviously, coding personnel cannot develop diagnosis codes for conditions that are not documented.

As previously noted, diagnosis coding for rule-outs, probable, suspected, and versus diagnoses is prohibited for clinics and outpatient services. This can create a significant medical necessity quandary and raise serious questions about timing of coding relative to claims filing. Consider the following situation.

Case study 14-13. Symptoms versus definitive diagnosis. An elderly patient presents to Acme Medical Clinic. An examination results in diagnoses of cough, fever, and congestion, and rule out pneumonia. An x-ray and several laboratory tests are ordered. The results arrive two days later and confirm pneumonia.

The diagnosis coding questions arising from such situations provide the mechanisms for medical necessity for the services and subsequent payment. Since third-party payers do not want to pay for unnecessary services, various compliance issues are also involved. Obviously, if the diagnosis of pneumonia is coded, the services will most likely be considered medically necessary. However, is it appropriate to code the pneumonia if the diagnosis was confirmed two days after the encounter? If the pneumonia is to be coded, is it appropriate to also code the cough, fever, and congestion? These symptoms are typically signs of pneumonia.

These and similar questions are not easy to answer and generally require the development of explicit coding polices and procedures that must be grounded in current official diagnosis coding policies and guidelines. However, personnel may have some latitude. For instance, are they willing to code the pneumonia if the doctor makes a note about the laboratory test results?

Claims development: CPT, modifiers, and ICD-9

Developing 1500 claims form for the professional component of billing is a complex task. Knowledge of surgical and E/M CPT coding is essential and a good understanding of modifiers is also important. Moreover, coding staff should fully understand the various physician payment systems, such as RBRVS and the included Medicare global surgical package (GSP). As discussed above, diagnosis coding is important for establishing the medical necessity of a procedure performed. Most third-party payers use a one-day window for physician services. Under CPT, if a physician places a patient in observation status, he or she must bundle other E/M services into this observation admission.

The GSP is a prime example of a payment system coding methodology that has many compliance overtones. For Medicare purposes, surgeries are divided into minor and major categories. The post-operative period for minor surgeries is 0 days or 10 days—the exclusive *or* means the period may be 0 days or 10 days and no number of days between 0 and 10. The distinction between 0- and 10-day surgeries is that surgeries "performed through an existing body orifice" are 0-day follow-up procedures. Major surgeries are permitted 90-day follow-ups. Post-operative periods are listed in the Medicare Physician Fee Schedule or RBRVS *Federal Register* that typically appears in November of each year.

CPT modifiers separate surgical procedures into three distinct areas:

- -56   Pre-operative
- -54   Intra-operative
- -55   Post-operative

Physicians may code for that portion of the surgery performed. Medicare generally recognizes only the intra-operative and post-operative components and divides payments between them.

Thus, a physician who plans to perform only an operation should code the surgical procedure with the -54 modifier. The physician assuming the post-operative care uses the -55 modifier. If the surgery has a 90-day post-operative period, the physician or physicians assuming post-operative care must determine how to bill properly for post-operative services.

Post-operative care can present significant compliance problems. For instance, if the surgeon transfers care, the transfer should be in writing. A transfer back to the surgeon should also be handled in writing. In some cases, a physician may provide post-operative care such as suture removal, and will have no idea what codes were used or who billed for the original service. Thus the ability to use the -55 modifier with surgical codes also becomes problematic.

Case study 14-14. Post-Operative suture removal. An elderly patient visited Apex Medical Center's ED to have a laceration repaired. The ER physician made the repair and instructed the patient to see her primary care physician in five or six days. She presents to Acme Medical Clinic for suture removal. The physician examines the repair and instructs the nurse to remove the sutures. How should the removal be coded and billed?

Primary care physicians have encountered problems with the circumstances delineated in Case study 14-14. In theory, the surgical code with the -55 modifier should be used. However, did the ER physician actually transfer the post-operative care? Did the ER physician use the -54 modifier to indicate that only the intra-operative portion was provided? Most primary care physicians tend to use a low level E/M for this type of service because no code exists for suture removal (except when anesthesia is used), but coding a low level E/M raises compliance concerns.

The pre-surgical situation comes into play even for the Medicare GSP. The basic idea is that if a surgeon performs services for a patient within the 1-day pre-surgery window, the services are bundled into the payment for the surgery. The exception is that a surgeon will always be paid for an initial assessment for a surgery. If the surgeon performs the initial assessment on the day of or the day before the surgery, the -57 modifier (decision to perform surgery) comes into play. This pre-surgery window can also be important relative to the pre-surgery history and physical (H&P). If the surgeon is to perform the pre-surgical H&P, he or she must perform it more than one day in advance of the surgery to receive additional payment. Otherwise another physician should perform the pre-surgery H&P.

Despite this discussion, coding considerations for pre-surgery H&Ps are complex for compliance purposes. In many cases, the pre-surgery H&P is performed by a primary care physician at the request of the surgeon. The primary care physician will issue a report and render advice or an opinion. More specifically, the primary care physician will indicate readiness of the patient to undergo surgery. However, the primary care physician will not take over care relative to the surgery. Thus the question becomes, can the primary care physician bill a consultation? This situation is deemed a reverse consultation—it is the reverse of a normal consultation request made by a primary care physician to a specialist or surgeon.

Some statistical measures should be noted in connection with coding. The first is the distribution of E/M codes. This issue was addressed earlier in the book. The relative frequency of E/M code utilization should be monitored and audited to ensure that coding documentation guidelines are met. A second issue is the need to meet time averages for E/M services. Since a number of E/M codes are associated with average times, it is possible to look at the pattern of E/M codes utilized by a physician on a single day or days and then determine whether the sum of the average times is reasonable relative to period in which the physician performed the services. While these time units are not to be used in this manner, auditors and investigators tend to use them as benchmarks.

Another area of concern related to physician coding is preventive medicine. In some cases, patients may present for what appear to be preventive medicine visits. A good example is an elderly patient requesting an annual physical examination. Since the patient intends to obtain preventive medical services that are not covered under Medicare, the physician must be vigilant about coding the services as preventive unless a new diagnostic condition is discovered. In this case, a portion of the visit can be coded and billed using the regular office visit E/M along with the preventive medicine visit. Care must be taken to adjust the charging process in this case by prorating part of the preventive care charge to the regular E/M level.

The range of modifiers used by physician coders is extensive. While a complete discussion of the all the modifiers is beyond the scope of this book, several merit attention in this section. The -25 modifier has been mentioned and another common modifier is -59 (distinct services), used in conjunction with CMS's correct coding initiative (CCI)—essentially the same set of some 200,000 code combinations hospitals use on UB-04s.*

Case study 14-15. Use of -25 modifier. Acme Medical Clinic physicians are tired of coding and billing staff queries about their use of the -25 modifier on claims involving both E/M level and a surgical or medical procedure. They directed coding staff to always attach the -25 modifier to E/M levels for all cases. Using the -25 modifier

when not necessary does not appear to affect claim adjudication.

Hopefully, coding and billing personnel will recognize that this is not a good practice. It is possible that a physician may see a patient, perform an E/M service and perform surgery on a subsequent day. Without compelling documentation to the contrary, no E/M level should be entered in connection with the surgery and the -25 modifier would not be used. Moreover, the -25 should not be used on the first day unless a surgical or medical procedure is performed. The OIG has indicated that the -25 modifier should only appear on a when its use is appropriate.†

Case study 14-16. Use of -59 modifier. The coding and billing staff at Acme Medical Clinic are concerned about the use of the -59 modifier to bypass certain correct coding initiative (CCI) edits. For hospital-based services in particular, the coding staff does not have easy access to the documentation that would establish the proper use of the modifier. Thus, the physicians must be queried regularly about the circumstances surrounding its use.

The -59 modifier should be used only when documentation supports its use. In this case, the coding and billing personnel require routine access to the documentation and/or access to hospital coding of the cases in question.‡

Case study 14-17. Physician versus hospital coding. Apex Medical Center is conducting an audit of outpatient surgical coding. The auditors request a review of both hospital and physician coding on a sampling of records. In addition, Acme Medical Clinic has been asked to provide copies of its coding and billing for the sampling generated during the audit. The physicians at Acme want to know whether this request is appropriate.

The correlation of physician and hospital surgical coding is a legitimate compliance issue. Certainly, if surgical services are provided by physicians in a hospital setting, the CPT coding for these services should generally be the same.

---

* There are minor differences. The CPT code for critical care includes a number of specific diagnostic or interpretive tests. Specific bundling of services is listed in the CPT manual. The technical component for these tests is not included in a hospital's billing for critical care services.

† See OIG's *Use of Modifier 25*, OEI-07-03-00470, November 2005.
‡ See OIG's report, *Use of Modifier 59* to Bypass Medicare's National Correct Coding Initiative Edits, OEI-03-02-00771, November 2005.

Key learning area: Physician coding is a complex technique that involves CPT coding for surgery and E/M, ICD-9-CM diagnosis coding, and the correct application of rules and regulations covering global surgical packages, consultations, CCIs, and preventive medicine among other issues.

Reciprocal and locum tenens physicians

In a physician clinic setting, whether free-standing or provider-based, physicians may be absent for several days. Absences may arise from continuing education, vacations, sick leaves, and/or other circumstances. To cover such absences, a clinic may contract with other physicians to "stand in the place of" the absent physician. The replacement is referred to as a *locums tenens* physician. If the period does not exceed 30 days, the clinic can code and bill under the absent physician's NPI and pay the locum tenens physician whatever is specified in their contractual arrangement. Note that the locum tenens physician is an independent contractor and not an employee.

Similar arrangements apply to reciprocal physicians, that is, physicians who cover for each other on a reciprocal basis. Note that recent changes to the 1500 claim form and complete development of NPIs now allow reporting if the performing physician is different from the billing physician.

> **Case study 14-18. Locum tenens physician.** One physician at Acme Medical Clinic is taking a leave of absence for 30 days. His mother has terminal cancer. He also indicated that he may not return to the clinic and is tentatively planning to relocate in another state. A temporary physician is contracted from a locum tenens service.

This case study illustrates the need for great care in using locum tenens billing arrangements. The clinic physician is taking an official leave of absence and locum tenens billing is correct during the 30 days when the clinic physician is on official leave. Of course, the clinic physician should agree to billing under his NPI. If, at the end of the 30 days, he does not return, the services of the contracted physician may no longer be billed as locum tenens because no further arrangement has been made and the clinic physician is no longer considered an official member of clinic staff.

Medical staff bylaw considerations

One key area a physician should understand fully is his or her relationships with other healthcare providers and other physicians. One area of concern is how such relationships affect (or are affected by) the medical staff bylaws at hospitals where they have been granted privileges. While this may appear to be routine, physicians are cautioned to be very aware of what the medical staff bylaws allow relative to privileges. Hospitals grant different levels of privileges and credentialing can be an issue. For instance, physicians may provide services in the emergency room. It is important to ensure they have the right to perform EMTALA screenings and/or that have the right to admit patients to inpatient status. Physicians should understand the formal processes cited in medical staff bylaws relative to disciplinary actions and steps for remediation.

In today's healthcare environment, medical staff is rapidly evolving into provider staff. More NPPs are performing extended services. The relationships of physicians and NPPs are important and should be addressed in medical staff bylaws. The relationships among physicians are also important. ER physicians, for example, do not generally have inpatient admitting privileges and may not have observation admitting privileges. In some situations they may not perform fracture care. The way an attending physician relates to ER physicians and/or other physicians providing services in the ER can raise compliance issues. This interface, generally governed by medical staff bylaws, should be carefully examined and fully understood.

The medical staff organization's standing orders represent another key issue. Physicians on the hospital staff may agree that certain tests and/or services must always be provided under certain circumstances or they may want to indicate that certain reflex testing can be performed by the laboratory or radiology without specific physician orders if certain prior tests are positive. In other words, based upon the results of a first test, a follow-up test is performed without a specific physician order.

Key learning area: The medical staff organization (MSO) area may be overlooked relative to CBR compliance. Qualification and credentialing of physicians and practitioners are vital. Establishing standing orders for certain tests and reflex testing situations must be carefully considered.

Medical directorships

Many physicians serve as medical directors in hospital settings. Medical directorships vary widely and each has its own set of responsibilities and obligations. Typically a medical director heads the medical staff. Medical directors also supervise laboratory and radiology departments, and other service areas such as emergency, pulmonary, oncology, etc.

Medical directorships are important both for the physician and the hospital and may be used as criteria for meeting quality, certification, and accreditation standards. Because physicians are paid for performing medical director services, some fundamental compliance concerns come into play. In particular, the services performed by a physician in his or her capacity as a medical director must be documented. Moreover, the nature of the services should be defined. Verification can appear in meeting minutes, special reports, and/or the development of care paths. The evidence should reasonably indicate the level and types of services provided and the consistency of payments to the physician.

Hospital-based clinic profitability

Hospitals and/or integrated delivery systems continue to purchase more clinics. Particularly with hospitals, the question of profitability arises after a clinic is acquired or developed. The simple fact is that many hospitals operate clinic systems at significant losses over a period of years. It is not unreasonable for federal regulators to ask why a business such as a hospital or integrated delivery system would continue to operate a clinic or system of clinics at a loss. The concern is whether a hospital is actually subsidizing physicians for the express purpose of gaining referrals—a question that has strong implications related to the Medicare fraud, abuse and anti-kickback regulations.

While this potential compliance issue affects mainly hospitals and integrated delivery systems, physicians should be aware of the potential ramifications. Physicians, as employees, should be careful to work with hospitals and other parent organizations to make certain that clinic operations generate profits for the overall organization.

Summary and conclusions

Medical clinics face a number of special compliance factors. Their organizational structures relative to hospitals and integrated delivery systems come into play. The compliance focuses on false claims and coding systems including CPT and ICD-9-CM. Special payment system considerations including the Medicare global surgical package also present compliance issues. Physicians work more frequently with a variety of NPPs and have a number of different types of relationships with hospitals and other physicians. The systematic process of addressing compliance extends to physician practices and medical clinics that should follow formal compliance programs and utilize manuals that cover various coding policies and procedures.

Key learning area: This chapter touches only on important areas for physician and clinic CBR compliance. Of particular concern are organizational structurings of physicians and associated relationships, particularly with hospitals.

---

fifteen

Special compliance audits and reviews

Introduction

Developing a roster of CBR audits and reviews *may* be relatively simple. For a small physician clinic, the main audits may involve proper surgical coding, use of modifiers, selection of E/M levels, diagnosis coding, and administrative concerns such as NPIs filing of CMS-855s. However, for a hopsital the addition of provider-based clinics and skilled nursing services to a modest hospital setting will result in a dramatic increase in the number of audit and review areas.

While both settings deal with standard issues such as proper CPT coding, proper E/M level selection in the ED, and proper diagnosis coding for inpatient and outpatient services, certain more specific or unusual CBR compliance concerns also arise. Two areas of concern are inpatient stays followed by skilled nursing admissions and discharge dispositions after inpatient admissions relative to the DRG transfer rule. Another concern surrounds the use of Condition Code 44 for changing an inpatient admission to an outpatient observation stay. Others may arise in connection with proper billing of pharmacy items, dates of services, and bill types.

Thus, as healthcare organizations become larger and the services they provide more varied, the potential number of CBR audit and review areas may grow well into a hundred or more categories. Routine audits, such as the annual inpatient DRG audit or APC audit, will be augmented with audits or reviews required by unusual circumstances including coding, billing, and claims filing errors. The challenge for healthcare organizations is to determine which areas to address and whether to use external resources, then prioritize the audits and reviews to be conducted.

The intent of this chapter is to continue the discussions of special compliance areas with emphasis on identifying audits and situations requiring reviews. The preceding chapters covered designing of audits and reviews. Standard approaches apply to well known compliance issues.

CBR compliance personnel must carefully identify a problem or issue, delineate the objectives of the audit, determine the scope and sample size, select cases, establish review templates for the specific steps, write reports, and implement and monitor solutions. Fundamentally, the greatest challenge is to identify specific circumstances requiring examination. This challenge requires careful thought and meaningful investigations of provider activities.

Case study 15-1. Condition Code 44. Apex Medical Center has been working on aspects of compliance surrounding observation services. Utilization review personnel must now carefully monitor potentially short-term inpatient admissions. If the services provided do not exceed 48 hours, a decision must be made whether to convert the case from inpatient to outpatient observation using Condition Code 44. This step appears to work well for private third-party payers because a case can be converted after a patient has been discharged. However, Condition Code 44 seems to be of little use for Medicare patients because a patient must be present for the status to change. How would you design an audit and select cases to see whether the code is used appropriately?

Key learning area: In addition to the common coding and billing audits and reviews, certain specialized areas must be considered. The number and type of specialized areas correlates directly to the size and complexity of a healthcare organization and services it provides. Healthcare providers must be prepared to prioritize scarce resources to perform meaningful audits and reviews. Many CBR- related audits and reviews require special designs.

Emergency department (ED)

The ED may merit a separate CBR compliance plan because it provides many different types of services and a wide range of unusual circumstances may arise. Chapter 12 briefly discussed EMTALA (Emergency Medical Treatment and Labor Act) as a special compliance area. As indicated, several coding, billing, and claims filing issues related to EMTALA arise through ED services.

EDs, or more correctly DEDs (dedicated emergency departments), under CMS and EMTALA, are hospital-based services, and thus fall into the general provider-based category. This triggers the provider-based rule (PBR) discussed in Chapter 12. The PBR requires professional component coding and billing along with technical component coding and billing, leading to concerns related to both the professional 1500 claim form and the UB-04 technical component claim form. ED physician coding and billing may be totally separate from hospital coding billing or a hospital may perform both professional and technical component coding and billing. A hospital may employ non-physician practitioners and the ED physicians may be under contract. Additionally, consideration must be given to the proper correlation of physician and hospital coding and associated billing for compliance purposes. This interface of professional versus technical component coding can become very complex.

As with other hospital-based healthcare services, several payment systems may be used. For the ED, the CMS RBRVS (Resource-Based Relative Value System) for *physician, professional services* is widely used, often in modified form. Payments on the *hospital, technical component* side, the payment systems are more variable. This chapter focuses on CMS's APC (ambulatory payment classification) system as it pertains to compliance concerns and associated audits and reviews. Other payment systems may require additional types of audits or reviews.

E/M coding and billing

Evaluation and management coding must be performed for both physician and hospital services. The bases for coding are distinct for physicians and hospitals. Physicians code for services provided while hospitals code for resources utilized. Thus, E/M levels for a physician and hospital for the same encounter may not match. Under Medicare, physicians must follow an extensive set of E/M documentation guidelines although their application the ED may be less than clear. Hospital guidelines are less precise. When CMS implemented APCs in 2000, hospitals were instructed to develop their own mappings of resources utilized into five ED E/M levels (CPT Codes 99281 through 99285). At the time this book was written, the national guidelines for EDs and provider-based clinics were under study and discussion by CMS.

Audits should be conducted to ensure that appropriate E/M levels are developed based on current guidelines. Internal and external auditing staffs will be very interested in the frequency distribution of the five CPT code levels. Distribution should be normal, i.e., conform to a bell-shaped curve. If the distribution seems skewed or unbalanced, auditing staff must determine whether the variance is reasonable.

Case study 15-2. Small hospital ED E/M levels. Apex Medical Center is located in a small Midwestern community. It has an active ED, but many encounters do not involve emergency medical conditions. Little primary care coverage is available locally during evenings and weekends. As a result, the center codes many more Level I and Level II ED visits than Level IV and Level V visits. Based on patient demographics and community circumstances, does the finding appear reasonable?

From an auditing perspective, the frequency of use of the five ED E/M levels should be represented by a bell-shaped curve. However, the frequency histogram of E/M levels may not conform to the normal curve. As a result, audits should consider external causes that may skew the anticipated normal curve (see Figure 15.1).

Auditing E/M level selection requires guidelines that may also document and handle selection of a particular E/M level. The *physician, professional* E/M coding has reasonably well-defined guidelines that are nonetheless controversial at times. No national guidelines cover the *hospital, technical* component although they are under development through Medicare. Hospitals are required to develop their own mappings of resources consumed and subdivide them into the five levels. Auditors reviewing hospital technical component coding, must assess whether the correct level was chosen based on documentation. If a hospital develops its own mappings, an assessment must be made to determine whether the mapping is appropriate.

Key learning area: CMS in connection with Medicare is developing national guidelines for technical component E/M level coding. Analysis of E/M coding involves reviewing the distribution of E/M levels, the mapping or coding guidelines used, and the appropriateness of such guidelines.

Surgical coding and billing

An ED physician may provide surgical services such as fracture care, splinting, laceration repairs, burn care, and foreign body removal. These services must be coded and billed both for the physician and the hospital. Coding for these services is complex and ED staff should work closely with coding and billing staff to make certain that appropriate coding and billing guidelines are in place. These guidelines will allow auditing staff to judge whether surgical coding is correct.

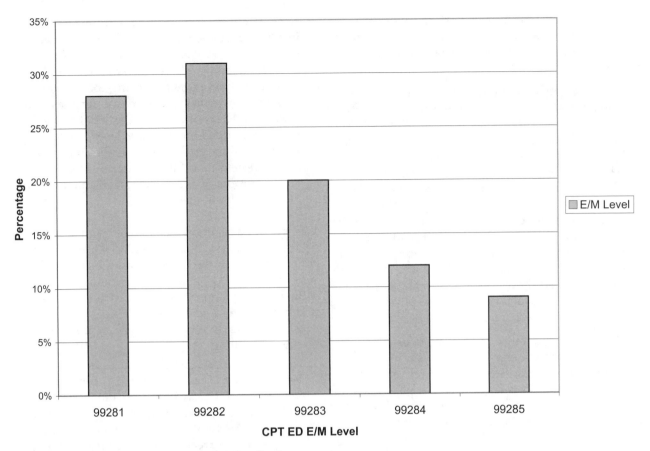

Figure 15.1 Emergency department E/M distribution.

Note that Medicare's global surgical package (GSP) applies to physicians so that certain pre- and post-surgery services are included in payments for surgical procedures. A hospital has no GSP. This difference represents a disconnect in the way coding, billing, and claims filing are handled for surgical services relative to post-operative care. See the discussion below concerning physician modifier -54 (intra-operative services only).

Another difference in surgical coding relates to the fundamental basis for procedure coding. Physicians code for work done. Hospitals identify and code resources utilized. This is especially evident for incident-to services. Since EDs are hospital departments and thus provider-based, physicians can code and bill only for services they perform. Direct supervision does not meet the requirement. This creates real concerns for auditors. The following case study illustrates this concept.

Case study 15-3. ED Surgical coding: Suture technician. Many of Apex Medical Center's ED patients have lacerations that require suturing. As a result, the hospital has hired a specially

trained suture technician who works with ED physicians to provide suturing. The technician is not a practitioner such as a PA or NP. Assume the ED physicians code and bill separately from the hospital. Typically the ED physician performs the EMTALA-mandated MSE, examines the laceration, refers the case to the suture technician, then checks the laceration care before the patient is discharged.

The issue in this case study is whether the physician can code and bill for the laceration repair. Since resources were utilized, the hospital will code for the laceration repair. From its perspective, the laceration was repaired, regardless of who performed the repair, and resources were consumed. However, the ED physician did not personally perform the services and most likely will not code for the service and no professional component payment for the surgery will result.* Although this seems incongruous, auditors

---

* If the suture technician is a non-physician practitioner (physician assistant, nurse practitioner, clinical nurse specialist), a professional claim can be made and the practitioner will be paid at 85 percent of the Medicare Physician Fee Schedule.

must carefully determine who performs what services and the proper way to code such services both on the hospital technical side and also on the professional physician side.

Note: The ability of a physician or practitioner to professionally code and bill only for services personally performed in a facility setting is covered by the Social Security Act. Section 1861(s) of the act (Medical and Other Health Services) addresses the incident-to concept but uses the phrase in two very different ways. In Section 1861(s)(2)(A), the phrase is used in the context of incident-to billing that allows a physician in a free-standing setting to code and bill for services under the direction of a physician. Section 1861(s)(2)(B) uses the phrase in the context of incident-to services, indicating that a hospital will be paid for all services incident-to those of a physician. Because the hospital is paid for such services in its facility setting, the physician cannot also bill professional fees for these services.

CMS issued guidance in this area for joint E/M services. If a physician and a non-physician practitioner jointly provide an E/M level service, only one of them may file a professional claim. The physician and patient must have some face-to-face contact although it can be minimal. See CMS Transmittal 1776 to the *Medicare Carriers Manual* dated October 25, 2002.*

Procedure coding guidelines are essential for both correct coding and also to enable auditing and review staff to verify that coding is correct. Of course, correct coding depends on the documentation that provides the justification to code and bill for a service. Fracture care and splinting services also represent surgical procedure coding challenges.

Case study 15-4. Simple leg fracture. A patient presents to Apex Medical Center's ED after an accident. X-rays indicate a non-displaced fracture of the leg. Because of the pain and swelling, the ED physician applies a splint and instructs the patient to follow-up with his primary care physician in three to five days.

The coding question in this case study is whether the physician provided definitive fracture care versus temporary care in anticipation of further definitive fracture care by another physician. Should the splinting be treated as a service or as fracture care? Coding and billing policies and procedures are needed to resolve such questions.

---

* This is a major CBR compliance issue that must be duly considered.

Case study 15-5. Bundling surgical services into E/M level. Auditors noted in a recent audit of surgical cases at Apex Medical Center's ED the absence of coding for fractured ribs, toes, and fingers. The auditors met with the coding staff to determine why these fracture care services were not coded. The coding staff indicated that the services were added into the E/M level by elevating the code by one level. However, the coding staff also indicated that this was not a written policy and the process was also not documented as part of the E/M level selection.

Clearly, the audit report included recommendations for addressing the situation. To audit coding and billing for procedures in the ED for physicians and practitioners or for the hospital technical component, coding, billing, and chargemaster policies and procedures; and also coding and billing policies and procedures must be in place to serve as metrics for judging correct coding and billing.

Key learning area: ED surgical coding is challenging. Based on available documentation, the coding, billing, and chargemaster staffs must determine the intents of ED physicians and staff. While correct coding is a major issue, so is proper correlation of codes used on professional claim forms and technical claim forms.

Modifiers

The two most common modifiers used for ED coding and billing are (1) -25 (significant, separately identifiable service) and (2) -59 (separate procedure). Both are used for physician and hospital services and serve as payment modifiers. Whenever they are used, the physician or hospital attests that the use is appropriate. This implicit attestation means that documentation on file supports the use of the modifier.

The -25 modifier indicates that an E/M service was provided along with another surgical or medical procedure. If this modifier is not used, the E/M level may be bundled into the surgical or medical procedure. The -59 modifier is used to indicate that a CCI (correct coding initiative) edit should be circumvented so that separate payments are made for more than one associated service. An audit may focus on the means of placing a modifier on a claim form instead of simply checking whether the modifier is used correctly.

Physicians should also consider the -54 modifier that indicates that a physician performed only intra-operative services and that no post-operative component is provided and/or anticipated.* The use of this modifier is a result of the GSP. Under RBRVS and other physician payment systems, post-operative services may be included in payments for surgical services.

Case study 15-6. Suture removal. An elderly patient presented to Apex Medical Center's ED on a Monday evening with an arm laceration. The laceration was cleansed and sutured. The ED physician instructed the patient to see her primary care physician to have the sutures removed. However, the patient returned on Saturday morning to have the sutures removed. An ED physician examined the wound and instructed a nurse to remove the sutures.

During the initial encounter, the ED physician instructed the patient to see her own physician for post-operative care. Thus, the ED physician claim would include a -54 modifier on the laceration repair code indicating that only intra-operative care was provided. The hospital would not use the -54 modifier since the GSP generally does not apply to the hospital technical component side. When the patient returned to the ED to have the sutures removed, the ED physician (assuming he or she is part of a group of ED physicians at Apex) should have used the laceration repair code with a -55 modifier.† It is problematic for an ED physician to code anything other than the E/M level for a medical screening examination.

This patient represented a new encounter for the hospital. Thus, the hospital would simply code an E/M level for nursing service because no CPT code covers suture removal. A technical component E/M level mapping must be established to handle cases of this type.

Auditing for correct use of modifiers for the ED can be a challenge because compliance issues in this area concern not using a modifier when it should be used. From an auditing perspective, it is not hard to generate a computer report of cases in which modifiers were used, but generating such reports when modifiers should have been used is a very different matter. Hospital CBR compliance staff should routinely check for the proper use of modifiers in the ED and other hospital areas, for example, in provider-based clinics and for surgical services.

---

* See current CPT manual for information about the triple set of modifiers: -54 (intra-operative only), -55 (post-operative), and -56 (pre-operative). These modifiers allow a physician to delineate services within these categories.

† This simple example illustrates the complexity in what can appear as a straightforward sequences of services. Technically, the -55 modifier should be used; in practice, it is not used as much as it should be. See the FY2008 OIG work plan.

> **Key learning area: Proper use of modifiers is a major compliance issue. The two modifiers of greatest concern are -25 (significant, separately identifiable service) and -59 (separate procedure). Both professional claims and hospital claims must be monitored for correct modifier use. ED physicians must consider additional modifiers in connection with Medicare's global surgical package.**

Correlation of physician and hospital coding

E/M coding is performed both for ER physicians and for hospital technical components. These E/M levels are based on completely different methodologies and do not need to correlate. However, some correlation of services as indicated by CPT codes should be present. If an ED physician codes the repair of a laceration or fracture care, the hospital reports the same services. For the ED, this is a special area of a more general compliance issue that effects an entire hospital, particularly for surgical procedures. If a surgeon performs surgical services and codes for them, the hospital should report the same codes for these services.

This issue was cited in an OIG annual work plan. (See *FY2003 OIG Work Plan*, page 7, Procedure Coding of Outpatient and Physician Services.) While this correlation of surgical coding has been identified as a compliance issue, the ability of hospital and external auditors to check for this correlation has been problematic. For Medicare claims, the professional component goes to the geographic carrier and the hospital; technical component claims go to the FI. Generally, the carrier and the FI do not have the ability to easily cross-reference claims, and thus conducting an audit is difficult. This situation is changing. Congress has directed CMS to utilize the services of regional Medicare administrative contractors (MACs) that will easily be able to cross-correlate professional and technical component claims.

Case study 15-7. ED Surgical coding correlation. Compliance auditing staff at Apex Medical Center want to perform an audit to see whether surgical coding in the ED is the same for physicians as it is for the hospital. The ED physicians are contracted. Billing and claims filing for the physicians are performed by the physician group outside the control of the hospital. The ED physicians are balking at providing a sampling of surgical claims, and the audit cannot be conducted.

This case study shows that hospitals should carefully craft their provider agreements so that the relationships do not impede audit activities. The audit in this case would benefit both the physicians and hospital, but audits often raise sensitivities. Because of the contractual relationship, the best approach would have been preventive by including a provision covering auditing arrangements in the contract. In the absence of such a provision, CBR compliance personnel must persuade the physicians to share such information on the basis of better compliance and better reimbursement.

Medical necessity

Medical necessity is an overarching compliance issue in all healthcare areas and is particularly critical for coding, billing, and reimbursement. The fact that services were provided does not necessarily imply that they were necessary. This concept is particularly troublesome in the ED. During an encounter with a patient, an ED physician will often will perform a number of diagnostic tests to rule out certain conditions. These tests and the assessment of patient condition are generally conducted under stressful circumstances. At the end of a complex assessment, everyone involved may look back and recognize that certain diagnostic tests were not really necessary for determining the final diagnosis.

Third-party payers including Medicare are particularly sensitive to what is perceived as excessive and unnecessary diagnostic testing in the ED. The OIG addressed this issue on page 6 of its *CY2003 Work Plan*. Congress even intervened via the Medicare Modernization Act (MMA). Section 944(a) indicates that the determination of services must be considered based on the information available at the time of service. Clearly medical necessity is an issue, particularly for diagnostic tests. For the ED, audits should assess the numbers, types, and medical necessities of diagnostic tests. While the decision about what tests to perform lies with physicians and practitioners, other personnel should be sensitive to compliance concerns and the potential for impact on coding, billing, and reimbursement.

> **Key learning area: The emergency department presents dozens of CBR audit and review concerns because it is a microcosm of hospital services involving both physician and hospital coding and billing. Development of a separate audit and review plan for the ED should be carefully considered. The discussion here is only a starting point for audit and review functions relative to the ED.**

Cardiovascular interventional radiology

Cardiovascular interventional radiology (CVIR), one of the most challenging and technical areas for documenting, coding, billing, and filing correct claims, uses a component coding approach combining surgical codes (catheter placements), therapeutic codes (balloon angioplasties, atherectomies, stent placements), and correlated radiological supervision and interpretation (S&I) codes. The conventions and guidelines are complicated and sometimes controversial. Services are typically separated into coronary versus non-coronary areas and the ensuing billing process and procedure codes and guidelines are very different for coronary versus non-coronary services. Combinations of both types of services may be provided and this further exacerbates the difficulties of properly coding and billing. The two major questions associated with CBR compliance audits in CVIR are:

- Are we coding and billing correctly based on the documentation?
- What system do we have in place to ensure correct coding and billing?

In an audit or review, both the claims generated (along with itemized statements and documentation) and the processes used to generate them must be considered. An additional concern is that physician coding and billing for these services should closely correlate with the hospital coding and billing for the same services. The following simplified case study reveals some of the complexities. The ensuing discussion will be general and readers are encouraged to consult with coding, billing, and chargemaster experts for more detailed information.

Case study 15-8. Vascular interventional radiology. A patient is brought to Apex Medical Center's catheterization laboratory. After conscious sedation of the patient, a puncture is made in the right femoral artery. The catheter is advanced into the aorta, and an abdominal aortography is performed with bilateral runoffs. A stenosis is noted in the left popliteal artery. The catheter is manipulated across the aortic bifurcation down into the left popliteal. A balloon angioplasty is performed, but the results are not satisfactory. The physician decides to deploy a stent that successfully addresses the stenosis as verified by follow-up angiography. A vascular plug is used to address the wound site and the patient is taken to recovery. Catheterization laboratory personnel enter charges for the radiological S&I

services that drive CPT codes statically placed in the chargemaster. Charges are also entered for the surgical procedures, but the chargemaster contains no surgical CPT codes. Professional coding staff codes the surgical procedures based on documentation of the physician.

This case study may appear complicated and it is to an extent. CVIR cases can become even more complicated. Two key issues must be considered: (1) the claim generated (professional and technical) and (2) the process used to generate the claim. First, consider the codes that should be on the claim. The sequence of services for coding purposes is:

1. From a right femoral puncture, a catheter is positioned in the aorta, and an abdominal aortography with bilateral runoffs is performed.
2. The catheter is manipulated to the left popliteal artery.
3. A balloon angioplasty is performed but fails to address the stenosis.
4. The physician decides to deploy a stent.
5. After the stent is successfully deployed, as verified by follow-up angiography, the catheter is withdrawn and a vascular plug addresses the femoral puncture.

CPT codes must be developed for the services. At Apex Medical Center, the radiology codes are devised by service area personnel inputting charges. The surgical codes will be developed by coding staff. Using 2007 codes and general CVIR coding guidelines, the following codes would probably be developed:

1. Catheter to Aorta plus Abdominal Aortography with Runoffs
   a. 36200—Catheter to Aorta (This non-selective code will be bundled into a selective catheter placement code.)
   b. 75630—Abdominal Aortogram with Bilateral Runoffs
2. Catheter to Left Popliteal
   c. 36247-LT—Third Order Selective Catheter Placement
3. Balloon Angioplasty of Left Popliteal Artery
   d. 35474-LT—Balloon Angioplasty
   e. 75962-LT—Balloon Angioplasty Radiological S&I
4. Stent Placement of Left Popliteal Artery
   f. 37205-LT—Stent Placement
   g. 75960-LT—Stent Placement Radiological S&I

Note: The follow-up angiography is not separately coded under general CVIR guidelines.* Both the balloon angioplasty and the stent placement are coded because the physician documented the angioplasty failure. Also, the physician coding will be the same except for the use of the -26 (professional component) modifier on the radiology S&I codes. Special C codes for catheters and guide wires, Q codes for low osmolar contrast media (LOCMs) and G or C codes for vascular plugs may also be utilized. The claim must be reviewed for proper coding and appropriate charges.

Because a stent is involved, consideration must be given to the charge for it. A third-party payer may insist on some variations. For Medicare, the charge would be developed using the cost divided by an appropriate CCR (cost-to-charge ratio). Another third-party payer contract may require that the actual cost be charged.

We must also consider the process by which codes are developed. Catheterization laboratory personnel enter charges based on what they observe. The professional coding staff will code from the documentation. This could lead to a disconnect. What if the physician does not state that the angioplasty failed? The documentation may seem to indicate that the angioplasty was in preparation for the stent placement and thus would not be separately coded.

This brief discussion illustrates the need for special audit and review considerations in the CVIR area. Since CVIR services will continue to grow in volume and scope as the baby boom generation matures, coding issues will be important for both inpatient and outpatient areas. It is critical for every healthcare facility to determine the exact flow for coding, charge capture, and documentation for CVIR services.

Key learning area: CVIR coding and associated billing are very complex on the outpatient side because a component coding approach is used. CVIR services represent high volume and high revenue. Special audits must be conducted to ensure both compliance and proper reimbursement. The claims and the processes used to generate them must be audited.

Technical component E/M coding

This chapter discussed E/M coding for the emergency department. Now we will expand this discussion to the rest of the hospital. Technical component E/M coding

---

* See Society of Interventional Radiology's *SIR Coding Manual*, www.sirweb.org.

involves two main factors: (1) the level of E/M code developed and (2) the decision to code and bill an E/M level.

In standard service areas such as the ED or a provider-based clinic, E/M services will certainly have to be coded and billed. For these areas, compliance involves selecting the correct level. Other concerns may relate to whether an E/M level should have been charged at all.

> **Case study 15-9. Injection by nurse.** A patient presents to an outpatient area to receive one of a series of injections ordered by a physician. The patient has not seen a physician or other practitioner for more than a week. The nurse performs a thorough assessment and determines that the injection can be safely provided. Nursing staff want to bill an E/M level along with the injection code. Is this proper? What if the nurse determined the patient was not ready for the injection and instructed him to return the next day?

This type of situation can occur in many settings around a hospital and can even be difficult to recognize. Services that are normally not performed by a formally recognized provider-based clinic are referred to as provider-based *clinical* services. For example, a patient may present for one of a series of blood transfusions or for infusion therapy of immune globulin. Another case might be a patient returning to the catheterization laboratory for a dressing change two days after a cardiovascular catheterization. If E/M levels are to be billed for these types of nursing provider-based clinical services, three compliance concerns must be considered:

- Was the nursing assessment provided above and beyond the normal E/M services provided in conjunction with a codeable and billable service?
- Did the nursing staff fully document the services?
- Were the services provided medically necessary and ordered by a physician?

The first issue arises from injections, infusions, chemotherapy, blood transfusions, and the like. The fundamental question is whether the services provided go beyond those that would normally be provided in conjunction with the associated service. Documentation is not normally an issue; nursing staff typically do a good job of documenting assessments. The main question is medical necessity. The service may be provided and documented, but was it medically necessary? And was it ordered by a physician or qualified practitioner?

Consider the patient mentioned above who returns to the catheterization laboratory for a dressing change on a femoral puncture. If the nursing staff provides

services such as a dressing change, a charge should be made because the visit is a separate encounter. However, no CPT code covers the service so an E/M level becomes appropriate. However, should patients return to the laboratory for such services? Should they not go to a clinic or the ED? The thrust of coding and billing E/M levels for provider-based clinical services is that hospitals must make policy decisions and carefully craft appropriate policies and procedures if such billings are to take place.

Now consider the choice of E/M level. Depending on the specific type of service, E/M codes fall into five levels. When CMS implemented the APC payment system, hospitals were instructed to develop their own mappings of resources utilized into the five levels for ED and provider-based clinics.* As this book was going to press, CMS was developing national guidelines for the ED, critical care, and provider-based clinics. Auditors must ensure that E/M levels developed for the ED and provider-based clinics meet relevant internal and external standards.

Key learning area: Technical component E/M coding for provider-based clinics is similar to that type of coding in the ED. However, a subtle variation arises when nursing staff provides services that should be billed with a low level E/M technical component code. Since these services are not typically provided in a formal clinic setting, they are referred to as provider-based *clinical* services.

DRG and inpatient audits

Inpatient audits are often synonymous with DRGs although various other inpatient payment mechanisms exist. Diagnosis-related groups (DRGs) represents the oldest prospective payment system (PPS) implemented by Medicare. The system was implemented on October 1, 1983, and has been evolving since then. For Fiscal Year 2008 a major change has been made to the MS (Medicare severity) DRGs. The change is more than evolutionary; it can be classified as revolutionary. DRGs will also be heavily affected when the change is made to ICD-10 or ICD-11.

Because the system has been in place for more than 20 years, its proper use and application should have been mastered long ago. However, the OIG annual work plan continues to list DRGs and potential upcoding as compliance issues almost every year. The work plan also lists associated matters such as same-day admits and discharges, one-day inpatient stays, skilled

---

* See April 7, 2000 *Federal Register*, page 18451 (65 FR 18451).

nursing discharge status, and special hospital status (sole community, Medicare-dependent, etc.).

Standard DRG audits

A typical approach to the Medicare DRG system and other third-party payers that use forms of DRGs, is to conduct annual DRG audits. While the targets of audits can certainly vary, a fairly typical approach is to have an external consulting firm acting as an independent review organization (IRO) perform an audit. In selecting cases, a combination approach may be used. Part of an audit may involve randomly chosen discharges; another part may concentrate on problem DRGs that are actually problem pairs, triples, or quadruples. These groupings of DRGs are related in that a change in the principal diagnosis can often move a DRG payment upward, sometimes significantly. The listing of problem DRGs shifts over time, but some seem to stay on the list forever.

One basic concern of Medicare and the OIG is that slight changes in the ICD-9-CM diagnosis and/or procedure coding can create a significant increase in the DRG payment. If such upcoding takes place systematically over a large number of discharges, significant overpayments could accrue to the hospital. Below is a representative listing of problem DRGs based on the previous CMS-DRGs. How these problem DRGs will eventually translate into the new MS-DRG categories will take several years to determine.

002	014	015	079	080	088
089	090	110	121	122	124
125	127	128	130	132	140
142	143	144	148	151	182
183	296	297	320	416	443
468	475	477	478	479	518

Certainly, as a starting point the *old* CMS-DRGs can be cross-walked to their new equivalents in the new system. For example, the CMS-DRG 88 (chronic obstructive pulmonary disease) has been divided into three separate MS-DRGs (190, 191, 192) based upon three severity levels:

- With MCC (major complication or comorbidity)
- With CC (complication or comorbidity)
- Without MCC/CC

Whether the 190–191–192 triple will turn into a problem area under the MS-DRGs remains to be determined. CMS-DRGs 89 and 90 (simple pneumonia and pleurisy) will map into a triple: MS-DRGs 193, 194, and 195. Again, whether the triple will become problematic

is unknown. The refinements into three classes may ease concerns about upcoding.

Because DRGs have been around for more than twenty years, hospital coding staffs have learned how to legitimately optimize reimbursement. The basic approach is to find the proper principal diagnosis and then look for a CC. This approach now requires searches for MCCs as well as CCs and auditors must adjust the way they conduct DRG audits accommodate the new MS-DRG system. Since private third-party payers often use DRGs in some form, they may impose additional changes.

In the course of converting to MS-DRGs, CMS also developed the POA (present on admission) one-position indicator to be attached to diagnosis codes on UB-04s. The basic idea is that Medicare does not want to pay for conditions acquired at hospital after admission. POA indicators will affect reimbursement and this creates a need to audit for the correct POAs on claim forms and also audit for a proper process of determining POA indicators.

Key learning area: CMS implemented major changes to the DRG system by introducing a third level of severity for Fiscal Year 2008. The new MS-DRGs were completely renumbered, the CC list was augmented by an MCC list, and the grouping process was altered. A new POA (present on admission) was implemented. Determining the impact of this change on DRG audits and reviews will take time and experience. Up-coding for DRGs will continue to be an issue.

Inpatient audits

Other inpatient audits can and should be performed regularly. One area of concern is the differentiation of inpatient admissions and observation admissions. The distinction becomes academic in cases of one-day inpatient stays, that is, a patient is admitted one day and discharged the next day. Such inpatient stays should be periodically audited to ensure that the inpatient admission and discharge are appropriate and that the involved inpatients were not actually observation patients.

CBR compliance personnel should be fully cognizant of other types of inpatient payment systems that involve case rates. They should thoroughly review inpatient coding, adherence to formal guidelines, and hospital-developed coding and billing policies and procedures. Concurrent inpatient coding can sometimes generate higher quality coding and documentation.

Finally, the entire inpatient coding process should be critically examined.

APC audits

On August 1, 2000, CMS implemented the long-awaited Hospital Outpatient Prospective Payment System (HOPPS) in the form of APCs (ambulatory payment classifications). This system was based on the precursor ambulatory patient group (APG) system, also developed by CMS.

Note: APCs represent the most complex payment system of the Medicare program. Payment for services under APCs is driven by CPT and HCPCS coding and many of the issues are highly technical. Thus, CBR auditing needs for APCs generally merit a separate compliance plan.

Performing a single, comprehensive audit of APCs at a hospital is unusual. Typically, APC audits focus on a particular department or service area (emergency, cardiovascular, interventional radiology, etc.) or occur in response to a particular coding issue (CPT coding or use of modifiers). The following discussion is an overview of auditing issues that should be considered.

CPT/HCPCS coding

The APC mantra is "no code, no payment." APC payment is driven by CPT and HCPCS coding. Of course, services must still be medically necessary and ordered by a qualified physician or practitioner. The CPT system was developed and extensively refined for the use of physicians. As a result, most CPT guidance is written for physicians, not for hospitals. CMS developed the CCI or correct coding initiative edits for physicians; a slightly modified set of edits is used for hospitals. From a compliance perspective, hospitals use a coding system not designed for hospital use and this creates additional compliance concerns.

Case study 15-10. Conscious sedation coding and billing. In 2005, the AMA introduced a new annotation to the CPT manual, namely the bull's eye (⊙) to indicate that conscious sedation is an inherent part of a procedure and should not be reported separately. The Chargemaster Coordinator at Apex Medical Center decides to completely remove conscious sedation from the chargemaster so that it cannot be separately reported. She understands that no charges will be made for procedures not annotated with the bull's eye, even though the conscious sedation service can be coded and charged.

Case study 15-10 Illustrates what often occurs when a hospital uses CPT guidance that applies to physicians. The immediate question related to this new annotation was whether it applied to hospitals.* CMS finally indicated that this guidance did indeed apply to hospitals and this led to the additional question of the exact meaning of *not reporting separately*. With rather oblique guidance, CMS indicated that this phrase or its equivalent, *to not separately bill*, meant that no CPT or HCPCS code was to be reported† and thus a separate charge could be made, but no code should be attached. This appears to concur with the no-separate-payment concept which for APCs would occur only if a CPT or HCPCS code was used. Of course, this situation is moot because the conscious sedation codes are packaged for APCs.

CPT/HCPCS coding audits are complex and depend upon other coding, billing, and chargemaster policies and procedures. As with other CBR auditing areas, the related concerns are (1) the final product (claim form) and (2) the process or flow that generates claim forms. Thus, the billing system, chargemaster, and coding considerations all come into play. The chargemaster may have codes statically placed, or codes may be developed dynamically outside the chargemaster. For certain service areas, the coding is performed by charge entry through the chargemaster. In other areas, professional coding staff develops codes from documentation. The coding interface to the chargemaster plays an important part in the coding process. Coding audits must address this process to determine whether it produces correct, complete, and accurate claims. As with other discussions of CPT/HCPCS coding, proper correlation of physician coding to hospital coding is an area of concern.

Many hospitals conduct annual CPT coding reviews that concentrate on surgical areas where codes are generally developed by professional coding staff. General outpatient claims quality issues can also be audited. These types of audits may also cover service areas that develop codes through charge entry.

Note: We discussed the technical component E/M coding for EDs, provider-based clinics, and provider-based clinical services. E/M coding is also a distinct APC compliance issue.

---

* CMS provided this guidance at its Question & Answer website, http://questions.cms.hhs.gov, #4869, June 9, 2005.

† See *CY2006 OPPS Drug Administration Questions Related to Pub 100-04*, Medicare Claims Processing Chapter 4, Section 230.2, published by CMS, February 2006, particularly Q&A #6. See CMS website at http://www.cms.hhs.gov/HospitalOutpatientPPS/Downloads/OPPSGuidance.pdf.

Modifier utilization

The -59 (separate procedure) payment modifier is used to circumvent CCI edits. Care must be taken to check whether this modifier is correctly used (documentation on file justifies its use) and that correct processes are in place to determine whether it should be used.

> **Case study 15-11. CCI Edit.** An audit at Apex Medical Center focuses on the use and non-use of the -59 modifier. While most of the claims using the modifier appear to be correct, a subset of claims reveals insufficient documentation to justify the use of -59. The problems appear to arise from codes driven through the chargemaster. The auditing staff checked the flow process used to place the modifier on claims. Basically, billing personnel note that a CCI edit is invoked and simply add -59 to the claim to move it through the process.

Apex Medical Center must modify this procedure. Any individual deciding to use the -59 modifier must verify the existence of documentation on file to support the use.

Another important payment modifier is -25 (significant, separate procedure), used only with E/M codes. In the APC payment system, use of an E/M level with most other service codes will result in bundling of the E/M level unless the -25 modifier is present. Technical component E/M levels are often determined by service area personnel in EDs, provider-based clinics, and possibly with provider-based clinical services. Because service area personnel input the E/M levels, a mechanism must be established to determine when to add and not add the -25 modifier.

> **Case study 15-12. Use of -25 Modifier in Chargemaster.** The Chargemaster Coordinator at Apex Medical Center, has decided to place the -25 modifier on *all* technical component E/M levels. Through experimentation, she found that use of the -25 modifier on claim forms seemed to cause no problems even if the modifier was unnecessary. The -25 modifier will automatically appear whenever an E/M level is charged.

From a compliance stance, this is not a good practice. Physicians have used the -25 modifier for many years. The OIG conducted audits of physician use of -25 and noted that it is used when not needed on some claims and that this practice is inappropriate.*

Many other modifiers are used in developing CPT and HCPCS codes for APCs. Some affect payments; many provide additional information but do not influence payments for CPT and HCPCS codes per se. For example, the -LT (left) and -RT (right) modifiers are basically informational. However, -LT and -RT have been used in place of the -59 modifier to bypass a CCI edit. Three additional payment modifiers that should be reviewed for correct utilization are:

-73—Discontinued Procedure before Anesthesia Administration

-74—Discontinued Procedure after Anesthesia Administration

-52—Reduced Service

Conscious sedation is considered anesthesia for billing purposes. If a procedure is discontinued before anesthesia is administered, a 50 percent payment results. If a procedure is discontinued after anesthesia administration, 100 percent payment for the planned procedure is made under APCs. However, concern may be raised if several procedures are planned or a procedure is interventional and requires more than one code. Coding and billing policies and procedures must be in place to delineate how claims are to be generated for combinations of services.

The -52 is also now a payment modifier.† Only a 50 percent payment is made if it is used. Generally, the -52 is used in areas such as radiology. Both the use of and the need for the -52 modifier are areas of concern. Another issue is how the modifier is entered into the billing system.

Special situations and special service areas

Abundant special situations have arisen around APCs and associated hospital outpatient services. Case study 15-10 illustrates concerns with conscious sedation. Discontinued procedures present another special situation. A concern on a far larger scale is outpatient cardiovascular interventional radiology.

In 2007, CMS adopted new CPT codes for injections, infusions, and chemotherapy administration. APCs provide payment for the administration, but generally package the associated pharmaceutical items. Of course, expensive chemotherapy drugs are paid separately. APCs pay for the vaccines and toxoid immunizations, but not their administration. CBR auditing staff should be particularly sensitive to how CPT/ HCPCS codes are developed in the areas of injections and infusions for which nursing staff may perform the coding through charge entry that then drives through

---

* See OIG Report, "Use of the 25 Modifier," November 2005, OEI-07-03-00470 and a companion report, "Use of Modifier 59 to Bypass Medicare's National Correct Coding Initiative Edits," November 2005, OEI-03-02-00771.

† See discussion in November 10, 2005 *Federal Register*, page 68710 (70 FR 68710).

the chargemaster. Codes developed by professional coding staff versus codes developed by service area personnel can invoke very different concerns, and audits should be adjusted accordingly.

Observation services represent another major APC issue. CMS maintains that hospitals have inappropriately billed for observation services and, as a result, CMS generally bundles payment for observation services into associated services. Starting in 2008 CMS developed two new separately payable composite APCs. These two composite APCs are used for observation admissions through the ED or a clinic. Observation services must be provided for at least eight hours and there must be no status indicator T services (i.e., surgical services). If there is a status indicator T surgery, then any payment for observation is bundled into the surgery payment. This type of grouping logic can lead to inappropriate situations as illustrated in the next case study.

Case study 15-13. Observation with minor surgery. An elderly man suffers from chest pains. His niece has driven him to Apex Medical Center's ED. While getting out of the car, the man suffers a laceration to his hand. He is worked up under the chest pain protocol and placed in observation. The laceration on his hand requires a single suture. He remains in observation for 36 hours and is discharged.

The correct conclusion is that no payment will be made for the observation services although all the requirements were met. Payment will be made for the laceration repair and the ED services, and the total is less than the payment for observation services.

Observation is another issue related to the APC payment interface to the DRG inpatient payment process. DRGs are typically concerned with one-day stays that should really be classified as observation services. Another payment system interface for APCs occurs with skilled nursing patients. SNF patient are often brought to the hospital to receive a variety of outpatient services before return to the SNF. Which services are covered by APCs? Which are covered by the SNF payment? See the CD accompanying this book for further information on APCs.

Key learning area: APCs were developed by CMS, but private third-party payers impose several deviations. Proper audit and review of all aspects of APCs requires a separate CBR compliance plan. The key feature of APCs is that payment is driven by proper CPT/HCPCS coding and the use of modifiers when justified.

Chargemaster audits

In recent years, the chargemaster has become a direct target of both statutory and contractual compliance. The chargemaster is a key element in developing itemized statements and associated claims. Hospital pricing and the way prices are set continue to fall under increasing public scrutiny.

Case study 15-14. Drug-eluting stent pricing. Apex Medical Center was the subject of a local newspaper article when a self-pay patient discovered that a drug-eluting stent was charged at $9000 when the stent manufacturer listed a price of $4000 on its website. The article was critical and claimed that Apex overcharged patients for drug-eluting stents.

The $9000 charge may be correct under Medicare due to Apex's cost-to-charge ratio (CCR). When the $4000 cost is divided by Apex's CCR, the result is $9000. On the surface, it appears that Apex must charge all such patients $9000 in order to not violate the so-called Medicare charging rule. Apex may also have a contract with a private third-party payer that requires the charge to be no more than the acquisition cost plus a 10 percent mark-up for administrative expenses. Thus, Apex may devise a set of different charges for the drug-eluting stent, with the highest charge made to the Medicare program.

A chargemaster audit should review charge formulas and overall pricing relative to statutory and contractual constraints and consider increased public visibility. Such audits basically address what is commonly called transparent pricing. See Chapter 13 for additional methods, i.e., strategic pricing, geographic pricing, and market pricing. All these concepts may come into play in a chargemaster review. Possibly a dozen different types of chargemaster reviews may be conducted as part of a CBR compliance program, but they are generally categorized as (1) static or (2) dynamic.

Static reviews involve looking at the chargemaster as a large, complex file. Concerns for static reviews involve updating CPT/HCPCS codes, proper revenue code assignment, appropriate descriptions, consistent pricing, and the like. For the most part, auditors who conduct these line-by-line reviews check the propriety of each item in the chargemaster. Because such audits are conducted in relative isolation, they are often called back-office reviews.

Dynamic reviews are more complex. They address the overall CBR flow relative to the chargemaster as an integral tool of a greater process. In other words, they determine how the chargemaster is used to generate itemized statements and claims. Issues such as charge capture, coding interface, cost reporting, and associated items must be considered. These reviews require auditors to visit service areas and involve coding and billing staff in the analysis and assessment of data flow.

Regardless of the type of chargemaster review, the goal is for the billing system to generate correct, complete, and accurate claims. Because the chargemaster is part of a larger process, many of the quality tools embedded in disciplines like Six Sigma can help refine and optimize the process that ultimately generates the claims. This is an area in which compliance personnel can assist the hospital in process improvement. Auditing personnel should also be concerned about the organizational structure that supports the development and maintenance of the chargemaster.

Case study 15-15. Third-party payer audit of chargemaster. The Chargemaster Coordinator at Apex Medical Center approached the compliance department about auditing the chargemaster. She has been informed that a contract with a large third-party payers allows the payer to audit the chargemaster. The coordinator wants to know what this type of audit involves and how she should prepare for it.

The type of audit depends on the payment system or systems used by the third-party payer. The audit will probably concentrate on charges and the chargemaster pricing process along with categorization of supplies, pharmacy items, and the like. Hospitals have difficulties meeting all the demands of multiple payment systems and specific third-party payer demands for chargemasters and have no easy ways to prepare for third-party audits. Development and maintenance of the chargemaster are ongoing processes requiring many design decisions. Preparation for audits should proceed on a long-term basis. The best answer to the situation in Case study 15-5 is to have the coordinator participate in contract negotiations related to chargemaster issues.

> **Key learning area: A hospital chargemaster is in essence a large complicated file that delineates all charges. Each line item represents a charge that may appear on an itemized statement and after further processing appear on a claim. chargemaster pricing has become a major issue with the advent of transparent pricing and consumer-drive health care. Several types of chargemaster audits and reviews may be performed. The chargemaster should serve as an integral part of a system generating compliant, complete, and accurate claims.**

Provider-based rule (PBR) reviews

Chapter 12 discussed the PBR. This chapter expands on several topics of compliance interest. The PBR is a Medicare concept (see 42 CFR §413.65) that typically applies to provider-based clinics, also known as hospital-based clinics. While hospitals are the main providers defined in this rule, other providers such as skilled nursing facilities (SNFs) can also establish operations as provider-based clinics.

Historically, this concept and associated rule have gone through a rather tortuous process spanning more than ten years. Hospital-based clinics became popular in the 1970s and 1980s. One specific form is the model ambulatory practice (MAP) clinic. Coincidental with the development of APCs, CMS finalized rules in this area. While hospital-based clinics provided the impetus for developing the PBR, the requirements in the proposed rule published in the April 7, 2000 *Federal Register* were expanded to include inpatient and outpatient situations. Thus, while this discussion focuses primarily on provider-based clinics, CBR compliance personnel should consider this issue more broadly. Basically, any services for which UB-04 (CMS-1450) forms are filed are considered provider-based.

As noted in Chapter 12, the basic benefit to be realized from a provider-based clinic is increased reimbursement resulting from filing two claim forms: a CMS-1450 (UB-04 for non-Medicare) for the hospital technical component and a CMS-1500 (1500 for non-Medicare) for professional services.* The two claims enable a provider-based facility to increase reimbursement relative to a free-standing clinic that files a single 1500 claim. Physicians at provider-based clinics receive decreased payments tied to the Medicare site-of-service (SOS) differential but the technical component payment more than compensates for the reduction. The application of the SOS reduction is driven by use of the place of service (POS) code on the CMS-1500. If this POS code is not correctly reported, the reduction may not be implemented and incorrect payment may result.

A single UB-04 claim is filed for certain hospital departments such as radiology, outpatient surgery, and physical therapy. However, with any department or service area that poses the potential of a payment differential if the services are provided in a free-standing analog, CMS is interested in ensuring that all PBR requirements are fulfilled. If they are not fulfilled, payments made by CMS may be subject to recoupment. 42 CFR §413.65(o)(2) states:

---

* A hospital may elect to split-bill (file both claim forms) only for Medicare patients and not for other types of patients. See April 7, 2000 *Federal Register*, page 18519. (65 FR 18519).

Inappropriate treatment as provider based or not reporting material change. Effective for any period on or after October 1, 2002 (or, in the case of facilities or organizations described in paragraph (b)(2) of this section, for cost reporting periods starting on or after July 1, 2003), if a facility or organization is found by CMS to have been inappropriately treated as provider-based under paragraph (j) of this section for those periods, or previously was determined by CMS to be provider-based but no longer qualifies as provider-based because of a material change occurring during those periods that was not reported to CMS under paragraph (c) of this section, CMS will not treat the facility or organization as provider-based for payment purposes until CMS has determined, based on documentation submitted by the provider, that the facility or organization meets all requirements for provider-based status under this part.

The penalties for non-compliance in this area involve recoupment of payments. However, read the language with care. The final implementation of the PBR places the burden of proof on the hospital or provider. A provider can seek a formal determination by submitting a formal request and supplying supporting documentation. A hospital may also file a simple statement of attestation for in-hospital or on-campus activities. For off-campus operations, the attestation should be accompanied by supporting documentation.

The following discussion divides the auditing concerns for two entities: (1) a hospital meeting PBR requirements for all departments, facilities, and/or service areas and (2) a provider-based clinic. The various inpatient and outpatient departments of a hospital can generally be addressed as a single project. A hospital may elect to file an attestation with its FI, indicating that the provisions of the PBR have been met and that the hospital has documentation on file to substantiate the attestation. Provider-based clinics present a special challenge, particularly those that are off-campus, for which it is generally recommended that an attestation with supporting documentation be filed or a formal determination requested from CMS via the FI and regional office (RO).

General provider-based compliance

While we generally think of provider-based status as an outpatient concept, the rule applies to all departments of a hospital, both outpatient and inpatient. Thus, any prohibitions and special billing requirements must be considered for inpatient and outpatient services. The four main concerns are (1) qualifying (including application and/or attestation), (2) prohibitions, (3) obligations, and (4) reporting. It is also help-

ful to separate a hospital into three distinct geographic areas: (1) in hospital, (2) out of hospital but on campus, and (3) off campus.

In matrix form (4 concerns × 3 geographic areas), twelve different areas must be considered for compliance purposes. The four main concerns will be briefly addressed and then examined as they relate to different hospital areas.

Hospitals must meet all the provider-based criteria to qualify as provider-based and thus file claims on CMS-1450 or UB-04 forms. For compliance purposes, documentation should be on file and readily available to verify that all criteria have been met. These criteria are delineated in Chapter 12 and discussed in some detail in the PBR. One of key issues in auditing is to verify that a hospital or provider meets PBR requirements.

One criterion covers the way a given facility or operation is presented the public. The basic idea is that patients who enter a provider-based facility, building, and/or service area must know they have entered a hospital (main provider). For in-hospital and on-campus situations, hospital entry is a foregone conclusion. However, patients entering an off-campus facility must know they have entered a hospital. Thus, names and signage become important because they confirm how a facility is presented or defined.

All required criteria must be met and a hospital should be fully prepared to prove that. A hospital can choose attest to this fact on record. For in-hospital and on-campus situations, an attestation is the only document filed and supporting documentation may be retained by the hospital. However, for much more sensitive off-campus situations, both the attestation and supporting documentation should be filed. The PBR imposes the responsibility for meeting the requirements on hospitals. A hospital may and in some cases should make a formal application to its FI and the RO for provider-based classification. This is generally recommended for off-campus provider-based clinics.

The PBR includes several prohibitions. One involves joint ventures although on-campus joint ventures constitute exceptions. While the rule is not explicit in this area, a fairly safe presumption is that the campus on which the joint venture is located is the main provider for the joint venture facility or organization.

A more disturbing prohibition involves services "under arrangements." How broadly or narrowly this prohibition is to be interpreted has not been determined. 42 CFR §413.65(i) states:

Furnishing all services under arrangement. A facility or organization may not qualify for provider-based status if all patient care services furnished at the facility or organization are furnished under arrangements.

All patient care is a key phrase. In essence, if a hospital is to file a technical component claim, at least a minimal amount of patient care must be performed by hospital employees. The next case study shows the potential for difficulties with this prohibition.

> **Case study 15-16. Hyperbaric oxygen therapy.** Apex Medical Center entered into an agreement with an outside company for the provision of hyperbaric oxygen therapy. Apex has a building about a block away from the hospital. The outside company will provide all the equipment, supplies, and service personnel. Apex will pay the company for all the services and then file technical component claims for the services.

The case study does not provide sufficient details, but the fact that Apex employees will not provide patient care under this arrangement is problematic and should raise immediate suspicion. Plans for participating in such an arrangement should be delayed pending further investigation and possibly a legal opinion.

The PBR also has a somewhat convoluted section on prohibitions relative to management contracts. This area should be audited for possible deficiencies. Special PBR requirements and obligations relate almost exclusively to off-campus provider-based clinics and facilities, and these are discussed in the next section. This leaves the reporting requirement. As with much of the PBR, the reporting requirement is very general:

> **Reporting of material changes in relationships.** *A main provider that has had one or more facilities or organizations considered provider-based also may report to CMS any material change in the relationship between it and any provider-based facility or organization, such as a change in ownership of the facility or organization or entry into a new or different management contract that would affect the provider-based status of the facility or organization.*

Auditing concerns present a challenge. The hospital is already reporting such changes by maintaining billing privileges under Medicare. Moreover, this PBR statement is not specific as to who should be notified and/or time periods during which such reporting is required.

Provider-based clinics

While different aspects of auditing are intended to assure that provider-based clinics operate appropri-

ately (use correct E/M levels and split-billing fees, etc.), this section focuses on conducting audits relative to meeting all PBR requirements. The special concerns revolve around three requirements:

- Physician supervision
- Notice of two co-payments (if applicable)
- EMTALA policies and procedures

Physician supervision means direct supervision as discussed in Chapter 13. Generally, a physician or qualified practitioner must be in the office suite and immediately available. For a provider-based clinic in a hospital or on a hospital campus, CMS presumes that a physician will be available.*

The notice of two co-payments is another requirement for off-campus clinics and other provider-based operations. In a clinic setting in which two claim forms are filed, the Medicare beneficiary must be informed of the two co-payments. For most hospitals, calculating exact co-payments in advance will be onerous. Thus, notices to patients usually include examples. While this requirement is an operational burden for a hospital, most Medicare beneficiaries have supplemental coverage that covers both copayments.

For some provider-based operations such as satellite radiology facilities, a single co-payment for the technical component will be involved. CMS changed the PBR requirements so that these operations do not have to give notice of two co-payments.

The EMTALA requirement relates back to the concept that a provider-based clinic or operation is part of a hospital. Thus, the EMTLA definition of "comes to the hospital" becomes important. Off-campus provider-based clinics are not typically equipped to act as dedicated emergency departments (DEDs). Policies and procedures must be drafted and properly approved to address emergency presentations. Probably the most typical policy is for staff to dial 911. Of course, a provider-based clinic may be an urgent care center, which, by definition, is a DED under EMTALA. See Chapter 12 for further discussion of EMTALA.

In summary, conducting an audit of a hospital's stance relative to the PBR involves review of qualifying criteria, checking for violations of the prohibitions, ensuring that all obligations are met, and ascertaining that all material changes are reported. All these tasks must be backed up by the assurance that appropriate documentation on file justifies provider-based status. Because of the special obligations, the greatest concern is for off-campus operations. These types of clinics and diagnostic testing facilities should be carefully examined.

---

* See April 7, 2000 *Federal Register,* pages 18524-18526 (65 FR 18524–18526).

> **Key learning area: The PBR developed by CMS over the last decade has a convoluted history. The impetus for developing the regulations was to address provider-based clinics and the increased payments that hospitals can generate by having provider-based rather than free-standing clinics. The current rule covers a hospital *in toto* and includes both inpatient and outpatient services.**

Billing privileges: CMS-855 reviews

Chapter 12 discussed the need for all healthcare providers that file claims with the Medicare program to gain billing privileges. This is accomplished by using the CMS-855 form. Other third-party payers impose similar, although generally less onerous, processes. The five CMS-855 forms cover all types of providers and situations:

CMS-855A—Institutional Providers
CMS-855B—Clinics/Group Practices and Certain Other Suppliers
CMS-855I—Physicians and Non-Physician Practitioners
CMS 855R—Reassignment of Medicare Benefits
CMS 855S—Durable Medical Equipment, Prosthetics, Orthotics and Supplies (DMEPOS) Suppliers

Recently, CMS decided to significantly increase the requirements relative to gaining and maintaining billing privileges. This initiative on the part of CMS was motivated by fraudulent activities by individuals and organizations that gained billing privileges and billed for services or products that were never provided.

For a solo physician organized as a sole proprietor, the CMS-855 process is fairly simple as is the process for obtaining an NPI (national provider identifier). However, for a hospital providing different types and levels of services, employing physicians, and maintaining provider-based clinics and other organizational structures, the CMS-855 situation can be very complex. Increasing organizational complexity makes the associated NPI situation more complicated. The entire Medicare provider-based situation triggers audits that are designed to make certain that compliance related to billing privileges is met and maintained.

Again, audit and review concerns involve the *accuracy and completeness of information* on the forms, i.e., information on file at the facility, the process or system used to maintain information transmitted to Medicare and other third-party payers, and the efficiency and accuracy of billing and claims filing. The process question involves the *organizational infrastructure* that maintains billing privileges and reports organizational changes.

For a solo practitioner, organizational structuring is almost non-existent. As the size and complexity of a healthcare provider increases, the need for a separately identified job function becomes important. In complex organizations such as hospitals, multiple initiatives and activities may require updating of CMS-855 forms. A significant question is whether any single person knows about every activity in a hospital or system and every event that affects billing privileges and other CBR functions.

Auditors should investigate the organizational structure used to develop and maintain the CMS-855 forms. Personnel performing these services may also be involved in credentialing, licensing, certification, and even the medical staff organization. Note that the extensive attachments to CMS-855 forms also require updating. Staff should be prepared for unannounced audits intended to verify information on file via CMS-855 forms. See the CD accompanying this book for additional information on CMS-855 forms and references to the rules for gaining and maintaining billing privileges.

> **Key learning area: CMS recently increased the regulatory burden for gaining and maintaining billing privileges under Medicare. CBR compliance staff should appropriately review the accuracy and completeness of CMS-855 forms and attachments, note changes in the organizational infrastructure, and update information appropriately.**

Summary and conclusions

Dozens, if not hundreds, of audits and reviews can and often should be conducted by healthcare providers. Reviews are minimal for solo physicians. The needs for formal audits and informal reviews increase dramatically for multispecialty clinics, hospitals, and hospital systems. While some audits are fairly standardized, most audits require specific design and implementation.

> **Key learning area: A long list of special audit areas can easily be developed. This chapter discussed only a handful. Due to the complexity of the payment systems of Medicare and private third-party payers, coding, billing, and associated reimbursement can become ensnared with problems and challenges that justify audits and reviews.**

References and bibliography

The following references are provided for those seeking additional information in a number of areas discussed in this book. Note the absence of specific references covering statutory healthcare compliance and associated payment systems. Most of the information in this area is far too dynamic to allow for publication in book form. Readers are encouraged to consult the *Federal Register, Code of Federal Regulations, United States Code,* CMS Transmittals, and various CMS program manuals. Additional information can be obtained from the Office of the Inspector General (OIG), Government Accounting Office (GAO), Office of Management and Budget (OMB) and similar federal and/or state publications.

A CD-ROM has been provided with this book to provide immediate reference resources for specific compliance-related areas such as, EMTALA, HIPAA, the provider-based rule, etc. The table of contents (in HTML format) on the CD provides hyperlinks to various documents.

Although many journal articles that can provide additional information can be cited, CBR compliance is also too dynamic to prevent references covering rules, regulations, and their interpretation from becoming outdated very quickly. Current information is better retrieved through the Internet and/or periodicals.

As discussed in this book, a great deal of information concerns statutory compliance relating to many different payment systems. On the private third-party payer (or contractual) side, variability increases dramatically. While managed care contracts certainly contain similarities based on established payment systems from government programs, they also differ. Contract provisions, particularly requirements, must be studied with great care. Because of contract variabilities, most references in book form concentrate on the *process* and types of *provisions* at a general level. A few references are provided below. Healthcare providers entering into managed care contracts should research newsletters, conferences and workshop offerings in this area.

Healthcare compliance organizations

Several organizations address healthcare compliance and/or auditing. Two are:

Association of Healthcare Internal Auditors: http://www.ahia.org
Healthcare Compliance Association: http://www.hcca-info.org

Other organizations whose domains include certain compliance issues:

Healthcare Financial Management Association (HFMA): http://www.hfma.org
American Health Information Management Association (AHIMA): http://www.ahima.org
The American Health Lawyers Association (AHLA) maintains significant resource materials both in written form and also with active listservs: http://www.abanet.org/health
The American Bar Association (ABA) Health Law Section covers healthcare CBR concerns and issues: http://www.abanet.org/health

Healthcare-related certifications

Healthcare certifications related to coding, billing, and reimbursement are becoming more common. For compliance purposes, certified, well trained, and properly educated personnel are significant assets. The proliferation of such certifications, particularly in coding, means that determining the value of a certifications may be challenging.

Healthcare compliance

While this book is dedicated to many aspects of healthcare coding, billing, and reimbursement, provider organizations face additional compliance concerns. The following references generally cover compliance and include information about CBR aspects of compliance. Aspen periodically publishes materials about healthcare compliance. Likewise, West Group publishes an annual health law handbook.

Aspen Health Law Center (2007) *Health Law and Compliance Update*. Gaithersburg, MD: Aspen Publishers.
Gosfield, A. G., ed. (2007). *Health Law Handbook 2007 Edition*. St. Paul, MN: West Group.

Managed care contracting

Fisk, R. (2007). *Top Managed Care Contracting Clauses: A Tool-Kit for Providers*. Marblehead, MA: HCPro, Inc.
Garofalo, W., E. Horwitz, and T. Reardon (1999). *Managed Care Contracting: A Practical Guide for Health Care Executives*. San Francisco: Jossey-Bass.
Knight, W. (1997). *Managed Care Contracting: A Guide For Health Care Professionals*. New York: Aspen Publishers.

Spoden, L., and J. Kersnery (2006). *Managed Care Contracting Survival Guide for Healthcare Providers: Negotiating, Contracting, and Operational Planning for Success.* Marblehead, MA: HCPro, Inc.

Tinsley, R. (1999). *Managed Care Contracting: Successful Negotiation Strategies.* Chicago: American Medical Association.

Todd, M. (1996). *Managed Care Contracting Handbook: Planning and Negotiating the Managed Care Relationship.* New York: McGraw-Hill.

Training and education

Ahier, J., and G. Esland (1999). *Education, Training, and the Future of Work.* London: Routledge.

Argote, L. (1999). *Organizational Learning: Creating, Retaining and Transferring Knowledge.* Boston: Kluwer.

Bourner, T., V. Martin, and P. Race (1994). *Workshops that Work: 100 Ideas to Make Your Training Events More Effective.* New York: McGraw-Hill.

Campbell, C. P. (1996). *Education and Training for Work.* Lancaster, PA: Technomic.

Charney, C., and K. Conway (2005). *The Trainer's Tool Kit.* New York: Amacom.

Ford, J., ed. (1997). *Improving Training Effectiveness in Work Organizations.* Mahwah, NJ: Lawrence Erlbaum Associates.

Grubb, W. N. (1996). *Learning to Work: The Case for Reintegrating Job Training and Education.* New York: Russell Sage Foundation.

Gunter, B. H. (1996). *Making Training Work: How to Achieve Bottom-Line Results and Lasting Success.* Milwaukee: ASQC Quality Press.

Johann, B. (1995). *Designing Cross-Functional Business Processes.* San Francisco: Jossey-Bass.

Kommers, P., R. Grabinger, and J. Dunlap (1996). *Hypermedia Learning Environments: Instructional Design and Integration.* Mahwah, NJ: Lawrence Erlbaum Associates.

Lawson, K. (2006). *The Trainer's Handbook.* San Francisco: Pfeiffer.

Robbins, S. P., and P. L. Hunsaker (1996). *Training in Interpersonal Skills: TIPS for Managing People at Work.* Upper Saddle River, NJ: Prentice Hall.

Rothwell, W. J. (2006). *Handbook of Training Technologies.* San Francisco: Pfeiffer.

Silberman, M. (1996) *Active Learning: 101 Strategies to Teach Any Subject.* New York: Allyn & Bacon.

Silberman, M. L., and C. Auerbach (1998). *Active Training: A Handbook of Techniques, Designs, Case Examples, and Tips.* New York: Pfeiffer.

Smith, P., and L. Kearny (1994). *Creating Workplaces Where People Can Think.* San Francisco: Jossey-Bass.

Van Kavelaar, E. K. (1998). *Conducting Training Workshops: A Crash Course For Beginners.* San Francisco: Jossey-Bass.

Vaughn, R. H. (2005). *The Professional Trainer: A Comprehensive Guide to Planning, Delivering, and Evaluating Training Programs.* San Francisco: Berrett-Koehler.

Wheeland, S. A. (1990). *Facilitating Training Groups: A Guide to Leadership and Verbal Intervention Skills.* New York: Praeger.

Facilitation, teams, and team development

American Society for Training and Development (1991). Developing and Managing Work Teams. In *Training & Development and Technical & Skills Training.* Alexandria, VA.

Becker-Reems, E. D. (1994). *Self-Managed Work Teams in Health Care Organizations.* Chicago: American Hospital Publishing.

Becker-Reems, E. D., and D. G. Garrett (1998). *Testing the Limits of Teams: How to Implement Self-Management in Health Care.* Chicago: AHA Press.

Capezio, P. (1996). *Supreme Teams: How to Make Teams Really Work: Team Process and Dynamics Handbook.* Shawnee Mission, KS: National Press Publications.

Davis, J. (1992). *Successful Team Building: How to Create Teams that Really Work.* London: Kogan Page.

Dyer, W. G., and J. H. Dyer. (2007). *Team Building: Proven Strategies for Improving Team Performance.* San Francisco: Jossey-Bass.

Fisher, K. (1993). *Leading Self-Directed Work Teams: A Guide to Developing New Team Leadership Skills.* New York: McGraw-Hill.

Fisher, K., and M. D. Fisher (1998). *The Distributed Mind: Achieving High Performance through the Collective Intelligence of Knowledge Work Teams.* New York: Amacom.

Grant, N. (1996). *Teams Work.* Oak Brook, IL: GCCG Books.

Hicks, R., and D. Bone (1990). *Self-Managing Teams: A Guide for Creating and Maintaining Self-Managed Work Groups.* Los Altos, CA: Crisp Publications.

Hill, C. E. (2004). *Helping Skills: Facilitating Exploration, Insight, and Action.* Washington, D.C.: American Psychological Association.

Hitchcock, D. E. (1994). *The Work Redesign Team Handbook: A Step-by-Step Guide to Creating Self-Directed Teams.* White Plains, NY: Association for Quality and Participation.

Hitchcock, D. E., and M. L. Willard (1995). *Why Teams Can Fail and What to Do about It: Essential Tools for Anyone Implementing Self-Directed Work Teams.* Chicago: Irwin.

Jackson, S. E., and M. N. Ruderman (1995). *Diversity in Work Teams: Research Paradigms for a Changing Workplace.* Washington, D.C.: American Psychological Association.

Jones, P. H. (1998). *Handbook of Team Design: A Practitioner's Guide to Team Systems Development.* New York: McGraw-Hill.

Justice, T., and D. Jamieson (2006). *The Facilitator's Fieldbook: Step-by-Step Procedures, Checklists and Guidelines, Samples and Templates.* New York: Amacom.

Katzenbach, J. R. (1998). *The Work of Teams.* Boston: Harvard Business School Press.

Katzenbach, J. R. (2006). *The Wisdom of Teams: Creating the High-Performance Organization.* New York: Collins.

Kayser, T. A. (1994). *Building Team Power: How to Unleash the Collaborative Genius of Work Teams.* Carlsbad, CA: Irwin.

Organizational Dynamics, Inc. (2001). *Making Teams Work.* Burlington, MA.

Orsburn, J. D., and L. Moran (1999). *The New Self-Directed Work Teams: Mastering the Challenge.* New York: McGraw-Hill.

Parker, G. (2003). *Cross-Functional Teams: Working with Allies, Enemies, and Other Strangers.* San Francisco: Jossey-Bass.

Rees, F. (1991). *How to Lead Work Teams: Facilitation Skills.* San Diego: Pfeiffer.

Robbins, H. (2000). *The New Why Teams Don't Work: What Goes Wrong and How to Make It Right.* San Francisco: Berrett-Koehler.

Robbins, H., and M. Finley (1995). *Why Teams Don't Work: What Went Wrong and How to Make It Right.* Princeton, NJ: Peterson.

Schrage, M. (1995). *No More Teams! Mastering the Dynamics of Creative Collaboration.* New York: Doubleday.

Schwarz, R. M. (2005). *The Skilled Facilitator Fieldbook: Tips, Tools, and Tested Methods for Consultants, Facilitators, Managers, Trainers, and Coaches.* San Francisco: Jossey-Bass.

Silberman, M. (1996). *Team and Organization Development.* New York: McGraw-Hill.

Silberman, M. (2005). *The 2005 ASTD Team and Organizational Development Sourcebook.* Bend, OR: ASTD Press.

Turniansky, B. (1998). *Individuals and Groups in Organizations.* London: Sage.

Vennix, J. (1996). *Group Model Building: Facilitating Team Learning Using System Dynamics.* Chichester: Wiley.

Wellins, R. S., et al. (1991). *Empowered Teams: Creating Self-Directed Work Groups that Improve Quality, Productivity, and Participation.* San Francisco: Jossey-Bass.

Zoglio, S. W. (1993). *Teams at Work: Seven Keys to Success.* Doylestown, PA: Town Hill Press.

Six Sigma and other quality programs

Andersen, B. (1999). *Business Process Improvement Toolbox.* Milwaukee: ASQ Quality Press.

Andersen, B., and P. Per-Gaute (1996). *The Benchmarking Handbook: Step-by-Step Instructions.* London: Chapman & Hall.

Armistead, C. G., and A. P. Rowland (1996). *Managing Business Processes: BPR and Beyond.* Chichester: Wiley.

Born, G. (1994). *Process Management to Quality Improvement: The Way to Design, Document and Re-Engineer Business Systems.* New York: Wiley.

Brown, M. , D. Hitchcock, and M. Willard (1994). *Why TQM Fails and What to Do about It.* Burr Ridge, IL: Irwin.

Brussee, W. (2006). *All About Six Sigma: The Easy Way to Get Started.* New York: McGraw-Hill.

Carreira, B., and B. Trudell (2006). *Lean Six Sigma that Works: A Powerful Action Plan for Dramatically Improving Quality, Increasing Speed, and Reducing Waste.* New York: Amacom.

Codling, S. (1998). *Benchmarking.* Brookfield, VT: Gower.

Cordata J., and J. Woods (1995). *The McGraw-Hill Encyclopedia of Quality Terms and Concepts.* New York: McGraw-Hill.

Coulson-Thomas, C. (1994). *Business Process Re-engineering: Myth and Reality.* London: Kogan Page.

Damelio, R. (1995). *The Basics of Benchmarking.* New York: Quality Resources.

Fischer, L. (1995). *The Workflow Paradigm: The Impact of Information Technology on Business Process Reengineering.* Lighthouse Point, FL: Future Strategies.

Fisher, S., and R. T. William (1995). *Personal and Organizational Transformations: The True Challenge of Continual Quality Improvement.* London: McGraw-Hill.

Harbour, J. L. (1994). *Process Reengineering Workbook.* White Plains, NY: Quality Resources.

Harrington, H. J. (1996). *The Complete Benchmarking Implementation Guide: Total Benchmarking Management.* New York: McGraw-Hill.

Harrington, H. J., E. K. C. Esseling, and H. Van Nimwegen (1997). *Business Process Improvement Workbook: Documentation, Analysis, Design, and Management of Business Process Improvement.* New York: McGraw-Hill.

Healthcare Financial Management Association (1997). *Financial and Clinical Benchmarking: The Strategic Use of Data.* Westchester, IL: HFMA.

Hino, Satoshi (2005). *Inside the Mind of Toyota: Management Principles for Enduring Growth.* New York: Productivity Press.

Kanji, G. K., and A. Mike (1996). *One Hundred Methods for Total Quality Management.* London: Sage.

Koch, H.C.H. (1992). *Implementing and Sustaining Total Quality Management in Health Care.* Harlow, U.K.: Longman.

McHugh, P., G. Merli, et al. (1995). *Beyond Business Process Reengineering: Towards the Holonic Enterprise.* Chichester: Wiley.

Melum, M. M., and M. E. Sinioris (1992). *Total Quality Management: The Health Care Pioneers.* Chicago: AHA.

Morgan, J. (2005). *Creating Lean Corporations: Reengineering from the Bottom Up to Eliminate Waste.* New York: Productivity Press.

Nash, M., S. Poling, and S. Ward (2006). *Using Lean for Faster Six Sigma Results: A Synchronized Approach.* New York: Productivity Press.

Omachonu, V. K. (1991). *Total Quality and Productivity Management in Health Care Organizations.* Milwaukee: American Society for Quality Control.

Ould, M. A. (1995). *Business Processes: Modeling and Analysis for Re-Engineering and Improvement.* Chichester: Wiley.

Pande, Peter S., et al. (2002). *The Six Sigma Way Team Fieldbook: An Implementation Guide for Project Improvement Teams.* London: McGraw-Hill.

Patterson, J. G. (1996). *Benchmarking Basics: Looking for a Better Way.* Menlo Park, CA: Crisp Publications.

Pyzdedk, T. (2003). *The Six Sigma Handbook: Revised and Expanded.* New York: McGraw-Hill.

Povey, B. (1996). *Continuous Business Improvement: Linking the Key Improvement Processes for Your Critical Long-Term Success.* London: McGraw-Hill.

Rolstada, A. (1995). *Performance Management: A Business Process Benchmarking Approach.* London: Chapman & Hall.

Sethi, V., and W. R. King (1998). *Organizational Transformation through Business Process Reengineering: Applying Lessons Learned.* Upper Saddle River, NJ: Prentice Hall.

St. Anthony Publishing and Healthcare Design Systems (1995). *Guide to Benchmarking Hospital Value: Evaluating Inpatient Cost & Quality.* Washington, D.C.

Stamatis, D. H. (2003). *Six Sigma Fundamentals: A Complete Guide to the System, Methods, and Tools.* New York: Productivity Press.

Taghizadegan, S. (2006). *Essentials of Lean Six Sigma.* Boston: Elsevier.

Tague, N. R. (1995). *The Quality Toolbox.* Milwaukee: ASQC Quality Press.

Tweet, A. G., and K. Gavin-Marciano (1998). *Guide to Benchmarking in Healthcare: Practical Lessons from the Field.* New York: Quality Resources.

Vonderheide-liem, D., and B. Pate (2004). *Applying Quality Methodologies to Improve Healthcare: Six Sigma, Lean Thinking, Balanced Scorecard, and More.* Marblehead, MA: HCPro.

Watson, G. H. (2004). *Six Sigma for Business Leaders: A Guide to Implementation.* Salem, NH: Goal/QPC.

Zairi, M., and P. Leonard (1994). *Practical Benchmarking: The Complete Guide.* London: Chapman & Hall.

Mind mapping, creative thinking, and related subjects

Bennett, J. G. (1998). *Creative Thinking.* Santa Fe, NM: Bennett Books.

Bierman, A. K., and R. N. Assali (1996). *The Critical Thinking Handbook.* Upper Saddle River, NJ: Prentice-Hall.

Buzan, T. (1991). *Use Both Sides of Your Brain: New Mind-Mapping Techniques to Help You Raise All Levels of Your Intelligence and Creativity, Based on the Latest Discoveries about the Human Brain.* New York: Dutton.

Buzan, T., and B. Buzan (1994). *The Mind Map Book: How to Use Radiant Thinking to Maximize Your Brain's Untapped Potential.* New York: Dutton.

Evans, J. R. (1991). *Creative Thinking in the Decision and Management Sciences.* Cincinnati: South-Western.

Frumker, S. C. (1994). *Mind Map: Your Guide to Prosperity and Fulfillment.* University Heights, OH: Health Associates.

Gelb, M. (2003). *Mind Mapping: How to Liberate Your Natural Genius.* Chicago: Nightingale-Conant.

Hall, L., and B. Bodenhamer (2000). *The User's Manual for the Brain Volume I.* Williston, VT: Crown.

Hall, L., and B. Bodenhamer (2003). *The User's Manual for the Brain Volume II.* Williston, VT: Crown.

Keeney, R. L. (1992). *Value-Focused Thinking: A Path to Creative Decisionmaking.* Cambridge: Harvard University Press.

Kim, J. C. S. (1994). *The Art of Creative Critical Thinking.* Lanham, MD: University Press.

Pesut, D. J., and J. Herman (1999). *Clinical Reasoning: The Art and Science of Critical and Creative Thinking.* Albany, NY: Delmar.

Peterson, W. A. (1991). *The Art of Creative Thinking.* Santa Monica: Hay House.

Ruggiero, V. R. (1998). *The Art of Thinking: A Guide to Critical and Creative Thought.* New York: Longman.

Wycoff, J. (1991). *Mindmapping: Your Personal Guide to Exploring Creativity and Problem-Solving.* New York: Berkley.

Facilitation and interpersonal communications

For those interested in a more extensive bibliography concerning neurolinguistic programming (NLP), sociolinguistics, and/or psycholinguistic programming (PLP), please contact the author.

Arnold, E., and K. Boggs (2006). *Interpersonal Relationships: Professional Communication Skills for Nurses, 5th ed.* Philadelphia: Saunders.

Bacon, T. R. (1996). *High Impact Facilitation.* Durango, CO: International Learning Works.

Bebee, S. A., et al. (2007). *Interpersonal Communication: Relating to Others, 5th ed.* New York: Allyn & Bacon.

Bodenhamer, B., and L. M. Hall. (2000). *The User's Manual for the Brain.* Cardiff: Crown House.

Cameron, E. (2005). *Facilitation Made Easy: Practical Tips to Improve Facilitation Techniques.* London: Kogan Page.

Caputo, J. S., et al. (1994). *Interpersonal Communication: Competency through Critical Thinking.* Boston: Allyn & Bacon.

DeVito, J. A. (1999). *Messages: Building Interpersonal Communication Skills.* New York: Longman.

Hall, M. L., and B. G. Bodenhamer (2003). *The User's Manual for the Brain Volume II.* Cardiff, U.K.: Crown House.

Hartley, P. (1999). *Interpersonal Communication.* London: Routledge.

Hunter, D., et al. (1995). *The Art of Facilitation: How to Create Group Synergy.* Tucson, AZ: Fisher Books.

Kinlaw, D. C. (1996). *Facilitation Skills: The ASTD Trainer's Sourcebook.* New York: McGraw-Hill.

Kiser, A. G. (1998). *Masterful Facilitation: Becoming a Catalyst for Meaningful Change.* New York: Amacom.

Knapp, M. L., and G. R. Miller (1994). *Handbook of Interpersonal Communication.* Thousand Oaks, CA: Sage.

McClelland, S. B. (1995). *Organizational Needs Assessments: Design, Facilitation, and Analysis.* Westport, CT: Quorum.

Muir, J. K. (1992). *Introduction to Interpersonal and Small Group Communication Handbook.* Dubuque, IA: Kendall Hunt.

Putz, G. B. (1998). *Facilitation Skills: Helping Groups Make Decisions.* Bountiful, UT: Deep Space Technology.

Rees, F. (1991). *How to Lead Work Teams: Facilitation Skills.* San Diego: Pfeiffer.

Schnell, J. (1996). *Interpersonal Communication: Understanding and Being Understood.* East Rockaway, NY: Cummings & Hathaway.

Stewart, J. R. (1999). *Bridges Not Walls: A Book about Interpersonal Communication.* Boston: McGraw Hill.

Trenholm, S., and A. Jensen (2007). *Interpersonal Communication.* Ann Arbor, MI: Oxford University Press.

Webne-Behrman, H. (1998). *The Practice of Facilitation: Managing Group Process and Solving Problems.* Westport, CT: Quorum.

Auditing, statistics, and related subjects

For most practical applications, CBR compliance personnel use the free RAT-STATS program from the OIG. See: http://oig.hhs.gov/organization/OAS/ratstat.html.

American Institute of Certified Public Accountants (1999). *Audit Sampling.* New York.

Bailey, L. P. (1981). *Statistical Sampling for Attributes.* New York: Miller Accounting Publications.

Cassel, C., C.-E. Särndal, et al. (1993). *Foundations of Inference in Survey Sampling.* Malabar, FL: Krieger.

Chaudhuri, A., and H. Stenger (1992). *Survey Sampling: Theory and Methods.* New York: Marcel Dekker.

Foreman, E. K. (1991). *Survey Sampling Principles.* New York: Marcel Dekker.

Guenther, W. C. (1973). *A Sample Size Formula for the Hypergeometric.* Laramie, WY: University of Wyoming Press.

Guenther, W. C. (1973). *Sample Size Formulas for Some Binomial Type Problems.* Laramie, WY: University of Wyoming Press.

Guy, D. M., and D. R. Carmichael (1986). *Audit Sampling: An Introduction to Statistical Sampling in Auditing.* New York: Wiley.

Guy, D. M. et al. (1998). *Audit Sampling: An Introduction.* New York: Wiley.

Guy, D. M., D. R. Carmichael, et al. (1998). *Practitioner's Guide to Audit Sampling.* New York: Wiley.

Kish, L. (1995). *Survey Sampling.* New York: Wiley.

Levy, P. (2004). *Sampling of Populations.* New York: Wiley.

Mace, A. E. (1964). *Sample-Size Determination.* New York: Reinhold.

Satin, A., et al. (1993). *Survey Sampling: A Non-Mathematical Guide.* Ottawa: Minister of Industry, Science, and Technology.

Scheaffer, R. L., et al. (1995). *Elementary Survey Sampling.* Belmont, CA: Duxbury Press.

Singh, R., and N. Singh-Mangat (1996). *Elements of Survey Sampling.* New York: Springer.

Snedecor, G. (1989). *Statistical Methods, 8th Ed.* Ames, IA: Iowa State University Press.

Internet, intranet, and related subjects

With the availability of relatively inexpensive technology based on Internet protocols, one effective way to make policies and procedures available is via an intranet—a localized application of the Internet. A few references to intranets are provided along with books that may facilitate searching the Internet via powerful search engines.

Asprey, L., and M. Middleton (2003). *Integrative Document and Content Management: Strategies for Exploiting Enterprise Knowledge.* New York: IGI Global.

Azad, A. (2007). *Implementing Electronic Document and Record Management Systems.* New York: Auerbach.

Bannan, J. (1997). *Intranet Document Management: A Guide for Webmasters and Content Providers.* Reading, MA: Addison Wesley.

Bernard, R. (1997). *The Corporate Intranet.* New York: Wiley.

Bodensiek, P. (1996). *Intranet Publishing.* Indianapolis: Queue.

Bort, J., and B. Felix (1997). *Building an Extranet: Connect Your Intranet with Vendors and Customers.* New York: Wiley.

Bremner, L. M., et al. (1997). *Intranet Bible.* Las Vegas: Jamsa Press.

Colby, J., et al.(2003). *Practical Intranet Development.* Berkeley: Apress Publishers.

Edwards, M. J. A. (1997). *The Internet for Nurses and Allied Health Professionals.* New York: Springer.

Glowniak, J. V. (1997). *Internet Guide for Allied Health Professionals.* Reston, VA: Society of Nuclear Medicine.

Goltzman, S. et al. (1999). *Internet in an Hour: Health and Medical Resources.* New York: DDC Publishing.

Griffin, A. D. (1999). *Directory of Internet Sources for Health Professionals.* Albany, NY: Delmar.

Guengerich, S. L. (1997). *Building the Corporate Intranet.* New York: Wiley.

Hogarth, M., and D. Hutchinson (1996). *An Internet Guide for the Health Professional.* Sacramento: New Wind Publishing.

Holloway, R., A. Kyselica, and S. Caravajal. (2007). *SharePoint 2007 and Office Development Expert Solutions.* Indianapolis: Wrox.

Hutchinson, D. (1998). *MEDLINE for Health Professionals: How to Search PubMed on the Internet.* Sacramento: New Wind Publishing.

Kiley, R. (2003). *Medical Information on the Internet: A Guide for Health Professionals.* Edinburgh: Churchill Livingstone.

Maier, R. (2007). *Knowledge Management Systems: Information and Communication Technologies for Knowledge Management.* New York: Springer.

McDermott, J. E., and J. E. Phillips (1997). *Administering Usenet News Servers: A Comprehensive Guide to Planning, Building, and Managing Internet and Intranet News Services.* Reading, MA: Addison Wesley.

Miller, M., et al. (1998). *Managing the Corporate Intranet.* New York: Wiley.

Oppliger, R. (1998). *Internet and Intranet Security.* Boston: Artech.

Sosa-Iudicissa, M. C., et al. (1997). *Internet, Telematics, and Health.* Amsterdam: Ios Press.

Tanler, R. (1997). *Intranet Data Warehouse: Tools and Techniques for Building Intranet-Enabled Data Warehouse.* New York: Wiley.

Health Insurance Portability and Accountability Act (HIPAA)

While HIPAA is embodied in the *Code of Federal Regulations*, the following volumes may be useful.

Barnes, J., P. Rothstein, and D. Barnes (2004). *Business Continuity Planning and HIPAA: Business Continuity Management in the Health Care Environment.* Brookfield, CT: Rothstein.

Beaver, K., and R. Herold (2003). *Practical Guide to HIPAZ Privacy and Security Compliance.* New York: Auerbach.

Burton, B. (2003). *Quick Guide to HIPAA for the Physician's Office.* Belmont, CA: Saunders.

Hartley, C., and E. Jones (2004). *HIPAA Plain and Simple: A Compliance Guide for Healthcare Professionals.* Chicago: AMA Press.

Krager, D. (2005). *HIPAA for Medical Office Personnel.* New York: Thomson Delmar.

Meyer, J., and M. Schiff (2003). *HIPAA: The Questions You Didn't Know to Ask.* Upper Saddle River, NJ: Prentice-Hall.

Pabrai, U. (2003). *Getting Started with HIPAA.* Boston: Course Technology.

Rada, R. (2002). *HIPAA in 24 Hours: Small Healthcare Entity HIPAA Manual.* Brooklyn: HIPAA.

Rada, R. (2002). *HIPAA IT Essentials: Health Information Transactions, Privacy, and Security.* Liverpool: Hypermedia.

Rockel, K. (2005). *Stedman's Guide to the HIPAA Privacy Rule.* Philadelphia: Lippincott Williams & Wilkins.

Withrow, S. (2001) *Managing HIPAA Compliance: Standards for Electronic Tranmission, Privacy, and Security of Health Information.* New York: Health Administration Press.

Wu, S. (2007). *A Guide to HIPAA Security and the Law.* New York: American Bar Association.

Note: As a part of the research efforts at Abbey & Abbey, Consultants, Inc., Dr. Abbey maintains several specialized bibliographies on CBR compliance. Please feel free to contact him for further information on current bibliographies.

Chargemaster information

Abbey, Duane C. 2005. *Chargemasters strategies to ensure accurate reimbursement and compliance.* Marblehead, MA: HCPro, Inc.

Abbey, Duane C. 2005. *Emergency department coding and billing a guide to reimbursement and compliance.* Marblehead, MA: HCPro.

Abbey, Duane C. 1996. *The ambulatory patient group operations manual.* Chicago: Irwin.

Abbey, Duane C. 2004. *Nonphysician providers guide to coding, billing, and reimbursement.* Marblehead, MA: HCPro.

Abbey, Duane C. 1999. *Compliance for coding, billing & reimbursement a systematic approach to developing a comprehensive program.* New York: McGraw-Hill.

Abbey, Duane C. 1998. *Outpatient services designing, organizing, and managing outpatient resources.* The HFMA healthcare financial management series. New York: McGraw-Hill.

Abbey, Duane C. 1997. *Charge master review strategies for improved billing and reimbursement.* The HFMA healthcare financial management series. New York: McGraw-Hill.

Acronyms

The ability to read, study, and decipher issues relating to coding, billing, and reimbursement compliance requires fundamental knowledge of acronyms and specialized terms. CBR compliance personnel must understand and communicate via acronyms from several disciplines, including healthcare, law, Internet, and computers. Additional references are provided as appropriate.

1500: Professional Claim Form (*See* CMS-1500)

6σ: Six Sigma (*See* Quality Improvement Techniques)

AA: Anesthesia Assistant

A/P: Accounts Payable

A/R: Accounts Receivable

ABC: Activity Based Costing

ABN: Advance Beneficiary Notice (*See also* NONC, HINNC)

ACC: Ambulatory Care Center

ACEP: American College of Emergency Physicians

ACHE: American College of Healthcare Executives

ACS: Ambulatory Care Services

ADA: Americans with Disabilities Act

AGPAM: American Guild of Patient Account Managers

AHA: American Hospital Association

AHIMA: American Health Information Management Association

AHRQ: Agency for Healthcare Research Quality

ALOS: Average Length of Stay

ALJ: Administrative Law Judge

AMA: American Medical Association or American Management Association

AMGMA: American Medical Group Management Association

AMP: Average Manufacturer Price

AO: Advisory Opinion

AOAA: American Osteopathic Association Accreditation

APC: Ambulatory Payment Classification(s)

AP-DRGs: All Patient DRGs

APG: Ambulatory Patient Group(s)

APR-DRGs: All Patient Refined DRGs

ASC: Ambulatory Surgical Center

ASCII: American Standard Code for Information Interchange

ASF: Ambulatory Surgical Facility

ASP: Average Sales Price

AWP: Average Wholesale Price

BBA: Balanced Budget Act (of 1997)

BBRA: Balanced Budget Refinement Act (of 1999)

BCA: Blue Cross Association

BCBSA: Blue Cross and Blue Shield Association

BIPA: Benefits Improvement and Protection Act (of 2000)

BPR: Business Process Reengineering

CA-DRGs: Consolidated Severity-Adjusted DRGs

CAH: Critical Access Hospital

CAP: Capitated Ambulatory Plan

CBA: Cost Benefit Analysis

CBR: Coding, Billing, and Reimbursement

CBRCO: CBR Compliance Officer

CC (Computer): Carbon Copy

CC: Coding Clinic

CCI: (HCFA's) Correct Coding Initiative

CCO: Chief Compliance Officer

CCR: Cost to Charge Ratio

CCs: Complications and Comorbidities

CCU: Critical Care Unit

CDM: Charge Description Master (*See* Generic Term: Chargemaster)

CENT: Certified Enterostomal Nurse Therapist

CERT: Comprehensive Error Rate Testing

CEUs: Continuing Education Units

CF: Conversion Factor

CfCs: Conditions for Coverage

CFO: Chief Financial Officer

CfPs: Conditions for Payment (*See* 42 CFR §424)

CFR: Code of Federal Regulations

CHAMPUS: Civilian Health & Medical Program of the Uniformed Services

CHAMPVA: Civilian Health & Medical Program of the Veterans Administration

CHC: Community Health Center

CHCP: Coordinated Home Health Program

CIA: Corporate Integrity Agreement (*See also* Settlement Agreements)

CIO: Chief Information Officer

CIS: Computer Information System

CM: Charge Master

CMI: Case Mix Index

CMP: Competitive Medical Plan

CMP: Civil Monetary Penalty

CMS: Center for Medicare and Medicaid Services

CMS-1450: UB-04 Claim Form as Used by Medicare

CMS-1500: 1500 Claim Form as Used by Medicare

CMS-855: Form Used to Gain Billing Privileges for Medicare

CNP: Certified Nurse Practitioner

CNS: Clinical Nurse Specialist

COBRA: Consolidated Omnibus Reconciliation Act (of 1995)

CON: Certificate of Need

COO: Chief Operating Officer

CoPs: Conditions of Participations (*See* 42 CFR §482 and 42 CFR §485.601)

CORF: Comprehensive Outpatient Rehabilitation Facility

CP: Clinical Psychologist

CPI: Consumer Price Index

CPT: Current Procedural Terminology (CPT-4 is current; CPT-5 anticipated)

CQI: Continuous Quality Improvement

CRNA: Certified Registered Nurse Anesthetist

CSF: Critical Success Factor

CSW: Clinical Social Worker

CT: Computer Tomographic

CWF: Common Working File (*See* CMS)

CY: Calendar Year

DBMS: Database Management System

DED: Dedicated Emergency Department (*See* EMTALA)

DHHS: Department of Health & Human Services

DME: Durable Medical Equipment

DMEPOS: DME, Prosthetics, Orthotics, Supplies

DMERC: Durable Medical Equipment Regional Carrier (*See* CMS MACs)

DNS: Domain Name System (Internet)

DOD: Department of Defense (*See* Electronic Shredding Standards)

DOJ: Department of Justice

DP: Data Processing

DRA: Deficit Reduction Act (of 2005)

DRG: Diagnosis-Related Group(s) (*See* AP-DRGs, APR-DRGs, SR-DRGs, CA-DRGs, MS-DRGs-FY2008)

DSH: Disproportionate Share Hospital

DSP: Disproportionate Share Payment

EACH: Essential Access Community Hospital

EBCDIC (Computer): Extended Binary Coded Decimal Information Code

ECG: Electrocardiogram

EDI: Electronic Data Interchange

EEO: Equal Employment Opportunity

EEOC: Equal Employment Opportunity Commission

EGHP: Employer Group Health Plan

EIN: Employer Identification Number (*See* TIN)

EKG: Elektrokardiogramm [German] (*See* ECG)

E/M: Evaluation and Management

EMC: Electronic Medial Claim

EMG: Electromyography

EMI: Encounter Mix Index

EMS: Emergency Medical Service

EMTALA: Emergency Medical Treatment and Active Labor Act (of 1986)

EOB: Explanation of Benefits

EOMB: Explanation of Medicare Benefits

EPA: Environmental Protection Agency

EPCs: Event-driven Process Chains

EPO: Exclusive Provider Organization

ER: Emergency Room (*See also* Emergency Department)

ERISA: Employment Retirement Income Security Act

ESRD: End Stage Renal Disease

FAC: Free-standing Ambulatory Care

FAQs: Frequently Asked Questions

FBI: Federal Bureau of Investigation

FDA: Food and Drug Administration

FEC: Free-Standing Emergency Center

FFS: Fee for Service

FFY: Federal Fiscal Year

FI: Fiscal Intermediary (*See* MACs)

FIN: Financial Identification Number (*See* TIN)

FL: Form Locator (*See* UB-04)

FLSA: Fair Labor Standards Act

FMR: Focused Medical Review

FMV: Fair Market Value

FP: Family Practice

FR: Federal Register

FRGs: Functional Related Groups

FRNA: First Registered Nurse Assistant

FTC: Federal Trade Commission

FTE: Full-time Equivalent

FTP: File Transfer Protocol (Internet)

FY: Fiscal Year (Federal and State may differ)

GAF: Geographic Adjustment Factor

GAO: Government Accountability Office

GI: Gastrointestinal

GMLOS: Geometric Mean Length of Stay

GPCI: Geographic Practice Cost Index

GPO: Government Printing Office

GSA: General Services Administration

GSP: Global Surgical Package

H&P: History and Physical

HCFA: Health Care Financing Administration (Now CMS)

HCO: Health Care Organization

HCPCS: Healthcare Common Procedure Coding System (Previously HCFA's Common Procedure Coding System)

HCRIS: Hospital Cost Report Information System

HFMA: Healthcare Financial Management Association

HHA: Home Health Agency

HHMCO: Home Health Managed Care Organization

HHS: Health and Human Services

HICN: Health Insurance Claim Number

HIM: Health Information Management (*See also* Medical Records)

HIPAA: Health Insurance Portability and Accountability Act (of 1996)
HIS: Health Information System
HIT: Health Information Technology
HL-7: Health Level 7 (*See* HIPAA TSC)
HMO: Health Maintenance Organization
HOPD: Hospital Outpatient Department
HPSA: Health Personnel Shortage Area
HRSA: Health Resources and Services Administration
HTML: HyperText Markup Language
HTTP: HyperText Transfer Protocol (Internet)
HURA: Health Underserved Rural Area
HwH: Hospital within Hospital
I&D: Incision and Drainage
ICD-9-CM: International Classification of Diseases, 9th Revision, Clinical Modification
ICD-10-CM: International Classification of Diseases, 10th Revision, Clinical Modification (Replacement for ICD-9-CM Volumes 1 and 2)
ICD-10-PCS: ICD-10 Procedure Coding System (Replacement for ICD-9-CM Volume 3)
ICD-11-CM: International Classification of Diseases, 11th Revision, Clinical Modification
ICD-11-PCS: ICD-11 Procedure Coding System
ICU: Intensive Care Unit
IDS: Integrated Delivery System
IG: Inspector General
IOL: Intraocular Lens
IP: Inpatient
IPA: Independent Practice Arrangement or Association
IPPS: Inpatient Prospective Payment System
IRF: Inpatient Rehabilitation Facility
IRO: Independent Review Organization
IRS: Internal Revenue Service
IS: Information Systems
ISP: Internet Service Provider
IT: Information Technology
IV: Intravenous
JCAHO: Joint Commission on Accreditation of Healthcare Organizations
KSAPCs: Knowledge, Skills, Abilities, and Personal Characteristics
LCC: Lesser of Costs or Charges
LCD: Local Coverage Decision (*See also* LMRP)
LMRP: Local Medical Review Policy (*See* LCD)
LOS: Length of Stay
LTCH: Long-Term Care Hospital
LTRH: Long-Term Rehabilitation Hospital
MA: Medicare Advantage
MAC: Medicare Administrative Contractor (*See* FI, Carrier and DMERC)
MAO: Medicare Advantage Organization

MAP: Model Ambulatory Practice
MAC: Medicare Administrative Contractor
MAC: Monitored Anesthesia Care
MCE: Medicare Code Editor (*See* DRGs)
MCO: Managed Care Organization
MDH: Medicare Dependent Hospital
MDS: Minimum Data Set
MedPAC: Medicare Payment Advisory Commission
MEI: Medicare Economic Index
MFS: Medicare Fee Schedule
MIEA-TRHCA: Medicare Improvements and Extension Act: Tax Relief Health Care Act (of 2006)
MIS: Management Information System
MMA: Medicare Modernization Act (of 2003)
Modem (Computer): MODulator-DEModulator
MOG: Medicare Outpatient Grouping
MPFS: Medicare Physician Fee Schedule
MRI: Magnetic Resonance Imaging
MSA: Metropolitan Statistical Area
MS-DOS (Computer): Microsoft Disk Operating System
MS-DRGs: Medicare Severity DRGs (CMS Established in FY2008)
MSOP: Market-Service-Organization-Payment
MSP: Medicare Secondary Payer
MUA: Medically Underserved Area
MVPS: Medicare Volume Performance Standard
NCCI: National Correct Coding Initiative (*See also* CCI)
NCD: National Coverage Decision
NCQA: National Committee for Quality Assurance
NCQHC: National Committee for Quality Health Care
NF: Nursing Facility
NLP: Neurolinguistic Programming
NM: Nurse Midwife
NP: Nurse Practitioner [Some variation, e.g., Advanced Registered Nurse Practitioner (ARNP)]
NPI: National Provider Identifier
NPP: Non-Physician Provider or Practitioner
NSC: National Supplier Clearinghouse
NTIOL: New Technology Intraocular Lens
NTIS: National Technical Information Service
NUBC: National Uniform Billing Committee
OAS: Office of Audit Services (*See* OIG)
OASIS: Outcome and Assessment Information Set
OBRA: Omnibus Reconciliation Act
OCE: Outpatient Code Editor
OEI: Office of Evaluation and Inspections (*See* OIG)
OIG: Office of Inspector General (*See* HHS)
OMB: Office of Management and Budget
OP: Outpatient
OPD: Outpatient Department

OPPS: Outpatient Prospective Payment System

OPR: Outpatient Payment Reform

OR: Operating Room

OSCAR: Online Survey Certification and Reporting (System)

OT: Occupational Therapy or Therapist

OTA: Occupational Therapist Assistant

P&P: Policy and Procedure

PA: Physician Assistant

PAM: Patient Accounts Manager

PBR: Provider-Based Rule (*See* 42 CFR §413.65)

PDP: Prescription Drug Plan

PERL (Internet): Practical Extraction and Reporting Language

PET: Positron Emission Tomography

PFS: Patient Financial Services

PHO: Physician Hospital Organization

PHP: Partial Hospitalization Program

PM: Program Memorandum

PMPM: Per Member Per Month

POS: Place of Service or Point of Service

PPA: Preferred Provider Arrangement

PPI: Producer Price Index

PPO: Preferred Provider Organization

PPP: Point-to-Point Protocol (Internet)

PPR: Physician Payment Reform

PPS: Prospective Payment System

PRB: Provider Review Board

PRM: Provider Reimbursement Manual

PRO: Peer Review Organization (*See* QIO)

ProPAC: Prospective Payment Assessment Commission

PRP: Pulmonary Rehabilitation Program

PRRB: Provider Reimbursement Review Board

PS&R: Provider Statistical and Reimbursement (Report)

PSN: Provider Service Network

PSO: Provider Service Organization

PT: Physical Therapy or Physical Therapist

PTA: Physical Therapy Assistant

Pub. L.: Public Law

QA: Quality Assurance

QFD: Quality Function Deployment

QIO: Quality Improvement Organization (*See* PRO)

RAPs: Resident Assessment Protocols

RAT-STATS: OIG Statistical Software Program

RBRVS: Resource-Based Relative Value System

RC: Revenue Code (*See also* RCC)

RCC: Revenue Center Code (from UB-04 Manual)

RFI: Request for Information

RFP: Request for Proposal

RFQ: Request for Quotation

RHC: Rural Health Clinic

RHHI: Regional Home Health Intermediary (*See* MACs)

RM: Risk Management

RN: Registered Nurse

RRC: Rural Referral Center

RVS: Relative Value System

RVU: Relative Value Units

S&I: Supervision and Interpretation

SAD: Self-Administrable Drug

SCH: Sole Community Hospital

SDS: Same-Day Surgery

SGML (Internet): Standardized General Markup Language

SI: Status Indicator (*See* APCs)

SIC: Standard Industrial Classification

SLIP: Serial Line IP Protocol (Internet)

SLP: Speech Language Pathology (*See also* ST)

SLP: Sociolinguistic Programming

SMI: Service Mix Index

SMTP: Simple Mail Transport Protocol (Internet e-mail)

SNF: Skilled Nursing Facility

SOC: Standard of Care

SOM: State Operations Manual

SR-DRGs: Severity Refined DRGs (HCFA Proposed in 1994)

SSA: Social Security Act ("The Act")

ST: Speech Therapy (*See also* SLP)

SUBC: State Uniform Billing Committee

TEFRA: Tax Equity and Fiscal Responsibility Act (of 1982)

TIN: Tax Identification Number

TLAs: Three-Letter Acronyms

TQD: Total Quality Deployment

TQM: Total Quality Management

TSC: Transaction Standard/Standard Code Set (*See* HIPAA)

UB-04: Universal Billing Form 2004 (Previously UB-92)

UCR: Usual, Customary, Reasonable

UHC: University Health System Consortium

UHDDS: Uniform Hospital Discharge Data Set

UNIX: Computer operating system; not an acronym; a play on the word *eunuch*

UPIN: Unique Physician Identification Number

UR: Utilization Review

URL: Uniform Resource Locator (Internet Address)

USC or U.S.C.: United States Code

VDP: Voluntary Disclosure Program

VSR: Value Stream Reinvention

W-2: Tax Withholding Form

WWW (Internet): World Wide Web

XML (Internet): eXtensible Markup Language

Appendix

Abbey & Abbey, Consultants, Inc. (AACI) websites

AACI maintains three websites with slightly different orientations.

www.AACIWeb.com—Corporate website addressing educational and general consulting activities.

www.APCNow.com—Website devoted to ambulatory payment classifications (APCs) and the provider-based rule (PBR).

www.HIPAAMaster.com—Website devoted to those aspects of HIPAA involving coding, billing, and reimbursement issues.

Dr. Abbey can be contacted at Duane@aaciweb.com. Additional e-mail addresses can be found at the corporate website, www.AACIWeb.com. Additionally, Dr. Abbey's PGP (Pretty Good Privacy) public key can be found at the main corporate website in cases where encrypted communications relative to sensitive compliance situations are required.

Accompanying CD and CBR compliance research

A CD-ROM accompanies this book. Many documents cited in the text are included on the CD for easy access. The CD is organized around key topics pertaining to CBR compliance issues. It should be considered only as a starting point because of the number of issues and thousands of pages of rules and regulations.

Working in the CBR compliance area requires a broad knowledge of healthcare compliance issues and an understanding of how to research issues at both formal and informal levels. As an example, preparing for a court appearance versus searching for ideas about a possible coding and billing policy and procedure are significantly different processes.

Over time, you will develop a personal database of *Federal Register* entries, CMS transmittals, *MedLearn Matters* documents, and a host of other reference materials. The CD accompanying this book can serve as a starting point for such a database. How to organize and categorize the huge amount of compliance material will be one of your greatest challenges. The objective, which is difficult to achieve, is to categorize topics so that you can easily retrieve them. In some cases, your database may be repetitive because information may fit into more than one logical category.

For example, you may have accumulated information about the present on admission (POA) indicator that may include coding guidelines, CMS transmittals, articles, and other information. The POA involves the UB-04 (CMS-1450) claim form and can also be categorized under inpatient services or under DRGs. Alternatively, this can be a top-level item in your database. How you categorize is a personal preference and will involve the degree of formality with which you design your document database.

For some documents, you may simply want to have a reference or link because the document is archived and readily available over the Internet. In other cases, you may want to a personal copy of a document, for example, you may have read, highlighted, and/or annotated a *Federal Register* entry that you wish to keep handy.

Also, some documents must be captured because they may disappear from Internet access. You may have established a policy and procedure based upon a question and answer published by CMS on its website. You should save a copy to justify the decisions embodied in your policy and procedure. CMS may suddenly remove the material from its website even though it has not changed its stance on the issue.

You may also have access to a more general knowledge base and, of course, we all have access to the giant database that encompasses the Internet. You must have some skill to find the items or documents that you may be seeking. Certainly search engines such as Google are very useful. At times an Internet search may be faster than accessing your personal database or even a specialized knowledge base. For example, if you can remember a CMS transmittal number, such as 1776 for the joint E/M services of a physician and non-physician practitioner, you may be able to access this transmittal quickly through a Google search. Here is a simple case study.

Case study—DRG Pre-admission window. A question arises about proper bundling of outpatient services within the DRG pre-admission window. Apex Medical Center established several new provider-based clinics. Patients are often seen at the clinics and admitted to the hospital a day or two later. Billing personnel manually check to see whether outpatient services were provided within the three-day window and, if so, all the charges are included on the inpatient claim. Because of the increase in volume with the new clinics, billing personnel want to automate this process and set up the new system correctly.

This case has more facets that might be realized initially. Embedded in the case study is the fact that with a manual system all services provided on an outpatient basis are bundled into the inpatient billing. Apparently, a policy decision was made to bundle the services. A careful review of this DRG billing provision will indicate that only certain services must be bundled. Questions also arise concerning diagnosis coding for services that are or are not bundled into the inpatient claim. These diagnosis codes can influence the DRG generated and the POA indicator may also be affected.

Thus, you may need to collect all of the documents that address this particular process. You may have already established a category in your personal database for this issue. If not, you may need to perform research.

The CD accompanying this book contains the following references:

42 CFR §412.2
63 FR 6864, February 11, 1998
CMS Publication 104, Chapter 3
Medicare Intermediary Manual §3610.3.

An Internet search may identify additional information and articles about specific issues surrounding the DRG pre-admission window. For example, by bundling the billing for certain services, the diagnosis assignments may also be affected and the assignments in turn may change the DRG assignment and subsequent payment. What should be a relatively straightforward issue can almost take on a life of its own, and CBR compliance personnel should keep references handy to address this and other issues. CBR compliance personnel must develop the skills necessary to research, analyze, and resolve many different kinds of issues. A generalized systems approach is discussed in the main text of this book.

CBR compliance officer

Throughout this book we have referred to CBR compliance personnel and more specifically to the CBR compliance officer. Depending upon the size of your hospital, hospital system, clinic, or healthcare organization, you or may not have a designated compliance officer position. A single employee or even a small group may devote time to CBR compliance issues, audits, and investigations. For small healthcare organizations, compliance may be addressed on a part-time basis, often in connection with financial functions.

Many technical issues and an enormous range of related concerns have been discussed in this book. General compliance personnel, such as a hospital's chief compliance officer, often will not have the detailed, technical background required to fully address CBR compliance. The following hospital job description is provided

as a general guide for the activities, knowledge base, and capabilities needed. Readers are encouraged to adapt all or any of the job description as appropriate.

Coding, Billing, and Reimbursement Compliance Officer
Apex Medical Center

Job Description: With limited supervision from the Chief Compliance Officer, identifies, investigates and resolves all compliance issues relating to coding, billing, documentation, and reimbursement activities. As appropriate, acts as team leader for special compliance investigations in coding, billing, and reimbursement, including formal and informal audits, cost reporting, chargemaster, computer billing system, and various compliance-related computer systems.

Typical Activities:

Reviews and studies all information published by CMS and the OIG via the *Federal Register*, fraud alerts, OIG advisory opinions, OIG reports, and other publications relative to coding, billing, and reimbursement compliance.

Reviews and studies all information including companion manuals from third-party payers relative to claims filing, coding, and adjudication.

Subscribes to and reviews various written and Internet publications relative to coding, billing, and reimbursement compliance.

Reviews, assesses, studies, analyzes the overall coding, billing, documentation, and reimbursement system for potential compliance problems and noncompliant activities.

Uses a systematic approach to identify and resolve complex compliance problems.

Works with health information management, patient accounts, information system, and other medical center personnel to solve problems and implement solutions to maintain a proper compliance stance.

Works with chief compliance officer and legal counsel relative to difficult coding, billing, and reimbursement compliance issues.

Works with chargemaster and cost report personnel to maintain proper compliance with rules and regulations.

Works with contract management personnel in the review of contracts and other reimbursement or payment arrangements.

Works with Chief Compliance Officer on the development of and ongoing activities involved in baseline and periodic compliance audits.

Conducts informal audits on various aspects of the coding, billing, documentation, and reimbursement system.

Designs and conducts formal audits of specific aspects of the coding, billing, and reimbursement system.

Develops and directs technical teams in the investigation and resolution of complex compliance problems.

Works with legal counsel in developing systems to meet requirements of compliance settlement agreements including training, reporting, and computer system utilization.

Provides training sessions for both general and specific problem resolution in the coding, billing, and reimbursement area.

Writes and assists others in drafting policies and procedures to maintain proper compliance.

Attends workshops and seminars to maintain high levels of knowledge and capabilities.

Recommends and coordinates the use of consultants for specialized activities related to the coding, billing, and reimbursement compliance area.

Coordinates and facilitates problem resolution sessions when multiple departments and/or service areas are involved.

Monitors overall compliance in the coding, billing, documentation, and reimbursement area.

Works with upper management and chief compliance officer to prepare presentations and briefings to the board of directors.

Works with upper management in planning and organization of new service areas and acquisitions of service providers.

Works with financial department to optimize reimbursement while maintaining proper compliance status.

Addresses special projects as assigned.

Knowledge, Skills, Abilities, and Personal Characteristics:

Extensive knowledge of compliance rules and regulations in the coding, billing, and reimbursement areas.

Extensive knowledge of sources and resources for information about compliance at federal, state, and local levels.

Extensive knowledge of various payment systems including DRGs, APCs/APGs, RBRVS, RUGs-III, and managed care and capitated arrangements.

Extensive knowledge of various coding systems used by hospitals and physicians including CPT, HCPCS, and ICD-9-CM.

Knowledge of chargemaster, its use, design, revenue center codes, relationship to CPT/HCPCS coding, and its impact on coding, billing, and reimbursement.

Knowledge of computer hardware and software, and their uses, functions, and designs relative to coding, billing, and reimbursement.

Extensive knowledge of computer software for both prospective and retrospective reviews of coding, billing, and reimbursement compliance.

Knowledge of statistics and processes for developing audit sample sizes and selection of cases for review.

Knowledge of auditing process including various techniques relative to problem resolution.

Knowledge of team dynamics and consensus building.

Overall understanding of healthcare financial management and reporting.

Overall knowledge of functions and activities of hospitals and medical clinics.

Ability to participate with upper management in a decision support mode through the development of appropriate management information.

Knowledge of charge development and the interrelationships of cost accounting, cost management, and related functions.

Ability to work effectively with and coordinate activities of outside consultants.

Ability to work with outside auditors relative to formal compliance auditing.

Ability and skill to influence personnel through a matrix organization rather than line management authority.

Ability to develop and lead teams to stated objectives and goals.

Skill in using personal computers for financial analysis (spreadsheets), database development, and report generation.

Skill in using personal computers for electronic mail communications, Internet access, and internal intranet utilization.

Skill in performing research with bibliographic databases and Internet access to associated information resources.

Skill in networking directly through colleagues and professional organizations and ability to utilize networking capabilities through Internet news groups and list servers.

Interpersonal communication skills for training and working with personnel in tense and sensitive situations.

Educational Background and Certifications:

Master's degree in healthcare administration or business administration highly desirable.

Appropriate certification in risk management and/or healthcare compliance highly desirable.

Five to ten years of progressive experience in financial management, information systems, and/or health information management required.

Applicable certifications by ACHE, HFMA, AHIMA, AGPAM, and/or associated organizations desirable.

Reports to: Chief Compliance Officer.

Subordinate Personnel: Provided as needed and/or may be provided on special project basis.

Note: This is a highly responsible position that requires both quantitative and interpersonal skills.

CBR compliance checklist

Depending upon the type of healthcare organization for which you address CBR compliance issues, developing a checklist of possible areas of concern can be useful. Such checklists may be refined further to cover specific audit areas and/or areas for developing formal policies and procedures. The following checklist is provided *only as an example.* You should develop your own list based on type of organization, experience, researching issues, articles, OIG audits, Medicare audits, and the like.

The primary emphasis is on hospitals and medical clinics. Other areas such as home health and skilled nursing are addressed as adjuncts. This listing is provided only as an example of areas for consideration.

Note that some concerns are repeated based on different perspectives. Also note that most of the areas listed can pose complex problems and related discussions could be expanded into books. As more cases are tested, litigation ensues, and additional information becomes available, more definitive treatises will be generated.

Medical Necessity

ED
Laboratory
Radiology
Other Diagnostic Tests
Medical Clinics
Diagnostic Coding
Signed Physician Orders
General Documentation
Use or Non-Use of ABNs and NONCs

Non-Covered Services/Supplies/Drugs

Self-Administrable Drugs
Self-Administrable Services
Take-Home Drugs
Take-Home Supplies

Physician Interfaces and Services

Medical Staff Bylaws
Medical Staff Dues
Medical Directorships
Hospital-Based Physicians
Face-to-Face, Personally Performed
Specialty Clinics, Rental versus UB-04, POS
Rental Agreements
Case Management Services and Billing
Private Contracts, Opting out of Medicare

False Claims

Variety of Situations and Circumstances

Medicare Fraud, Abuse and Anti-Kickback Law

Numerous Interpretations (See OIG Fraud Alerts)
Safe Harbors, Investment Interests
Safe Harbors, Space Rental
Safe Harbors, Equipment Rental
Safe Harbors, Personal Services and Management
    Contracts
Safe Harbors, Sale of Practice
Safe Harbors, Referral Services
Safe Harbors, Warranties
Safe Harbors, Discounts
Safe Harbors, Employees
Safe Harbors, Group Purchasing Organizations
Safe Harbors, Waiver of Beneficiary, Co-insurance,
    and Deductibles
Safe Harbors, Increased Coverage, Reduced Cost-
    Sharing Amounts, or Reduced Premium Amounts
    Offered by Health Plans
Safe Harbors, Price Reduction Offered to Health Plans

Non-Physician Service Providers

Practitioner Status
Credentialing
Organization
Billing Status
Employer Definition
Supervisory Status
Physician Relationships
1500 versus UB-04 Billing
Scope of Practice, State Laws
Provider-Based Clinical Services

Organizational Structuring

Licensing
Certification
Accreditation
Provider-Based Status
Acquisitions
Mergers
Integrated Delivery Systems
Special Forms: RHC, FQHC
Splitting Certification

Billing, Billing Services, and Management Service Companies

MSO Arrangements
Third-Party Billing Companies (See OIG Guidance)
Duplicate Billings
Credit Balances
Services and Items Not Provided
Medically Unnecessary Services
Late Charges
Billing under Arrangements
Outlier Payments

Billing Privileges

CMS-855 Forms, Submission and Updating
National Provider Identifiers (NPIs)
Private Third-Party Payers, Contracts
Physician and Non-Physician Practitioner Recognition

Medicare Charging Rule

Charge Development Formulas
Multiple Fee Schedules
Discounting
Price Reductions
Professional Courtesy
Cost Report
Cost-to-Charge Ratios (CCRs)

Documentation Guidelines

Formal Guidelines, CPT/HCPCS
Formal Guidelines, ICD-9-CM (ICD-10)
Quality, Legibility, Completeness, Accuracy
Ordering and Attending Physician
Documentation System
Location of Documentation Development
Specialized Areas (Laboratory, Radiology, Home Health, SNF)
Present-on-Admission (POA)

Coding Systems, Guidelines, and Issues

CPT
CPT Modifiers
HCPCS

HCPCS Modifiers
ICD-9-CM (ICD-10-CM)
Revenue Center Codes (RCCs)
Encoders and Automated Systems
Sequencing of Codes
Correlation of Codes (UB-92 to HCFA-1500)
Correlation of Codes (ICD-9-CM to CPT)
HCFA's Correct Coding Initiative

Chargemaster

Charge Development Formulas and Pricing
Line Item Billings
Supply Categorization
Nursing Services
Equipment
CPT/HCPCS Codes
Proper Descriptions
Proper Revenue Center Codes (RCCs)
Static versus Dynamic Coding
Correlation of Descriptions, CPT/HCPCS, and Revenue Codes
Charge Explosion
Bundling and Unbundling
Consistency and Reasonableness of Charges
Durable Medical Equipment (DME) Classification

Cost Reports

False Cost Reports
Non-Allowable Costs
Incorrect Chargemaster Interface
Incorrect Categorization of Costs and Charges
Improper Cost-to-Charge Ratios (CCRs)
Improper Cost Outlier Payments

Assignment/Reassignment Issues

Employer Status
Conditions for Payment (CfP)
CMS Form 855-R
Non-Physician Practitioners

Investigational Services

Experimental Devices
Experimental Drugs
Experimental Services

Transfers and Discharges

Transfer versus Discharge
Acute Care to Skilled Nursing
Acute Care to Subacute Care
Observation to Home
Observation to Acute Care
Acute Care to Home Care

Special Classifications and Special Situations

Home Health
Skilled Nursing (and Swing Beds)
Rehabilitation Facilities
Hospitals within Hospitals (HwHs)
Hospice Care
Respite Care
Partial Hospitalization
Ambulatory Surgery Centers (ASCs)
Independent Diagnostic Testing Facilities (IDTFs)
Medicare-Dependent Hospitals (MDHs)
Sole Community Hospitals (SCHs)
Rural Referral Centers (RRCs)
Critical Access Hospitals (CAHs)

Teaching/Residency Program Considerations

PATH Project
Documentation
Use of Modifiers
Allied Health Education
Indirect Medical Education (IME)

Diagnosis-Related Groups (DRGs)

Case Mix Index Creep
Upcoding
Pre-Admission Window
Discharge Status, Transfer Rule
Quality Improvement Organizations (QIOs)

Ambulatory Payment Classifications (APCs)

Upcoding
Use of Modifiers

Payment System Interfaces

DRGs to APCs
APCs to RBRVS
DRGs to RUGs-III
PPS to Cost-Based
Pre- and Post-Admission Windows

Provider Agreements, Third-Party Payer Contracts, Managed Care

Contractual Requirements
Secondary Payer Interfaces
Discounted Reimbursement Schemes

Corporate Integrity Agreements and Settlement Agreements

Standard
Special

False or Misleading Information, Patient Status

Transfer versus discharge
Inpatient versus outpatient

Physician Incentive Programs

Physician Employment Contracts
Physician Ownership (*See* Stark Laws)
Joint Ventures

Software Programs: Claim Adjudication, Tracking, and Correlation

Provider Understanding of Adjudication Software
  Logic

Software Programs: Retrospective Analysis and Review

Quality and Completeness of Assessments
Ability to Analyze Databases
Observations Services
Medical Necessity
Documentation
Coding (1500 versus UB-04)
RCC Utilization
Care Paths

Emergency Department Services

Face-to-Face Services
Critical Care versus CPR
Medical Necessity and Level of Service
Documentation
1500 to UB-04 Code Correlation
Use of RBRVS and APCs Modifiers
Post-Operative Care (GSP under RBRVS)
Use of Non-Physician Providers (NPPs)

Ambulance Services

Restocking
Alternative Billing Rules

Psychiatric Services

Individual versus Group Psychotherapy
Psychological Testing
H&P on Admission

Newer Prospective Payment Systems

APCs for Outpatient
RUGs-III Skilled Nursing (Consolidated Billing)
PPS for Home Health
PPS for Rehabilitation
PPS for Long-Term Care

HIPAA Rules

HIPAA Privacy
HIPAA Transaction Standard/Standard Code Set
HIPAA Security
HIPAA NPI

Audits and Auditing

Standard Audits
Special Problem-Driven Audits

Sample size determination

While the use of the OIG's RAT-STATS program is certainly a good way to determine samples size for certain situations, you can perform some relatively straightforward calculations that will produce similar results. The following discussion can easily be implemented through a spreadsheet program such as MS Excel. Assume for example, that

N_p = size or number of cases in universe population
n = size of required sample
π = proportion of estimated errors
z = confidence interval
E = proportion relative to error rate

The basic formula is:

$$N = N_p \left(\frac{z^2 \pi (1 - \pi)}{E^2(N_p - 1) + z^2 \pi (1 - \pi)} \right)$$

Value of z for Given Confidence Level

	99%	98%	95%	90%	80%	50%
z =	2.575	2.330	1.960	1.6450	1.280	0.675

If other values of z are required, i.e., for a confidence level not on the chart, consult the standard normal curve table found in statistics references to determine precise values.

Value of Proportion (π) for Initial Choice

π =	0.1	0.2	0.3	0.4	0.5	0.6	0.7	0.8	0.9
$\pi(1-\pi)$ =	0.09	0.16	0.21	0.24	0.25	0.24	0.21	0.16	0.9

Note that the value of $\pi(1 - \pi)$ is both maximized and symmetric about $\pi = 0.5$. Thus, in the absence of better information, the worst case can be assumed and the value of the estimated proportion set at 0.5.

These formulas allow a number of variations. See a standard statistics textbook for additional information. See also RAT-STATS documentation that includes a more advanced and lengthy discussion. In formal situations such as legal proceedings, you may want to retain a statistical expert to handle these types of determinations and/or to respond to governmental auditor concerns.

Note: The formulas utilized can present variations and thus lead to small variations in sample sizes developed with such formulas.

Table A.1 Sample Sizes for Confidence Level of 90% Worst Case—Proportion at 0.5

Universe Size	Error Rate 5%	Error Rate 3%	Error Rate 1%
250	130	188	241
500	176	301	466
750	199	376	675
1000	213	429	871
1500	229	501	1228
2000	238	547	1544
3000	248	601	2079
4000	254	633	2514
5000	257	654	2875
10000	263	699	4035

Table A.2 Sample Sizes for Confidence Level of 90% Medium Case—Proportion at 0.3

Universe Size	Error Rate 5%	Error Rate 3%	Error Rate 1%
250	119	179	240
500	156	279	460
750	175	343	663
1000	185	387	850
1500	198	445	1187
2000	204	480	1480
3000	211	522	1964
4000	215	545	2348
5000	217	561	2660
10000	222	594	3624

Table A.3 Sample Sizes for Confidence Level of 90% Good Case—Proportion at 0.1

Universe Size	Error Rate 5%	Error Rate 3%	Error Rate 1%
250	70	130	227
500	82	176	415
750	86	199	574
1000	89	213	709
1500	92	229	929
2000	93	238	1098
3000	94	248	1344
4000	95	254	1514
5000	96	257	1638
10000	96	263	1959

Table A.4 Sample Sizes for Confidence Level
of 80% Worst Case—Proportion at 0.5

Universe Size	Error Rate 5%	Error Rate 3%	Error Rate 1%
250	99	162	236
500	124	239	446
750	135	283	634
1000	141	313	804
1500	148	349	1098
2000	152	371	1344
3000	155	395	1732
4000	157	409	2024
5000	159	417	2252
10000	161	435	2906

Table A.5 Sample Sizes for Confidence Level
of 80% Medium Case—Proportion at 0.3

Universe Size	Error Rate 5%	Error Rate 3%	Error Rate 1%
250	89	151	233
500	108	217	437
750	116	253	616
1000	121	277	775
1500	126	305	1045
2000	129	321	1265
3000	132	339	1603
4000	133	349	1850
5000	134	355	2038
10000	136	368	2560

Table A.6 Sample Sizes for Confidence Level
of 80% Good Case—Proportion at 0.1

Universe Size	Error Rate 5%	Error Rate 3%	Error Rate 1%
250	48	99	214
500	53	124	374
750	55	135	497
1000	56	141	596
1500	57	148	744
2000	57	152	849
3000	58	155	989
4000	58	157	1078
5000	58	159	1139
10000	59	161	1285

Table A.7 Sample Sizes for Confidence Level
of 95% Worst Case—Proportion at 0.5

Universe Size	Error Rate 5%	Error Rate 3%	Error Rate 1%
250	152	203	244
500	217	341	475
750	254	441	696
1000	278	516	906
1500	306	624	1297
2000	322	696	1655
3000	341	787	2286
4000	351	843	2824
5000	357	880	3288
10000	370	964	4899

Table A.8 Sample Sizes for Confidence Level
of 95% Medium Case—Proportion at 0.3

Universe Size	Error Rate 5%	Error Rate 3%	Error Rate 1%
250	141	196	243
500	196	321	471
750	226	409	686
1000	244	473	890
1500	266	561	1265
2000	278	619	1603
3000	291	690	2187
4000	299	732	2674
5000	303	760	3087
10000	313	823	4465

Table A.9 Sample Sizes for Confidence Level
of 95% Good Case—Proportion at 0.1

Universe Size	Error Rate 5%	Error Rate 3%	Error Rate 1%
250	89	152	233
500	109	217	437
750	117	254	616
1000	122	278	776
1500	127	306	1046
2000	129	322	1267
3000	132	341	1607
4000	134	351	1855
5000	135	357	2044
10000	136	370	2569

Table A.10 Sample Sizes for Confidence Level of 98% Worst Case—Proportion at 0.5

Universe Size	Error Rate 5%	Error Rate 3%	Error Rate 1%
250	171	215	245
500	261	376	482
750	315	501	711
1000	352	602	931
1500	399	752	1351
2000	427	860	1743
3000	460	1004	2457
4000	478	1095	3090
5000	490	1159	3654
10000	515	1311	5758

Table A.11 Sample Sizes for Confidence Level of 98% Medium Case—Proportion at 0.3

Universe Size	Error Rate 5%	Error Rate 3%	Error Rate 1%
250	162	209	245
500	239	359	479
750	284	471	704
1000	313	559	919
1500	350	687	1326
2000	372	776	1702
3000	396	891	2375
4000	409	962	2961
5000	418	1011	3476
10000	436	1124	5328

Table A.12 Sample Sizes for Confidence Level of 98% Good Case—Proportion at 0.1

Universe Size	Error Rate 5%	Error Rate 3%	Error Rate 1%
250	110	171	238
500	141	261	454
750	155	315	650
1000	164	352	830
1500	173	399	1148
2000	178	427	1419
3000	184	460	1859
4000	186	478	2200
5000	188	490	2471
10000	192	515	3283

Table A.13 Sample Sizes for Confidence Level of 80% Worst Case—Proportion at 0.5

Universe Size	Error Rate 5%	Error Rate 3%	Error Rate 1%
250	99	162	236
500	124	239	446
750	135	283	634
1000	141	313	804
1500	148	349	1098
2000	152	371	1344
3000	155	395	1732
4000	157	409	2024
5000	159	417	2252
10000	161	435	2906

Table A.14 Sample Sizes for Confidence Level of 80% Medium Case—Proportion at 0.3

Universe Size	Error Rate 5%	Error Rate 3%	Error Rate 1%
250	89	151	233
500	108	217	437
750	116	253	616
1000	121	277	775
1500	126	305	1045
2000	129	321	1265
3000	132	339	1603
4000	133	349	1850
5000	134	355	2038
10000	136	368	2560

Table A.15 Sample Sizes for Confidence Level of 80% Good Case—Proportion at 0.1

Universe Size	Error Rate 5%	Error Rate 3%	Error Rate 1%
250	48	99	214
500	53	124	374
750	55	135	497
1000	56	141	596
1500	57	148	744
2000	57	152	849
3000	58	155	989
4000	58	157	1078
5000	58	159	1139
10000	59	161	1285

Index

Note: Page numbers in **bold** indicate figures or tables.